WITHDRAWAL
        SILENCE
                LONELINESS

WITHDRAWAL
SILENCE
LONELINESS

Psychotherapy of the Schizoid Process

Richard G. Erskine

With contributions from
Silvia Allari, Leigh Bettles, Dan Eastop, Amaia Mauriz Etxabe,
Linda Finlay, Ray Little, Lynn Martin, Marye O'Reilly-Knapp,
Eugenio Peiró Orozco

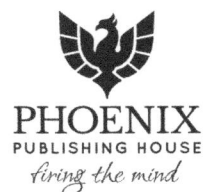

PHOENIX
PUBLISHING HOUSE
firing the mind

First published in 2023 by
Phoenix Publishing House Ltd
62 Bucknell Road
Bicester
Oxfordshire OX26 2DS

Copyright © 2023 by Richard G. Erskine
Illustrations copyright © Emily Mitchell

The right of Richard G. Erskine to be identified as the author of this work has been asserted in accordance with §§ 77 and 78 of the Copyright Design and Patents Act 1988.

Individual authors retain the copyright of their contributions.

All rights reserved. No part of this publication may be reproduced, stored in a retrieval system, or transmitted, in any form or by any means, electronic, mechanical, photocopying, recording, or otherwise, without the prior written permission of the publisher.

British Library Cataloguing in Publication Data

A C.I.P. for this book is available from the British Library

ISBN-13: 978-1-800131-87-3

Typeset by Medlar Publishing Solutions Pvt Ltd, India

www.firingthemind.com

I met a man along the way,
and we had many words to say,
because he too had known
a sorrow I have born alone.

—Lucille Erskine Koniecki (1908–1992)

Contents

Acknowledgments	xi
About the author and contributors	xiii
Foreword	xvii
Amaia Mauriz Etxabe (Basque Country, Spain)	
Preface	xxiii
Richard G. Erskine (Canada)	

Part I: Psychotherapy of the schizoid process

1. The schizoid process: an introduction — 3
   Richard G. Erskine (Canada)

2. Relational withdrawal, internal criticism, social facade: attunement to parts of the self — 9
   Richard G. Erskine (Canada)

3. Relational withdrawal, attunement to silence: psychotherapy of the schizoid process — 31
   Richard G. Erskine (Canada)

4. Engaging with the schizoid compromise 45
    Ray Little (Scotland)

 5. Silence, withdrawal, and contact in the schizoid process 65
    Marye O'Reilly-Knapp (USA)

 6. Relational needs and schizoid phenomena 79
    Dan Eastop (Ireland)

Part II: A five-year case study and colleagues' reflections

 7. Allan: depression or isolated attachment? 101
    Richard G. Erskine (Canada)

 8. Allan: internal criticism and shame, physical sensations, and affect 111
    Richard G. Erskine (Canada)

 9. Allan: isolation, loneliness, and a need to be loved 123
    Richard G. Erskine (Canada)

10. Allan: therapeutic withdrawal and painful memories 131
    Richard G. Erskine (Canada)

11. Allan: my mother's voice—psychotherapy of introjection 139
    Richard G. Erskine (Canada)

12. Reflexively exploring the "therapeutic use of self": a response to Richard Erskine's five-chapter case study of Allan 151
    Linda Finlay (UK)

13. The role of shame in the development of the schizoid process 177
    Lynn Martin (UK)

Part III: Clients' perspectives on the psychotherapy

14. "Come closer … but keep your distance": a client's perspective on the psychotherapy of schizoid process 189
    Leigh Bettles (UK)

15. From inner safety to contact-in-relationship: analyzing the psychotherapy
    of the schizoid process   209
    Silvia Allari (Italy) and Eugenio Peiró Orozco (Spain)

Part IV: Theory into therapeutic practice

16. Louise: social facade, depression, relational withdrawal   225
    Richard G. Erskine (Canada)

Index   243

Acknowledgments

Several chapters in this book were originally published in two professional journals. They are presented in this book with the permission of the original publications: the *International Journal of Integrative Psychotherapy*, published by the International Integrative Psychotherapy Association, and the *International Journal of Psychotherapy*, published by the European Association of Psychotherapy. The original citations for the articles are listed below.

Bettles, L. (2021). "Come closer … but keep your distance." *International Journal of Integrative Psychotherapy, 12*: 142–162.

Eastop, D. (2021). Relational needs and the schizoid phenomena. *International Journal of Integrative Psychotherapy, 12*: 89–113.

Erskine, R. G. (2020). Relational withdrawal, attunement to silence: Psychotherapy of the schizoid process. *International Journal of Integrative Psychotherapy, 11*: 14–28.

Erskine, R. G. (2021a). Depression or isolated attachment? Part 1 of a 5-part case study of the psychotherapy of the schizoid process. *International Journal of Integrative Psychotherapy, 11*: 28–40.

Erskine, R. G. (2021b). Internal criticism and shame, physical sensations and affect. Part 2 of a 5-part case study of the psychotherapy of the schizoid process. *International Journal of Integrative Psychotherapy, 11*: 41–55.

Erskine, R. G. (2021c). Isolation, loneliness, and a need to be loved: Part 3 of a 5-part case study of the psychotherapy of the schizoid process. *International Journal of Integrative Psychotherapy, 11*: 56–65.

Erskine, R. G. (2001d). Therapeutic withdrawal and painful memories: Part 4 of a 5-part case study of the psychotherapy of the schizoid process. *International Journal of Integrative Psychotherapy, 11*: 66–74.

Erskine, R. G. (2001e). My mother's voice: Psychotherapy of introjection: Part 5 of a 5-part case study of the psychotherapy of the schizoid process. *International Journal of Integrative Psychotherapy, 11*: 75–88.

Erskine, R. G. (2022). Relational withdrawal, internal criticism, social façade: Psychotherapy of the schizoid process. *International Journal of Psychotherapy, 26*: 1, 75–93.

Finlay, L. (2021). Reflexively exploring the "therapeutic use of self": A response to Richard Erskine's five-chapter case study of Allan. *International Journal of Integrative Psychotherapy, 12*: 163–192.

Little, R. (2020). Engaging with the schizoid compromise: Response to Erskine's "Relational withdrawal, attunement to silence: Psychotherapy of the schizoid process." *International Journal of Integrative Psychotherapy, 11*: 29–54.

O'Reilly-Knapp, M. (2020). Engaging with the schizoid compromise: Response to Erskine's "Relational withdrawal, attunement to silence: Psychotherapy of the schizoid process." *International Journal of Integrative Psychotherapy, 11*: 69–84.

Martin, L. (2020). The role of shame in the development of the schizoid process. *International Journal of Integrative Psychotherapy, 11*: 85–96.

Chapter 1 is based on Erskine, R. G. (2001) The schizoid process. *Transactional Analysis Journal 31*(1): 4–6. doi.org/10.1177/036215370103100102. Copyright © International Transactional Analysis Association, reprinted by permission of Taylor & Francis Ltd, http://tandfonline.com on behalf of the International Transactional Analysis Association.

About the author and contributors

Author

Richard G. Erskine, PhD (Canada) is a licensed psychoanalyst, a certified transactional analyst, and internationally recognized Gestalt therapist. He is the training director, Institute for Integrative Psychotherapy and is currently professor of psychology at Deusto University, Bilbao, Spain. Each year Richard Erskine teaches formal courses and experiential workshops on the theory and methods of integrative psychotherapy in several countries. He is the author of ten books and numerous articles on the theory and methods of psychotherapy. His writings have been translated into a dozen languages. Some of his articles are available on his website at www.IntegrativePsychotherapy.com.

Contributors

Silvia Allari (Italy) is an individual and group psychotherapist in Milan. Her theoretical orientations include transactional analysis, integrative psychotherapy, and bioenergetics. She provides training and supervision in psychotherapy. Website: www.silviaallaripsicoterapia.it.

Leigh Bettles (UK) is an accredited member of the British Association for Counselling and Psychotherapy with twenty-plus years of experience. She is a certified psychodynamic counselor and a certified integrative psychotherapist with the International Integrative Psychotherapy Association. She conducts a private practice and provides psychotherapy for an employee assistance program with the National Health Service in the UK.

Dan Eastop (Ireland) is a relationally focused integrative psychotherapist certified by the International Integrative Psychotherapy Association, the United Kingdom Council on Psychotherapy, and the Irish Council of Psychotherapy. He currently works in the National University of Ireland, Galway Counselling Service. He maintains a private practice in psychotherapy and supervision in the west of Ireland.

Amaia Mauriz Etxabe (Spain) is a clinical psychologist, certified psychotherapist trainer and supervisor in integrative psychotherapy, transactional analysis, psychodrama, and group analysis. She is professor on the Faculty of Psychology and codirector of the Postgraduate Master Program in Relational Integrative Psychotherapy at Deusto University in Bilbao. For the past thirty years she has been the director of BIOS Integrative Psychotherapy Institute, Bilbao (Basque Country), Spain. Website: https://bios-psicologos.com/.

Linda Finlay, PhD (UK) is an existentially oriented relational integrative psychotherapist in private practice in the United Kingdom. She teaches psychology and counseling at the Open University, UK. She has published numerous articles and books. Her most recent books are: *Phenomenology for Therapists* (Wiley), *Relational Integrative Psychotherapy* (Wiley), *Practical Ethics: A Relational Approach* (Sage), and *Therapeutic Use of Self* (Sage). She is currently editor of the *European Journal for Qualitative Research in Psychotherapy* (www.EJQRP.org). Website: http://lindafinlay.co.uk/.

Ray Little (Scotland) practices psychotherapy and supervision in Edinburgh and London. He is interested in incorporating psychodynamic theory into a relational transactional analysis and has published several articles exploring these ideas. In 2019 he received the Eric Berne Memorial Award for his contribution to theory and practice of TA. He is a founding member of the International Association of Relational Transactional Analysis and is a visiting tutor at several training institutes in Europe. Website: www.enderbyassociates.co.uk.

Lynn Martin (UK) is a certified integrative psychotherapist supervisor and trainer, a certified transactional analysis psychotherapist, and a registered child psychotherapist with the United Kingdom Council for Psychotherapy. Following twenty years in teaching and youth work, she has been in private practice in Devon for the past thirty years and has spent several years delivering training to therapists working with children and young people. Website: https://lynnmartinpsychotherapy.co.uk/.

Marye O'Reilly-Knapp, PhD (USA) is a founding member and certified psychotherapist trainer and supervisor in the International Integrative Psychotherapy Association, certified transactional analyst, certified clinical nurse specialist in psychiatric nursing, professor emerita of Widener University, and author of publications in psychotherapy and nursing journals and books.

Eugenio Peiró Orozco (Spain) provides psychotherapy to children, adolescents, and adults in his private practice in Valencia and Alicante, Spain. He has trained in cognitive behavioral therapy, transactional analysis, and integrative psychotherapy.

Foreword

Amaia Mauriz Etxabe

It is a privilege to introduce you to *Withdrawal, Silence, Loneliness: Psychotherapy of the Schizoid Process*. As I was reading the draft of this book, an event that occurred some years ago came to mind. Richard Erskine and I were leaving a workshop on a windy autumn afternoon. As we walked along the path to the parking area, Richard pointed to a group of birds flying in intricate patterns. I looked at the flock of birds but I didn't notice anything unusual. Then Richard pointed out the changing contours of the birds' flight patterns and said, "They are playing with the air waves. The updrafts of warm air under their wings have thrust them upward in circle after circle." I was amazed. Where I only saw common birds, Richard was admiring the complex patterns of the birds' flight paths and predicting how the flight path would alter as the wind changed.

In this book about the *Psychotherapy of the Schizoid Process* you will be introduced to this same type of observation about the various patterns and homeostatic functions underlying the psychological dynamics that lead people to establish a social facade, suffer from internal criticism, and withdraw from interpersonal relationships. You are also going to discover the subjective experiences of both client and psychotherapist as they engage in the intricacies of the psychotherapy.

While describing the schizoid process in detail, each author in this book writes of their own investment in the psychotherapy as well as the uniqueness of their clients. Each author stimulated me to think about my clients, to evaluate what I have been doing, and to consider options in our psychotherapy. The challenge for me—as it is for each psychotherapist—is to keep in mind the distinct history of each client, to decipher what they may need, and to choose how and when to provide the interpersonal qualities essential in a healing relationship.

Clients who struggle with the schizoid process also face a challenge to either risk being involved with others or to withdraw into a safe inner world of fantasy and potential loneliness. On the surface their struggle is like the children's game, "Here I am; now I'm not here," played by toddlers as they put their hands over their eyes while saying, "You can't see me, I'm not here." When children are a little older, they learn to hide in the house and may call out, "You can't find me." They are full of hope, the hope of being searched for and eventually found. Our clients who engage in a schizoid process may have only an inkling of hope that someone will find them and understand what they need; yet, at the same time, they may be filled with dread that they will be invaded, misdefined, and controlled.

I have read this book with pleasure and admiration because in each chapter the schizoid process is described through the appreciative eyes of psychotherapists who are committed to the journey of discovering their clients' internal processes, psychological functions, complex affects, and silent quest for security. An essential part of each chapter are the various recommendations for how to therapeutically engage with each of our clients' sense of self, whether it be a vital and vulnerable self, a social self, an internal critic, or a sequestered self.

Some years ago, I was invited to make a presentation about depression so I decided to discuss it in a supervision session with Richard. Although he began with, "I don't know much about depression," he quickly guided the conversation into my describing one of my clients' internal struggles: his intense self-criticism, his lonely despair, his fear of close interpersonal contact, and his belief that all relationships ended in a disaster. As Richard and I talked it became clear that my client's internal dynamics included more than depression. He had many parts to his sense of self; it was as though he was split into various selves and deeply ashamed that he was different than other people. That supervision session was an eye-opener; I could then see the schizoid process in other clients who described themselves as living with internal criticism and depression.

In this book you will find a treasure trove of ideas that may guide your understanding of the schizoid process and provide you with new options in how to time your therapeutic interventions, and how to use the prosody of your voice to establish secure therapeutic relationships that allow a sequestered self to emerge and engage in interpersonal contact. This book highlights the profound damage that comes from cumulative relational neglect, the devastating effects of criticism, and the trauma of what never happened but should have happened. The concept of therapeutic attunement, the importance of patience and respect, the significance of a non-pathological attitude are all part of the necessary therapeutic ingredients in creating a healing relationship (Erskine, 2021a, 2021b).

Through vividly described case examples Richard and his clients, Marianne, Violet, Allan, and Louise, illustrate the fine points of a developmentally based, relationally focused, integrative psychotherapy. These case presentations are written to illustrate two different intersubjective encounters between client and therapist wherein they mutually learned from the other. In this same personal way Richard engages the reader by describing his countertransference, self-awareness, and how his internal experiences interlace with what is happening inside his clients.

Through a detailed description of his psychotherapy with Allan, Richard takes us on a multi-year therapy journey where he illustrates the slow revealing of his client's secret life. Interwoven in the story of Allan's psychotherapy Richard divulges his worry and soul-searching, an internal questioning that should happen inside every psychotherapist in order to understand "the puzzle" of our clients' internal life.

Richard's initial chapters describe a therapeutic metaphor of various selves—a vital and vulnerable self, a social self, a self-sabotaging self, and a sequestered self—that has influenced his understanding and creation of a treatment map. His descriptions of psychotherapy provide a model in how to listen to our clients' silences, how to make sense of our clients' reluctance to express themselves, how to appreciate their coping strategies, and how to inquire about the homeostatic functions underlying their behaviors. The foundation of this psychotherapy is non-pathological. The clients' isolation, depression, shame, internal criticism, and withdrawal are all symptoms of previous relational disruptions; they are all ways of coping with relational failures.

All of the authors in this book share this non-pathological perspective. They offer us their own views on the schizoid process and how they engage in the practice of psychotherapy. Ray Little provides a unique view of the internal dynamics of his clients. He focuses on the clients' mental schemas and child–parent ego state relational units and how they reflect implicit memories that unconsciously influence behavior. The ego state relational units that Ray Little describes are related to the clients' internal world, where relationships occur in fantasy, attachments can be controlled, and fears are managed through emotional distancing.

Marye O'Reilly-Knapp's writings highlight the relevance of listening to our clients' silences as a means of maintaining contact with their withdrawn self. Marye emphasizes that interpersonal interaction is central to the discovery of one's self and that the client who engages in a schizoid process has lost contact with themselves. Through her case examples Marye identifies her clients' "isolated attachment" pattern. This is a relevant contribution to the general knowledge of psychotherapy and to an understanding of the schizoid process.

Dan Eastop normalizes the experience of the schizoid process and makes us consider our own "compartmentalized self" as a useful way to organize some of life's experiences. Dan also helps us realize that we cannot know what actually happens in the inner world of our clients; we can only have a glimpse, only surmise. Through his work with Helen, he teaches us how to respect the vulnerability and the importance of going with the client into her world instead of challenging or trying to shape it. Central to Dan's practice of psychotherapy is his attunement and involvement.

I found Leigh Bettles's chapter to be a marvelous presentation of her personal therapy experience. She writes about her internal experience and the impact of the psychotherapist's involvement. In this chapter the client is our teacher, a teacher who articulates what it is like to feel intense fear and loneliness and yet risks engaging in a cocreated endeavor of two persons involved in the process of healing. Leigh says, "That session helped me to know, not just cognitively, but deeply, in the depths of my body, that I am not alone."

Lynn Martin's chapter introduces us to Carmen, a depressed woman dependent on medication. Through Lynn's descriptions we learn of her parallel process with the client's entangled sense of self-blame, shame, and withdrawal. Lynn's explanations of her practice of psychotherapy provide a model from which we can each learn.

A discussion about the importance of the use of the therapist's self is the central theme in Linda Finlay's humanistic perspective. In her chapter, Linda challenges us to open our eyes and to commit to keeping them open as we engage with our clients, particularly when they may be "in hiding." Linda encourages us to maintain an attuned inquiry. She describes how a sustained inquiry respects our clients' experience and sense of identity.

Silvia Allari and Eugenio Peiró Orozco's chapter describes a single session research project where the authors record the transactions between therapist and client in their attempt to identify what is effective and what may be ineffective in the psychotherapy. This is the kind of research that each of us can do in our own therapeutic practice to enhance our understanding of both the client's experience and what types of interactions are beneficial to the client.

The last chapter, written by Richard Erskine, puts the theory of the schizoid process into therapeutic practice. He vividly describes a client whose habitual relational withdrawal was hidden by her self-aggrandizement and social activities. Throughout the chapter Richard reveals his countertransferential responses (perplexity, being challenged, tenderness, patience, gratification, and sorrow) as he takes us step-by-step into understanding the client's social facade, her internal criticism, the relational neglect of her childhood, and her constant schizoid withdrawal.

The case studies presented throughout this book provide us with a unique form of research into our clients' phenomenological experiences and what is needed to create a healing relationship.

As I finish reading this book, I realize that it has been thirty years since I attended my first lecture with Richard Erskine at a conference in Siena, Italy. At that time Richard was teaching about an in-depth psychotherapy of childhood sexual abuse and dissociation. I did not understand English then, but the Italian translator helped me comprehend the attunement, tenderness, and therapeutic involvement that was evident in how Richard presented the various cases. I was captivated by the profound respect he showed as he talked about the relational disruptions that were encoded in each behavior—behaviors that on the surface may seem strange and incomprehensible to many of us.

Since that conference I have attended many of Richard's training workshops where I have had the opportunity of observing his way of working with a variety of "diagnoses." I have been, and still am, impressed by Richard's wisdom and his many ways of relating to various clients from a respectful, non-pathological attitude. That wisdom is evident in his psychotherapy cases presented in this book.

Richard has, in previous writings (2013, 2015), described the philosophical foundations of a developmentally based, relationally focused integrative psychotherapy. These philosophical principles are relevant with all clients and they are particularly significant in our work with clients who struggle to emotionally stabilize themselves via a schizoid process. If we want to create significant therapeutic connection with a client who is hidden in their private place, we have to appreciate their unique way of experiencing the world with respect, patience, and compassion. Three of the philosophical principles that are most evident in the case studies and theoretical discussions throughout the chapters in this book are:

- Humans suffer from relational disruptions not psychopathology
- The intersubjective process of psychotherapy is more important than the content of psychotherapy, and
- Humans have an innate thrust to grow.

I want to express my gratitude to each author for sharing their understanding and stories about working with clients who can be described as relying on a schizoid process to manage interpersonal relationships. I have learned much from reading your contributions.

With appreciation, Amaia Mauriz Etxabe
Clinical psychologist and professor, Deusto University, Bilbao, Spain

References

Erskine, R. G. (2013). Vulnerability, authenticity, and inter-subjective contact: Philosophical principles of integrative psychotherapy. *International Journal of Integrative Psychotherapy*, 4(2): 1–9.
Erskine, R. G. (2015). *Relational Patterns, Therapeutic Presence: Concepts and Practice of Integrative Psychotherapy*. London: Karnac.
Erskine, R. G. (2021a). *Early Affect Confusion: Relational Psychotherapy for the Borderline Client*. London: nscience.
Erskine, R. G. (2021b). *A Healing Relationship: Commentary on Therapeutic Dialogues*. Bicester, UK: Phoenix.

Preface

Richard G. Erskine

It is an honor to present the concept of the *schizoid process* to you. I have spent many years thinking about, teaching, and having productive discussions concerning the psychotherapy for clients who struggle with internal criticism, shame and silence, relational withdrawal, and loneliness. During the late 1980s I read a lot of the psychoanalytic literature, primarily from both the American self-psychology and the British object relations schools of psychoanalysis. These psychoanalytic writings provided the foundation for understanding many of my clients and particularly the clients who relied on a schizoid process to manage their lives.

My transactional analysis and Gestalt therapy training provided me with the therapeutic skills to attend to the clients' internal criticisms and adaptation of a social facade. My client-centered background gave me a deep appreciation of the importance of empathy in psychotherapy. The time I spent in my personal psychoanalysis and my psychoanalytic training provided me with an appreciation of the silent moments in psychotherapy—the silent moments that I refer to as a *pregnant pause*—that quiet time when implicit memories emerge and affects germinate. The integration of the theories and methods from these different approaches to psychotherapy are reflected in this book that portrays a relationally focused, integrative psychotherapy perspective on the treatment of clients who rely on a schizoid process to stabilize their affect.

Over the past thirty-five-plus years I have continued to investigate the methods that are effective in the psychotherapy of the schizoid process. I have spent countless hours with clients, sitting in silence, yet fully present. I have listened to clients' attempts to articulate their lethal internal criticisms. I have challenged their social facades and I have encouraged them to express their vitality and vulnerability. It has been a fascinating and informative journey—a journey that is chronicled in the case presentations in this book. But I have not journeyed alone.

Many colleagues have been actively involved in lengthy discussions about the therapeutic work they do with their clients. I am always fascinated by how psychotherapists change their therapeutic involvement when they understand the internal dynamics of the schizoid process and the qualities of therapeutic contact necessary for a healing relationship. I have invited eight colleagues to write about their therapeutic experiences; the results form informative and therapeutically useful chapters. Therefore, it is an honor to present the writings of these colleagues who have accompanied me on this professional journey—a journey of refining our understanding and our practice of psychotherapy of the schizoid process.

As I organized this book, I reflected upon the camaraderie and enthusiasm that several colleagues and I experienced as we discussed our psychotherapy with clients who self-stabilized their intense affect through internal criticism, presentation of a social facade, and reliance on relational withdrawal. We shared the articles and books we found enlightening; we discussed the difficulties in doing psychotherapy with clients who were emotionally isolated; and, we explored various ways of being therapeutically effective with clients who did not respond well to either our phenomenological inquiry or our attempts to be interpersonally contactful. Some of these discussions about our therapeutic endeavors with reticent clients culminated in a two-day "Symposium on the Schizoid Process" in San Francisco in August, 1999.

I want to particularly acknowledge Marye O'Reilly-Knapp (USA) for the professionally enriching years we spent discussing the schizoid process. Both Ray Little (Scotland) and Gary Yontef (USA) have offered valuable insights into working with clients who struggle with interpersonal contact, internal criticism, shame, and emotional withdrawal. Marye O'Reilly-Knapp's (2001) article entitled "Between Two Worlds: The Encapsulated Self" has become a classic reference point when psychotherapists are discussing our work with clients who engage in relational withdrawal to stabilize their intense affect. Gary Yontef's (2001) article "Psychotherapy of the Schizoid Process" provides a Gestalt therapist's perspective and a necessary discussion of the schizoid process. Ray Little's (2001) chapter on "Working with the Defenses of the Withdrawn Child Ego State" offers a transactional analyst's approach to working within the various forms of transference that may emerge in psychotherapy with clients who engage in a schizoid process.

Each of these three authors published their ideas and therapeutic findings in the January, 2001, *Transactional Analysis Journal*, a special issue devoted to the psychotherapy of the schizoid process. Although these articles were written more than twenty years ago, they remain fresh and informative today.

I recommend that you read each of their articles to enrich what is presented in this book. Also published in that same issue is a roundtable discussion on the psychotherapy of the schizoid process entitled, "Withdrawal, Connection, and Therapeutic Touch" (Erskine et al., 2001). The roundtable members included Helena Hargaden (UK), Lynne Jacobs (USA), Ray Little (Scotland), Marye O'Reilly-Knapp (USA), Charlotte Sills (UK), Thomas Weil (Germany), and Gary Yontef (USA).

In this book

Chapter 1 is entitled "The schizoid process: an introduction." It contains excerpts from an article I wrote entitled, "The schizoid process," published in the *Transactional Analysis Journal* (2001, pp. 4–6). I hope it lays the foundation for your reading the rest of the book.

Chapter 2 is a distillation of concepts and therapeutic interventions that I have found useful with my clients who rely on relational withdrawal to manage socially intense situations. These concepts are illustrated through vignettes from psychotherapy sessions with a client, Maryann, whose internal processes and external relationships reflect a schizoid style. As I wrote this chapter, I realized that it is a mere outline of therapeutic ideas but I hope it will stimulate you to read the rest of this book, particularly the longer case presentations about Violet's (Chapter 3) and Louise's (Chapter 16) psychotherapy.

It is in the detailed descriptions of the psychotherapy that the concepts and therapeutic interventions come alive. Ray Little (Chapter 4), Marye O'Reilly-Knapp (Chapter 5), and Dan Eastop (Chapter 6) elaborate on these ideas in each of their chapters. They provide a further expansion on the seminal ideas of psychotherapy with clients who are caught within a schizoid compromise.

The heart of this book lies in Part II: "A five-year case study and colleagues' reflections." These chapters provide a longitudinal case study of Allan, a client whose psychotherapy revealed a schizoid pattern of affect and social behavior. In writing these chapters I focused on the narrative of our psychotherapy sessions while interweaving several salient concepts throughout the story of Allan's psychotherapy. Some readers may want to begin this book by reading Chapters 7 through 11 first; these chapters illustrate a patient, nonjudgmental, caring relationship that is so essential in the psychotherapy. Linda Finlay's (Chapter 12) and Lynn Martin's (Chapter 13) writings provide significant observations on the process of the psychotherapy. Their chapters represent the important aspects of our professional dialogue that are so central to our refining the practice of psychotherapy.

Part III of this book is titled "clients' perspectives on the psychotherapy."

We are very fortunate to have chapters that reflect two clients' personal views on their internal experience of their psychotherapy. Chapter 14, entitled, "Come closer ... but keep your distance," is authored by Leigh Bettles. She describes her psychotherapy from the inside out by narrating her lifelong internal experience of being terrified by interpersonal contact. She reports how even though she was inundated with fear she responded to the therapist's rhythm and affect—to the caring prosody of how he spoke with her. Her story offers psychotherapists an opportunity to question our own rhythm and desire to accomplish a cognitive or behavioral outcome.

Chapter 15, written by Silvia Allari and Eugenio Peiró Orozco, presents another description of a client's internal reactions to the therapist's way of being with the client. Both Chapters 14 and 15 represent the type of phenomenological research that is necessary in our profession because they reveal the client's subjective experiences in response to the psychotherapist's attunement to their affect and rhythm, how they process various inquiries about their memories and thought processes, as well as the subtle qualities of the therapeutic relationship. There is much for all of us to learn through this type of phenomenological research.

The book concludes with Chapter 16, a case study of my client's five-year psychotherapeutic journey entitled, "Louise: social facade, depression, relational withdrawal." This chapter demonstrates how the theory of the schizoid process is put into therapeutic practice.

Thank you

This book is dedicated to the members of the professional development seminars of the Institute for Integrative Psychotherapy who have listened to my lectures and discussions about the psychotherapy of the schizoid process. Your continued interest and professional challenges leave me with a richer understanding of the unique nature of our profession of psychotherapy. Your enthusiasm stimulates my desire to learn more.

I am grateful to Kate Pearce, editor at Phoenix Publishing House, for encouraging me to publish the concepts and methods about a relational psychotherapy for clients with a schizoid process. Working with you and your team of editors at Phoenix is a pleasure.

I am a terrible speller. This book would not be publishable without Karen Hallett's dedicated proofreading. I am grateful to you, Karen, for your editorial assistance, your inspiration, and for your constant support.

And, a "Thank you" to each of you who are reading this book. I feel honored by your choosing to read the ideas expressed in these pages. This book is not meant to be a definitive description of the psychotherapy of the schizoid process. Rather, this book is a description of my professional journey and involvement with my clients, as well as the rewarding cooperation with colleagues. I wish you well as you read about the psychotherapy of the schizoid process.

References

Erskine, R. G. (2001). The schizoid process. *Transactional Analysis Journal*, *31*(1): 4–6. doi.org/10.1177/036215370103100102.

Erskine, R. G., Hargaden, H., Jacobs, L., Little, R., O'Reilly-Knapp, M., Sills, C., Weil, T., & Yontef, G. (2001). Withdrawal, connection, and therapeutic touch: A round table on the schizoid process. *Transactional Analysis Journal*, *31*(1): 24–32. doi.org/10.1177/036215370103100104.

Little, R. (2001). Schizoid processes: Working with the defenses of the withdrawn child ego state. *Transactional Analysis Journal*, *31*(1): 33–43. doi.org/10.1177/036215370103100105.

O'Reilly-Knapp, M. (2001). Between two worlds: The encapsulated self. *Transactional Analysis Journal*, *31*(1): 44–54. doi.org/10.1177/036215370103100106.

Yontef, G. (2001). Psychotherapy of schizoid process. *Transactional Analysis Journal*, *31*(1): 7–23. doi.org/10.1177/036215370103100103.

Part I

Psychotherapy of the schizoid process

CHAPTER 1

The schizoid process: an introduction

Richard G. Erskine

In the 1950s my mother and stepfather owned a large Victorian house. To meet their expenses, they converted the upper rooms into rental apartments. As a boy I was often interested in the stories the various tenants would tell. One of the tenants was a psychiatric nurse who periodically told me captivating stories about her patients. One day she gave my mother an article that had been in the *Chicago Tribune*'s Sunday Magazine about people who withdrew from interpersonal relationships. The nurse said, "This article describes the *schizoid syndrome*. It will help you understand your husband's split personality."

As my mother and I read the article together I could recognize many of my stepfather's behaviors. Although he was superficially friendly to neighbors, he had neither friends nor contact with his many brothers and sisters. Each evening he spent many hours quietly reading. He often avoided conversation and any social gathering. From time to time, he would binge on alcohol. When semi-drunk he was punishingly self-critical and would tell me stories of how in his early life he had drifted aimlessly from one job to another. When completely drunk he would tearfully tell stories about witnessing the work demands and physical punishment that his father inflicted on his older brothers and sisters but never on himself. He was seldom overtly angry; instead he found some solace when he withdrew into prolonged silence. I was fascinated by how this man with whom I lived could have such different personalities. Each personality seemed real even though they were so dissimilar.

Throughout my various trainings in clinical psychology and psychotherapy the concept of "schizoid personality disorder" was referenced but no serious attention was given as to how to work with such clients. My initial experience of the *schizoid process* emerged from working with children who withdrew from social contact, were non-communicative, and were sometimes described as having autistic-like behaviors. Under the supervision of Robert Neville and Georgia Baker I learned to use non-directive, child-centered play therapy to create a safe environment for my young clients to express their internalized conflicts. The writings of Virginia Axline (1947, 1964), Dorothy Baruch (1952), Clark Moustakas (1953, 1959), and Bruno Bettelheim (1950, 1959, 1967) were influential in shaping my understanding of how to conduct psychotherapy with children who are withdrawn and wary of people.

Later in my professional life I applied these same child therapy concepts and relational methods with some of my adult clients who used dissociation as an ongoing coping mechanism to manage their internalized histories of profound physical and sexual abuse (Clark, 1986; Erskine, 1993). Many of these clients also employed shame as a primary way of organizing their internal processes (Erskine, 1994). They were often self-critical, sometimes charming, and at other times relationally withdrawn. Originally I thought that these clients were engaging in psychological dissociation, the result of acute trauma—a split between "me" and "not me." Yet, some of the clients did not have childhoods replete with acute physical or sexual abuse. Rather, they struggled with a history of relational neglect, repeated criticism, and an absence of parental tenderness.

I eventually came to realize that what at first appeared to be dissociation was better described as a subjective perception of "me," "me," and "also me." With these clients I found that I needed to refine my approach to psychotherapy in order to gain greater comprehension and appreciation of their subjective experience. Whenever I emphasized cognitive understanding or behavior change it seemed to disrupt our therapeutic relationship. They required consistent sensitivity to their unspoken forms of communication.

Clients such as Violet (Chapter 3), Allan (Chapters 7 to 11), and Louise (Chapter 16) taught me a lot about working within the client's schizoid process. It was evident that such clients require the psychotherapist's patient presence. Psychotherapy with these clients called for consistent attunement to their affective states: meeting their fear with security, their sadness with compassion, and their anger with a response of being taken seriously (Erskine & Trautmann, 1996). I became acutely interested in the clients who required a sensitive responsiveness to the fear-laden affect state that is so dominant in the schizoid process, one often related to a nonverbal experience.

My interest in refining psychotherapy for clients who rely on a schizoid process to manage their intense affect has been supported and enhanced by the therapy case presentations and discussions at the Institute for Integrative Psychotherapy. We found that such clients also need the therapist's attunement to their developmental level of functioning (Erskine, 2019), especially to what Daniel Stern (1985) described in his writings as the emerging self, the core self, and the intersubjective self—those levels of developmental functioning that are pre-language. Many schizoid clients regress to prelinguistic developmental functioning as a safety zone in the presence of threat (Guntrip, 1968).

Much of our therapeutic work and research has shown the importance of validating the client's subjective experience. When therapy emphasizes change, not as the primary goal but as a by-product of therapy, when the therapeutic focus is not on behavior but on the client's internal process, we wind up with a slower form of therapy but one that can fill the psychological void the schizoid individual experiences internally. What becomes evident in a phenomenologically focused psychotherapy is the sequestered, hidden, encapsulated affects of the client's self.

With many schizoid individuals, the affects of terror and rage have never found their way into verbal dialogue with another person. We know from treating trauma victims that without a healing relationship from an attuned and protective other person the physical and emotional distress of the trauma remains for years. Many people have traumatic experiences but do not remain traumatized because someone was there in a healing, supportive, and clarifying way that allowed the trauma to be integrated within the individual's experience (Erskine, 1993).

The schizoid process is defined in Eric Berne's (1961) description of the states of the ego—a sense of self fragmented by trauma—and how the fixation of child ego states interferes with here-and-now neopsychic functioning. Berne defined ego fragmentation and boundary issues—such as loss of reality, estrangement, and depersonalization—as "schizoid in character" (p. 67). Each of these child ego states, fragmented by trauma, requires a responsive, healing relationship. Berne described the therapeutic process: "The ego state can be treated like an actual child. It can be nurtured carefully, even tenderly, until it unfolds like a flower" (p. 226). Clients who engage in a schizoid process need the therapist to create a therapeutic relationship that allows each child ego state to emerge and be met with a safe, attuned response.

Ronald Fairbairn (1952) was among the first psychoanalysts to describe thoroughly the relational dynamics of early childhood—of a child in relationship from the first moments of life—and the damage to the child when there is a failure in those primary relationships. Thus, he articulated the etiology of the schizoid process. These relationship failures are not the acute traumas that we think of in, for example, our work with clients struggling with dissociative identity disorder. Rather, they are what Masud Khan (1963) referred to as "cumulative trauma" (p. 286)—the little missed attunements, discounts, punishments, and rejections—like grains of sand that pile up until they form a dune. The accumulation of missed attunements and missed connections creates the conditions wherein the child hides more and more in his or her own sequestered world while adjusting his or her behavior to provide what the other demands (Lourie, 1996). For clients engaging in a schizoid process, intimacy and interpersonal connections are a threat to the sense of self. They experience a great fear of contact; for such individuals, a genuine relationship is dangerous.

Bob Goulding (1974) described the schizoid process as a third-degree impasse. It is the split in a child's ego that occurs when the individual's natural organismic functioning is repressed and denied—split off—and the child becomes the social facade required by the grown-ups around them. The adaptive, social facade becomes "me," and the natural, fundamentally human part becomes "another me." What is natural may be lost or split off so intensely that the person experiences no other way of being in the world. Both my own clinical experience and the contemporary psychotherapy literature have led me to believe that a patient, consistent, respectful, and attuned therapeutic relationship allows those hidden aspects that were made into "another me" to become "me" (Bollas, 1987; Erskine et al., 1999; Mitchell, 1993; Stolorow et al., 1987).

Harry Guntrip (1961, 1968, 1971; Hazell, 1994) wrote extensively on the treatment of the schizoid process. He described how the person is driven into hiding by fear and then experiences a deep, sequestered loneliness that drives him or her out of hiding back into an adaptive interface with the world. Such a person is constantly caught in the struggle between hiding or connecting to others, but in an adaptive way. Guntrip (cited in Hazell, 1994) defined the psychotherapy of the schizoid process as:

> the provision of a reliable and understanding human relationship of a kind that makes contact with the deeply repressed traumatized child in a way that enables one to become steadily more able to live, in the security of a new, real relationship, with the traumatic legacy of the earliest formative years, as it seeps through or erupts into consciousness.... It is a process of interaction, the function of two variables, the personalities of two people working together towards free spontaneous growth. (p. 366)

Donald Winnicott also had extensive experience in treating the schizoid process (Hazell, 1994; Little, 1990). He (Winnicott, 1965) described the essential ingredients of an in-depth psychotherapy as providing a respectful, understanding, reliable environment, one that the client never had and needs if they are to resolve their inner conflicts and inhibitions. Such an environment allows the person to find out what is natural for themselves. Both Guntrip and Winnicott encouraged a psychotherapy that focuses on the client's internal process and not specifically on behavioral outcome, a psychotherapy that provides a healing relationship to a traumatized self.

In closing this introduction, it may be fitting to again quote Guntrip's beliefs about the psychotherapy of the schizoid process—an attitude that one of his clients described as providing a "cherishing" of her.

> It is the psychotherapist's responsibility to discover what kind of parental relationship the patient needs in order to get better.... The child grows up to be a disturbed person because he is not loved for his own sake as a person in his own right, and as an ill adult he comes to the psychotherapist convinced beforehand that this "professional man" has no real interest or concern for him. The kind of love the patient needs is the kind of love that he may well feel in due course that the psychotherapist is the first person ever to give him. It involves taking him seriously as a person in his difficulties, respecting him as an individual in his own right even in his anxieties, treating him as someone with the right to be understood and not merely blamed, put-off, pressed and molded to suit other people's convenience, regarding him as a valuable human being with a nature of his own that needs a good human environment to grow in, showing him genuine human contact, real sympathy, believing in him so that in the course of time he can become capable of

believing in himself. All these are ingredients of true parental love (agape not eros), and if the psychiatrist cannot love his patients in that way, he had better give up psychotherapy. (Guntrip, cited in Hazell, 1994, pp. 401–402)

References

Axline, V. M. (1947). *Play Therapy*. Oxford: Houghton Mifflin.
Axline, V. M. (1964). *Dibs: In Search of Self*. New York: Ballantine.
Baruch, D. W. (1952). *One Little Boy*. New York: Dell.
Berne, E. (1961). *Transactional Analysis in Psychotherapy: A Systematic Individual and Social Psychiatry*. New York: Grove Press.
Bettelheim, B. (1950). *Love Is Not Enough: The Treatment of Emotionally Disturbed Children*. Glencoe, IL: Free Press.
Bettelheim, B. (1959). Joey: A "Mechanical boy." *Scientific American, 200*(3): 116–127.
Bettelheim, B. (1967). *The Empty Fortress: Infantile Autism and the Birth of the Self*. Glencoe, IL: Free Press.
Bollas, C. (1987). *The Shadow of the Object: Psychoanalysis of the Unthought Known*. New York: Columbia University Press.
Clark, N. H. (1986). *Shatter: The True Story of Kathy Roth's Eight Separate Personalities and Her Struggle to Become Whole*. New York: Bantam.
Erskine, R. G. (1993). Inquiry, attunement, and involvement in the psychotherapy of dissociation. *Transactional Analysis Journal, 23*(4). doi.org/10.1177/036215379302300402.
Erskine, R. G. (1994). Shame and self-righteousness: Transactional analysis perspectives and clinical interventions. *Transactional Analysis Journal, 24*(2). doi.org/10.1177/036215379402400204.
Erskine, R. G. (2019). Child development in integrative psychotherapy: Erik Erikson's first three stages. *International Journal of Integrative Psychotherapy, 10*: 11–34.
Erskine, R. G., Moursund, J. P., & Trautmann, R. L. (1999). *Beyond Empathy: A Therapy of Contact-in-relationship*. New York: Brunner/Mazel.
Erskine, R. G., & Trautmann, R. L. (1996). Methods of an integrative psychotherapy. *Transactional Analysis Journal, 26*(4). doi.org/10.1177/036215379602600410.
Fairbairn, W. R. D. (1952). *An Object-relations Theory of the Personality*. New York: Basic Books.
Goulding, R. (1974). Thinking and feeling in transactional analysis: Three impasses. *Voices: The Art and Science of Psychotherapy, 10*: 11–13.
Guntrip, H. (1961). *Personality Structure and Human Interaction*. London: Hogarth.
Guntrip, H. (1968). *Schizoid Phenomena, Object Relations and the Self*. New York: International Universities Press.
Guntrip, H. (1971). *Psychoanalytic Theory, Therapy, and the Self*. New York: Basic Books.
Hazell, J. (Ed.) (1994). *Personal Relations Therapy: The Collected Papers of H. J. S. Guntrip*. Northvale, NJ: Jason Aronson.

Khan, M. M. R. (1963). The concept of cumulative trauma. In: R. S. Eissler, A. Freud, H. Hartmann, & M. Kris (Eds.), *Psychoanalytic Study of the Child* (Vol. XVIII, pp. 286–306). New York: International Universities Press.

Little, M. I. (1990). *Psychotic Anxieties and Containment: A Personal Record of an Analysis with Winnicott.* Northvale, NJ: Jason Aronson.

Lourie, J. (1996). Cumulative trauma: The non-problem problem. *Transactional Analysis Journal, 26*: 276–283. doi.org/10.1177/036215379602600402.

Mitchell, S. A. (1993). *Hope and Dread in Psychoanalysis.* New York: Basic Books.

Moustakas, C. (1953). *Children in Play Therapy.* New York: McGraw-Hill.

Moustakas, C. (1959). *Psychotherapy with Children: The Living Relationship.* New York: Ballantine.

Stern, D. N. (1985). *The Interpersonal World of the Infant: A View from Psychoanalysis and Developmental Psychology.* New York: Basic Books.

Stolorow, R. D., Brandchaft, B., & Atwood, G. E. (1987). *Psychoanalytic Treatment: An Intersubjective Approach.* Hillsdale, NJ: The Analytic Press.

Winnicott, D. W. (1965). *The Maturational Processes and the Facilitating Environment: Studies in the Theory of Emotional Development.* London: Hogarth.

CHAPTER 2

Relational withdrawal, internal criticism, social facade: attunement to parts of the self

Richard G. Erskine

> *Solitude is independence.*
> *It had been my wish*
> *and with the years I had attained it.*
> *It was cold. Oh, cold enough!*
> *But it was also still, wonderfully still*
> *and vast like the cold stillness of space*
> *in which the stars revolve.*
> —Hermann Hesse

In one of Maryann's early psychotherapy sessions she cried, "I'm so confused. Sometimes I am two people or even three. I'm split inside. I can be nice to people but then I get so scared that I can't talk. I just hide. Then I beat up on myself for being so stupid. I don't know which is really me. I'm so tired of it all." Maryann's anguish touched my heart as she struggled to speak about her "split inside." Her words were an apt portrayal of the internal struggle that we call the *schizoid process*.

Schizoid is the Greek word for scissors: it means "to split." When I use the terms "schizoid process" or "schizoid syndrome," I am describing a person's tendency to withdraw from relationship, to live with an internal sense of personal isolation and self-criticism in order to avoid the potential stress of interpersonal contact. People who rely on a schizoid process to stabilize and manage internal stress are often introverted and live primarily in an internal world without much emotional contact with others, even family. They may have a well-rehearsed social presence, but the essence of who they are, their vulnerability, is hidden.

Many people who seek psychotherapy may exist somewhere on the schizoid spectrum—from *schizoid style*, to *schizoid pattern*, to *schizoid disorder*. Yet for many of these people their schizoid process may go unnoticed, even in their psychotherapy. The schizoid syndrome is prevalent in the lives of many psychotherapy clients, but it is often not attended to because both a schizoid style and a schizoid pattern are subtle; the clues are not obvious as they are with a schizoid disorder. After we had established a consistent working relationship, my client Maryann revealed, "I was an expert at hiding in plain sight. I simply told my former therapist what she wanted to hear."

Schizoid disorder

With clients who have a clear diagnosis of schizoid disorder, their relational difficulties are often evident in the first session because they are unable to engage in interpersonal contact. Their tendency to withdraw emotionally is pervasive throughout all their relationships, as well as in their relationship with the psychotherapist. They may have a number of acquaintances, but they are usually without any meaningful relationships. People with a diagnosable schizoid disorder are more likely to avoid psychotherapy mainly because it is too personal and intersubjective. If they do come for psychotherapy, they are reluctant to talk about their internal process and prefer to talk instead about their day-to-day activities. They often want specific solutions to a problem. Novels that portray a protagonist with a schizoid disorder provide us with insight about both their relational discombobulation and internal turmoil.

Hermann Hesse's novel, *Steppenwolf* (1927) tells the story of Harry Haller, a man with a schizoid disorder, who wanders through his encounters with people like a bewildered alien, always a stranger in his community. He is prone to intellectualization; but he cannot tolerate interpersonal contact. As a result, his relational isolation and despair plague him with thoughts of suicide. In Damon Galgut's (2010) autobiographical novel, *In a Strange Room*, Damon reveals his personal anguish in a mix of first and third person voices, as he wanders from country to country, split between his longing to be in relationship with the various people he encounters and his desperate efforts to withdraw into his internal sanctuary. In Conrad Aiken's 1934 short story "Silent Snow, Secret Snow," Paul, a sensitive adolescent boy finds solace in daydreaming. He distances himself from the demands of school and family by withdrawing into a fantasy world of pure white snow—a world of silent snow that he must keep a secret. The first-person story of Paul, as well as each of the other two protagonists, provides us with a glimpse into their emotional and relational struggles. Unfortunately, none of these three stories addresses the qualities of relationship that the principal characters needed to heal from their internal distress.

Most psychotherapists are likely to have had some clients who we can identify as having either a schizoid style or a schizoid pattern. The distinction between a style, a pattern, or a disorder is in the *frequency*, *duration*, and *intensity* of their tendency to engage in relational withdrawal, to suffer from internal criticism, and to maintain superficial relationships. The intrapsychic and behavioral manifestations are the same. The term *schizoid process* refers to an entire continuum of internal and social dynamics. It is used to describe the psychological process of anyone struggling within the schizoid syndrome.

Schizoid pattern

Evidence that a client has a *schizoid pattern* is often apparent early on in their psychotherapy, as the client tends to talk about current events while avoiding displaying any of their affect. They may talk about the people in their lives, but it is often without any emotional connection. For the first year of her therapy, Maryann used most of our therapy hours recounting—in great detail—the many novels she had read. She disregarded any inquiry that I made about her feelings or personal experiences, while continuing to tell me about the stories in her books. It took me many months to decipher a pattern in the themes of her stories—authority, betrayal, and loneliness—that were metaphors about her life.

Clients with a schizoid pattern may not show evidence of it in the first few sessions, but the pattern will gradually become more evident as the therapeutic dialogue explores the quality of interpersonal contact in the client's life. A schizoid pattern will certainly become evident if the contact with the psychotherapist becomes emotionally close and intense. Clients with a schizoid pattern will usually struggle to escape being emotionally involved in any intersubjective relationship.

I have found that a client's schizoid pattern is often first apparent through examining my own countertransference. Such clients often leave me with a sense that something important is missing between us. With such clients, my countertransference reaction is to drift toward more cognitive and behavioral interventions. I may lose my relational perspective, or I start watching the clock to see how soon the session will be over. My loss of interpersonal contact is probably being engendered both by the clients' superficial conversation and their fear (often unconscious and unexpressed) of a meaningful interpersonal relationship. Colleagues working with similar clients report that they feel inadequate, bored, or sleepy, and/or that they have to work harder and harder trying to make something happen.

Schizoid style

In contrast, it may be difficult to identify clients with a *schizoid style* early on in the psychotherapy. At first, they may have a compatible social presentation with a tendency to be shy, quiet, or introverted. However, when the client is stressed, or after they have been in psychotherapy for a while, the client with a schizoid style will display a tendency to withdraw from relationships, to be plagued by internal criticism, or to put on a social facade. They will talk about preferring to be alone, rather than being with people. They may find solace in reading, video games, or some solitary activity; alternatively, they may be constantly busy with many energy-consuming activities.

Clients with a schizoid style often come to psychotherapy saying that they are depressed. As the psychotherapy unfolds with these clients, I have found that it is necessary to attend to the intense shame that they experience—a shame that is intrinsic to their depression. They are often afraid of being criticized and rejected for what they think, or how they behave; they report therefore constraining themselves in social situations. They may be sad about past rejections, but compensate by anticipating further denigrating comments; hence, they do not reveal any vulnerabilities. Clients with a schizoid style struggle to comply with what others expect of them. They make efforts at fitting into what other people, including the psychotherapist, require. They disavow any possible anger at how they have been treated, because any protest may produce further criticism and rejection. The result of disavowing their anger and complying with others' expectations is their conviction that "there is something wrong with me."

In my practice of psychotherapy, I have found that it is necessary to provide sufficient attention (often repeated over many sessions) to five focal points that I consider essential in the therapeutic resolution of shame (Erskine, 1994, 1995). I will briefly spotlight them here. Shame is usually composed of:

- Hurt in not being accepted for **who I am**: i.e., *"My worth as a human being is of less value"*
- Fear of rejection for **how I am**: i.e., *"My behavior means I'm not acceptable as I am"*
- Disavowal of anger at not being accepted **as I am**: i.e., *"I'll criticize myself so that you can never criticize me"*
- Compliance with how **others define me**: i.e., *"I will be what you say I am,"* and
- A belief that **something is wrong with me**: i.e., *"I have nothing useful to say."*

Schizoid process

The term *schizoid process* depicts a "splitting" of the self into various entities. The concept of "splitting" is borrowed from the early psychoanalytic literature and is used as a metaphor to explain our client's experience that their sense of self is internally divided into diverse parts. Ronald Fairbairn (1954) used the term "splitting" to portray an archaic, self-protective polarization of a sense of self that is the result of overwhelming and conflicting affects (Rubens, 1996). R. D. Laing (1960) also used this concept in his book titled, *The Divided Self*. Although the concept of splitting is not theoretically consistent with a physiological and relational perspective of psychotherapy, it serves as a useful metaphor in describing the client's internal sense of being segmented into various selves.

Therefore, I use the concept of splitting as a metaphor to describe how a child will struggle in their attempt to preserve their vitality and protect their vulnerability by dissecting their natural, whole self into several manageable parts. My clients seldom use terms like "splitting" or "schizoid"; they simply say, "I have different parts," or "I'm split inside." It is my conviction that each "part" requires its unique form of psychotherapy.[1]

---

[1] This has similarities with the treatment of "Sybil" in the 1973 book of that name by Flora Rheta Schreiber and also in *Shatter: The True Story of Katy Roth's Eight Personalities* by Nancy Clark in 1986. However, the clients featured in both of these books were fragmented into different personalities as a result of traumatic dissociation.

However, when we use the term splitting, we are describing a different dynamic than dissociation. As clients describe it, dissociation is a sense of "me" and "not-me," whereas splitting has a sense of "me" and "me" and "also me." Dissociation is often the result of physical and/or sexual trauma, persistent abuse, and a disorganized family environment. The splitting of a sense of self seems to occur when children have parents who are consistently experienced as simultaneously being neglectful and controlling. The result may be an implicit fear of invasion.

Maryann described her mother as: "a bee hovering around a flower, helping to pollinate, but always buzzing, pestering … and with a potential stinger. So, I learned to shut her out. I told her nothing. I wouldn't accept her pestering me and I didn't accept her helping me. I learned to live on my own."

Clients who rely on a schizoid process to manage their affect report that—in their childhood—significant caretakers were constantly misinterpreting their emotional expressions while—at the same time—controlling their sense of identity. In general, they report that their parents:

- Were constantly misattuned to their affect and rhythm
- Were overprotective and authoritative
- Were critical of their behavior and their sense of "who I am," and
- Failed to provide the tenderness and security necessary to heal from these traumatic relational ruptures.

As a result, they are left with an implicit and intense fear of invasion. In response, they learned to "split off" any affective connection with their caretakers; they distanced themselves, as a way to manage the confusing relationship; and they removed themselves from the intensity of this fear by splitting off their own sense of vulnerability, intimacy, and contact with self.

After a few years of psychotherapy, Maryann was able to summarize her schizoid process in her own words: "Even before I went to school, my natural need to depend on my mother was continually met with a lot of fussing and smothering. She continually misinterpreted any emotions that I had. She was always controlling and invasive." Maryann went on to describe how, as a very young child, she sensed that "to be vulnerable was risky." She told several stories about how she developed patterns of relationship marked by a social facade and the absence of emotional expression.

When "splitting" is used as an attempt to self-stabilize, the vital core of the personality is withdrawn from the self that lives in the external word (Guntrip, 1971). The driving force is fear (Guntrip, 1961). Harry Guntrip, in a significant article about the schizoid process, says that a child: "is capable of fear so intense that it can amount to fear of death in the absolute sense of annihilation" (Guntrip, cited in Hazel, 1994, p. 161). Because of repeated criticism, control, and relational conflicts, a child under such stress may deny their need for security-in-relationship. Security may then be pseudo-accomplished through fantasies of being in a safe hiding place: a cave, wardrobe, closet, or womb.

People with a schizoid process may engage in *relational withdrawal,* a blankness or fantasy that does not involve real people. These clients described how they created a sense of security for themselves—a pseudo-security that requires no interpersonal relationship. They talk about their preoccupation in a world of constant work projects, excessive reading, video games, or TV. Some clients have described how they imagine being alone in their safe hiding place where their affect is diminished, "All is quiet," "there are no conflicts," "the rhythm of life is slowed down," and, "the conflicts with my mother are forgotten." Marye O'Reilly-Knapp writes about her clients' relational withdrawal: "In the withdrawn and hidden places there is only existence, with no true sense of self, and no sense of self with another. The person remains uninvolved, unintegrated, and lives in quiet desperation" (2001, p. 48).

It seems to me that many clients, struggling with their schizoid process, bring into their relationships with their psychotherapist a twin desperation: the desperate fear that they will be invaded once again, and the desperation of profound loneliness. Donald Winnicott (1988) summarized his patients' schizoid process as an attempt to regain psychological stability by creating "isolation in quiet." Guntrip summarizes the schizoid dilemma with: "*They are caught in a conflict between equally strong needs for and fears of close good personal contacts, and in practice often find themselves alternatively driven into a relationship by their needs and then driven out again by their fears*" (Hazel, 1994, p. 164; italics in the original).

Our clients' relational withdrawal may be stimulated by several different factors:

- When there is external criticism and/or aggression. For example, one of my clients hides in her bed after her husband criticizes or shouts at her. She stabilizes herself by imagining that she is in her baby-crib with padded sides all around her.
- When the pressure of internal criticism becomes oppressive. Another client struggling with his schizoid process suffered from constantly saying to himself, "I'm worthless" and "I don't deserve anything." In response, he felt a constant urge to hide from people.
- When the psychotherapy relationship is perceived as consistently providing protection; when there is sufficient security to be able reveal their secret place. This withdrawal is for the purpose of physiological repair. The client's therapeutic withdrawal is motivated by hope for healing contact but at the same time this relational withdrawal is laden with fear. There is a flickering sense of hope that the psychotherapist will understand their desperation, provide safety, and be attuned to their rhythm and affect. Simultaneously, they are afraid of possible criticism and invasion, a speed of interpersonal interaction that they cannot manage, and a demand that they be in a close relationship. Hidden beneath all of this is a deep fear of abandonment, so they are often the first to disrupt the therapeutic relationship.

Whenever I made inquiries about Maryann's feelings, I noticed that she would look toward the window. At first, I asked about what had occurred just before she averted her eyes, but she was unable to answer. My attempts to get any answer were followed by her looking at the floor. She shrugged her shoulders and offered what seemed to be a superficial answer. Sometimes, she would tell me the details about a book she had read. I was left not knowing what was happening in her internal world.

Many clients who engage in a schizoid process will not reveal their relational withdrawal, or talk about their secret hiding place, especially if the psychotherapist lacks attunement to their rhythm and affect, or if the psychotherapist is focused on interpretations, behavior change, or uses confrontation. With such therapeutic interventions, the client will just turn away and will subtly withdraw. The child psychoanalyst, Selma Fraiberg (1982) identified how infants will "turn away" from interpersonal contact after they have experienced relational disruptions with their significant caretakers. The "turning away" from a parent who is invasive or controlling, when used repeatedly in early life, may become a pattern used in other significant relationships. Clients who rely on a schizoid process will internally "turn away" if there is a hint of control or invasion.

I eventually realized that Maryann's "turning away" was a clear indication that she experienced some uncomfortable disruption between us whenever I made a phenomenological inquiry. Over time, she was able to tell me that my inquiries, such as: "What are you feeling now?" or, "What do you remember about…?" were understood by her to mean: "You are wrong for feeling what you are feeling" or, "You always exaggerate." She could not hear the caring and interest in my inquiry; she only imagined ridicule. Hence, she turned away or talked about one of the books she read.

Clients who use a schizoid process to self-stabilize often come into psychotherapy because they feel depressed. They may appear to be adaptive, with socially appropriate behavior, but internally they have a vulnerable, frightened self that is deeply hidden from interpersonal contact.

They are secretly very lonely. Their relational needs force them to come out of hiding in order to make some (usually superficial) contact with people. Maryann's description of herself provides a good example: she was active in two charities; she organized fundraising social events for hundreds of people; she was an active board member in her professional association; and she attended many dinner parties—but she was often "secretly depressed." She said, "I prefer to just be left alone to read, but then I make all these social obligations that must get done."

Some clients who use a schizoid process have a social facade wherein their vulnerability is secret. Their *vital and vulnerable self* is withdrawn and in hiding and they have a *social self* that is well rehearsed. Some clients may be able to engage in business and social activities effortlessly because they are able to present themselves with a "social mask." This social facade helps them navigate a variety of interpersonal situations—but on only a superficial level. Harry Guntrip (1968) referred to this duality as the "schizoid compromise," where the person lives half in the external world and half in a secret hidden world.

Clients who have a schizoid process are perplexing to many therapists because they may:

- Have difficulty talking about needs, physiological sensation, and affect
- Forget what was discussed in previous sessions
- Be self-critical of any vulnerability, emotions, or the idea that they may have relational needs
- Be overwhelmed by shame
- Be frightened by phenomenological inquiry
- Fear dependence on the psychotherapist
- Have no memory of the interpersonal contact between self and the psychotherapist.

This list of symptoms may apply to many clients who would not be diagnosed with either a schizoid *pattern* or *disorder* but who may rely periodically on a schizoid *style* especially when they are under stress.

Ronald Fairbairn (1954) described how children, who have their affect and relational needs responded to with attunement and vitality, will develop a "whole self." He used the term "libidinal ego" to describe the child's liveliness. This is what John Bowlby (1988) called a "secure self." This "whole self" is *vital* and *vulnerable*, sensitive to both over- and under-stimulation, with a desire to explore, learn, and grow.

As I mentioned at the beginning, Fairbairn used the metaphor of "splitting" to describe his clients' internal struggles. "Splitting" is not real. People don't actually split their self, but they may suffer with internal criticism and shame; they may actively keep significant feelings, needs, and internal dynamics a secret. The concept of "splitting" is a metaphor and, as a metaphor, it is a useful way for us to think about our clients and what is therapeutically needed in their relationship with us. In the section that follows, I will illustrate four types of "splitting" and share with you some of what I know about working with each aspect of the self.

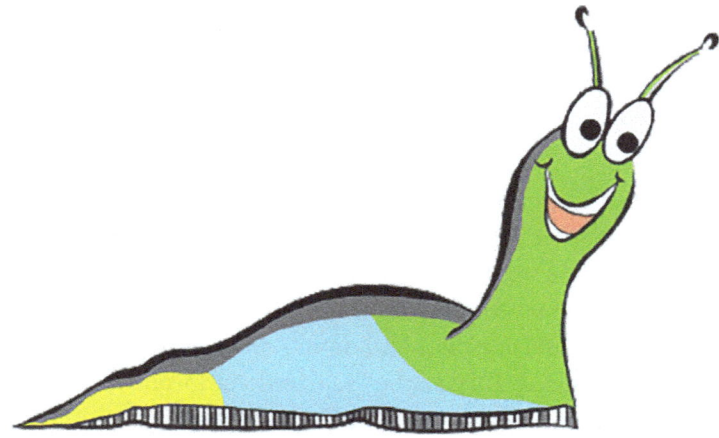

The vital and vulnerable self

"Splitting": a useful metaphor

First split

With repeated physical, rhythmic, and affect misattunements, developmentally unreasonable demands, and/or unrelenting criticism, a split may occur in the child's sense of self. In response, a *social self* may be formed that hides the *vital and vulnerable self*. This first split is an attempt to be accepted, validated, and attached to caregivers. The child learns to adapt to what is expected because any form of self-expression or protest could be dangerous. Without the intellectual development to comprehend the ramifications, the child may conclude, "I will be what you want me to be."

Donald Winnicott refers to this split as "organisation towards invulnerability" (1967, p. 198), the creation of a *social self*. It is as though the child is deciding, "If I am compliant, I am less likely to get hurt." Selma Fraiberg (1982) described how very young children, even prior to the acquisition of language, learn to transform affect and behavior in order to be accepted, validated, and loved. Anger, fear, or unacceptable behavior may be split off and replaced with a social mask of cooperation. This newly created *social self* maintains superficial relationships with people while the *vital and vulnerable self* is hidden behind a social mask. Donald Winnicott called this social self a "false self" (1960), while Eric Berne called it an "adapted child" (1961).

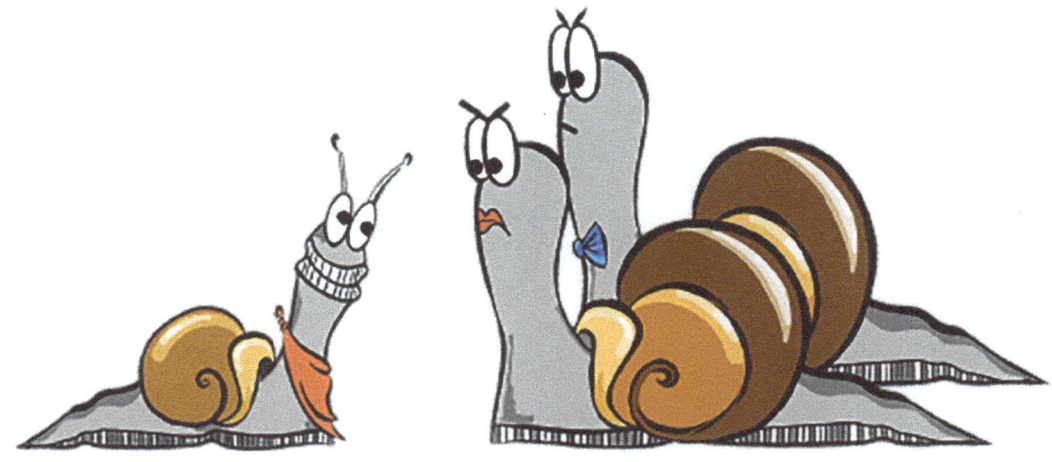

The first split: the social self

My client, Maryann, described this first split articulately:

> "I know I am segmented into parts because I'm not authentic with people. I am always acting smart and helpful, even when I don't know what is happening. I am always feeling pressured when I am with people. I work hard to please them but, at the same time, I long to be alone. But when I am alone, I'm either nervous or I just want to sleep. I don't know what I really want."

While some pseudo-security is achieved by displaying a social self, the child remains anxiously attached, because their emotional stability is always threatened. Sometimes, the vital and vulnerable self's natural feelings, desires, and needs leak through the split and are expressed. The child then runs the risk of disapproval, rejection, and punishment. The fear of punishment leads to a second split.

Second split

As a way to maintain some attachment to their primary caretakers, the child will introject the thoughts, feelings, and behaviors of their significant others. Introjection is a self-stabilizing, unconscious identification with a significant caretaker that occurs in the absence of need-fulfilling contact (Erskine, 2003). Introjection functions to provide a false sense of attachment when the secure attachment is threatened.

With introjection, vital aspects of the self are replaced with characteristics of the significant other person. The introjected thoughts, feelings, and behaviors dominate the child's sense of self. Vitality is lost and the vulnerable child refrains from full self-expression.

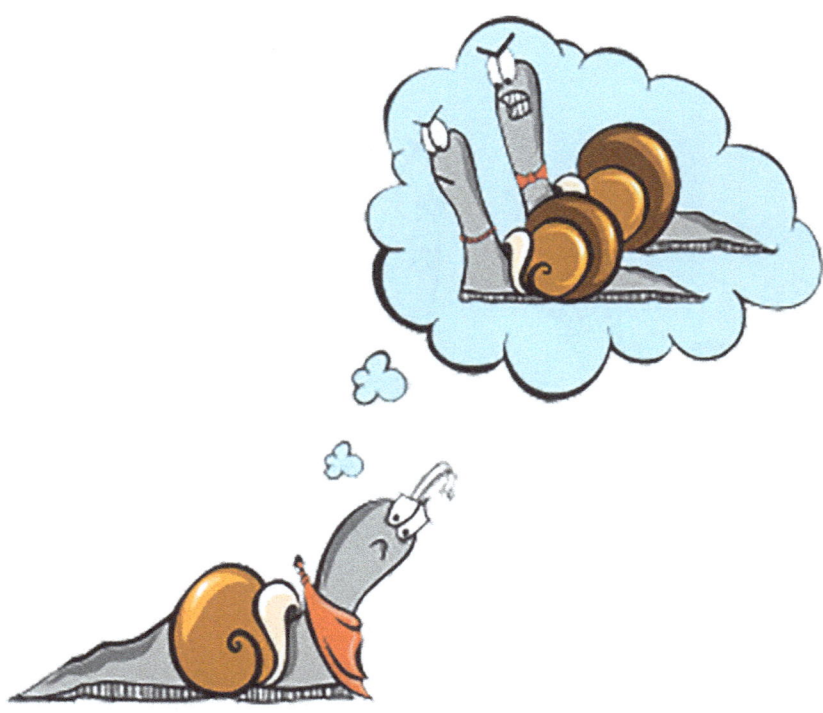

The second split: introjected others

Unfortunately, since the parents have become internalized, these introjected others follow the child wherever the child goes. Instead of vitality, the child feels shame and disappointment.

Maryann said,

> "I cannot remember my mother's actual words, but I just know that she wanted me to be perfect. She was always correcting the way I talked or looked so that her family and friends would think that she was a good mother. Right now, I can feel a pressure in my head to be social and happy looking the way mother always wanted me to appear."

Third split

As children mature, they become increasingly aware of the introjected attitudes of their parents. In order to stay attached to the parents, a child will deny the effects of the parents' criticisms and controls. As a self-protective strategy, they learn to criticize themselves. This self-criticism may be more demanding, intense, and continuous than the original criticism. With some clients, we refer to this self-critical part as an *internal strategist*. With other clients, we call this the *saboteur* because its purpose is to be more powerful than the introjected voices in order to maintain an illusion of attachment and an identity separate from the introjected criticism.

Maryann had volunteered—for a third time—to organize a large function to raise money for a charity. For the next several weeks she was plagued by a loud internal voice that repeatedly said, "I won't do it right"; "I'll look foolish"; "I can't produce what they need"; "Stop being so tired and just push through it." She described the harsh bitter tone as her own internal voice.

As we examined what she felt and remembered, she realized that these were the same admonishments that she "had lived with all the time in high school and at university. They are what made me get good grades, trying to be perfect."

This self-created saboteur is clever in that it takes preemptive control by criticizing the vital and vulnerable self. The person becomes their own oppressor—the vital and vulnerable self is frightened and goes into hiding; self-expression is perceived to be dangerous. Self-created criticism functions as both a deflection from awareness of the introjections and also as a way to have some control over difficult interpersonal situations. One client described their self-criticism as a "ghost that follows me everywhere," while another called it a "monster that hangs over me all the time."

The internal criticizer is controlling and despising of one's own relational needs, desires, and feelings. The constant self-criticism ensures that the person does not receive, seek, or even become aware of needs and feelings, except for the shame of having feelings and needs. It protects the vital and vulnerable self from the criticisms of others but it destroys the very vitality it is trying to protect. Both the *saboteur* and the *social self* function to anticipate—and avoid—real dangers of interpersonal conflict by inflicting an even more severe criticism on themselves.

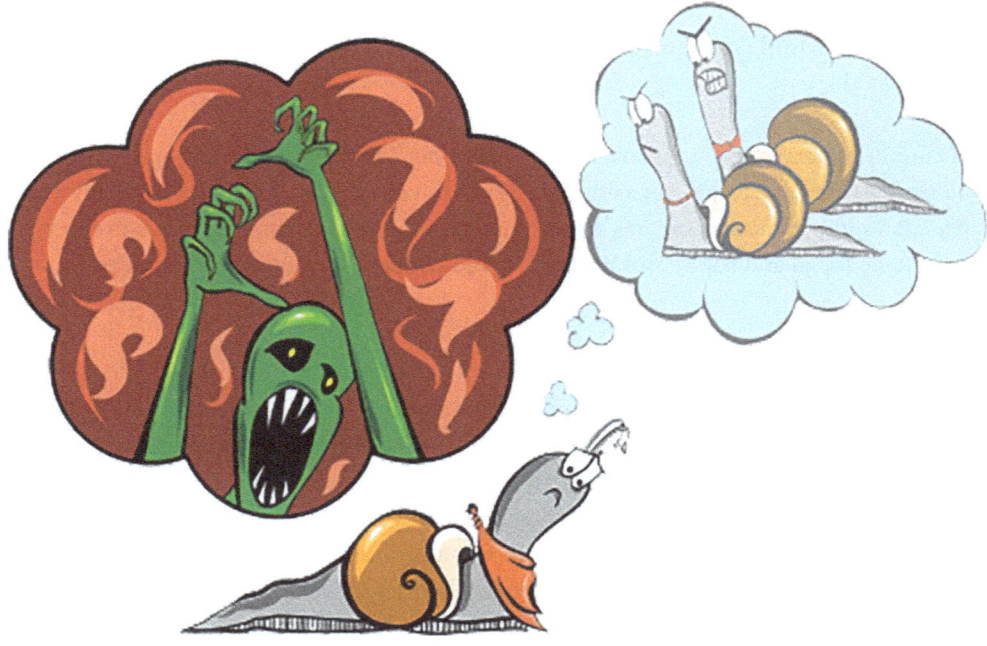

The third split: internal saboteur

During the second year of her psychotherapy, Maryann revealed some of her internal criticisms: "I'm not worth anything"; "I don't dare make mistakes"; "No one likes a depressive like me." Maryann often concluded her social activity stories with, *"I'm just not good enough."* These self-criticisms preceded and superseded any possible criticism from other people because Maryann strategically neutralizes any potential disapproval before it is ever made. However, rather than protecting her, each of these self-inflicted criticisms increased her sense of "feeling pressured when I am with people."

Fourth split

Under the intense pressures of either external criticism, introjected criticism, or the oppression of the *internal saboteur*, there may be a fourth split in the person's sense of self. They may withdraw to a *sequestered self*, where their vitality and vulnerability is completely disconnected from all human contact in a search for peace and quiet. Marye O'Reilly-Knapp (2001) calls this fourth split the "encapsulated self," where the person withdraws into their internal world because they are convinced that there is no security-in-relationship. This withdrawal is like living in a secret and protective closet, cave, or castle where the client can hide from demanding relationships.

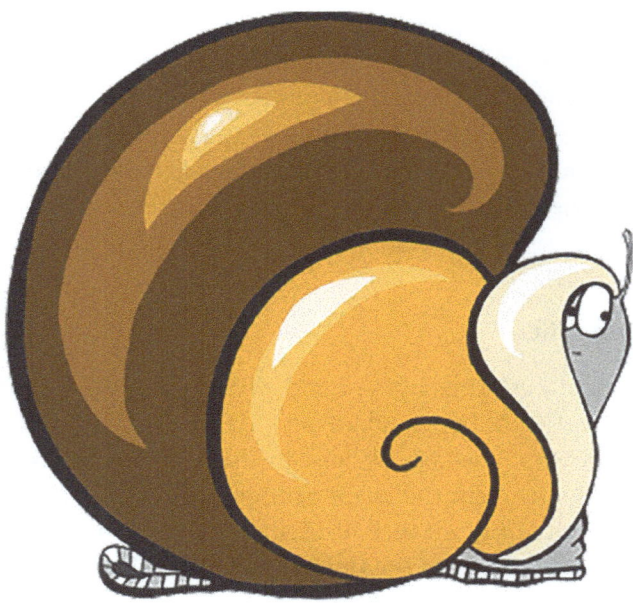

The fourth split: the sequestered self

As our therapy relationship progressed, Maryann put into words her strong urge to withdraw from any human contact. "I hate the pressures I have always lived with. I don't want to be social. I just want to find a quiet place. Often I go to a toilet and sit there for ten or fifteen minutes just to escape people." On another day, she added, "Even though I am lonely I never want to be in relationship with a partner. I don't want them messing with my life. I just want to be left alone to read my books. Books never invade me."

Considerations for psychotherapy

A unique form of psychotherapy is needed for the self that emerges from each split. Some clients will require that we attend to the social self first. Other clients will require relief from introjected messages, attitudes, or criticisms of significant others before we can proceed. Usually, later in the psychotherapy, it will be necessary to address the functions of the self-created criticisms, and most will require careful attention to the sequestered self. The various methods are not sequential. The focus of the psychotherapy may flow from one aspect to another and then back again. Some clients may be burdened by internal criticism and have a compulsion to maintain a social facade, while others will be secretly hiding from interpersonal involvements. Adjusting the psychotherapy for each individual—and their unique split of the self—requires that we think and work multidimensionally.

Each part of the self has its unique pattern of relational attachment. In creating an effective in-depth psychotherapy it is essential that the psychotherapist respond to the style of relational attachment unique to each part. The vital and vulnerable self reflects securely attached relationships where parents were predictably responsive to the child's various needs. As a result, the person is interpersonally contactful and excited about exploring and learning. Even secure individuals need acknowledgment, validation, and ongoing responsiveness to their emerging relational needs.

Working with the first split

The social self is relationally attached by *hope* and *anxiety,* because significant caretakers were *unpredictably responsive.* Out of hope and anxiety, they cling to dysfunctional relationships; they will adapt to the other at any cost. When our therapeutic work is focused on the social self, I find myself wanting to help the client acknowledge the various ways that they have adapted. I try to validate the significance of their compliance. I help the client explore the advantages of a social self, such as: maintaining attachment; less possibility for humiliation; less punishment; or, achieving some comforting attention. I also help the client recognize the various disadvantages of a social self, such as: loss of joy; loss of vitality; emotional numbness; or, loss of physical sensations.

I strive to help the client discover the vital aspects of the self that have been lost such as joy, anger, excitement, exploration, and their uniqueness. Much of our therapy time may be devoted to helping the client become more aware of their body sensations, becoming sensitive to their various affects, and validating the importance of vulnerability. This includes helping the client discover their relational needs—both the needs of childhood as well as today's relational needs.

When working with the split between the vital and vulnerable self and the social self, I often use the Gestalt therapy "empty chair" method to enable the client's vital and vulnerable self to express their body sensations, affects, and the homeostatic functions of splitting. I want to support the client's natural protests and to facilitate him or her in identifying and expressing their physical and relational needs.

I might also use the "two-chair" method to externalize and resolve the intrapsychic conflict between the social self and the vital and vulnerable self. It may be necessary for the client to physically express retroflected feeling and to actively protest to the introjected other(s) by defining their self. Any of the methods that invite clients into interpersonal contact are effective in working with this first split. The Gestalt therapy methods of the "empty chair" and "two-chair" techniques are designed to clarify and resolve the intrapsychic conflict between a person's natural desires and the introjected attitudes of significant others (Perls, 1969, 1973; Perls & Baumgardner, 1975).

The vital and vulnerable self is often confused, like a frightened child. Many of my clients learned to be compliant at several developmental stages. I find it necessary to talk to the child in my client about what they might have needed from an attuned parent. I want them to become aware of how they managed the criticisms and demands placed upon them. I aim to provide the quality of relationship that is protective of the client's exploration of change. I provide permission to be authentic, self-expressive, and intimate. However, I always want to assess the level of internal punishment before giving encouragement to change.

When working with the split between the vital and vulnerable self and the social self, I tend to encourage the client to express their relational need for self-definition and their need to make an impact. The expression of these vital needs can occur relationally between the client and a receptive psychotherapist, or to an imagined other by using the "empty chair" method.

After several sessions in which I talked with Maryann about the absence of any joy in her life, her physical and emotional numbness, and her constant urge to either read or sleep, we contracted to do some two-chair work. I asked her to imagine her social self in one chair and her vital and vulnerable self in the other. My role was to function like a film director, to suggest when she might change positions. We began with the social self boasting about having many friends and activities, how she received lots of attention and praise from acquaintances, and admonishing the other part of her for "hiding from people." Then, I suggested that she change chairs, so as to give her vital and vulnerable self a chance to express what she was holding inside.

The vulnerable self talked about how burdened she felt with all the social activity, with "putting on a good face." As I encouraged her to put her inner sensations into words, she detailed her loss of hope and desire and then added, "I have no pleasure in life because you are always playing a role." At this point, I asked her to change chairs. We continued the dialogue, back and forth, from one chair to another, for another fifteen minutes, until the vital and vulnerable self became a strong voice and proclaimed that, "I have the right to be me. If I want to be social I will do it and if I want to be alone I will be alone. … And, I appreciate how you can adapt to any situation; you are successful with people. I don't want to lose that skill but I also need to be alone, the freedom to be me." With this two-chair dialogue we were facilitating an integration of these two divergent parts of herself.

Working with the second split

In the second split, the child has unconsciously identified with some significant others in order to disavow the child's needs and feelings and, importantly, to maintain a semblance of a relationship. Although they struggle to maintain attachment, their pattern is *avoidant* because significant caretakers were *predictably unresponsive*. They are attached via *neglect* and *aggression*—two sentiments that are often turned against the vital and vulnerable self.

When the internal conflict is between the introjected other and the social self, I use phenomenological inquiry to identify how the client complied with messages and demands. I use historical inquiry to identify any criticism and control that may have been a part of their life—and I encourage them to talk about their fears, the lost opportunities, or punishments that they may have received for being authentic.

Sometimes, I might use a two-chair dialogue to externalize the introjected criticism and to facilitate the person becoming aware of the importance of a social self, or I may use myself as an *interposition* between the introjected other and my client's social self or vital and vulnerable self. I may engage my client in actual psychotherapy with the introjected other (see Erskine, 2015, chapters 16 and 17, for a detailed description of these methods).

In the second year of Maryann's psychotherapy, once she seemed reasonably secure with me, I asked Maryann to imagine her mother sitting in a chair across from the two of us. I talked with Maryann about how I would support her, both as a child and as an adult. I encouraged her to tell her mother what she had never said aloud. At first, Maryann was hesitant in talking to the image of her mother. After a few fearful interruptions, she was able to say aloud, "You have always controlled me. I was never allowed to be me." I coaxed her to say it with the full intensity that she felt inside and she exploded with, "I want to be me. I want to make my own mistakes. I want to be me. But being me was not good enough for you." She stood up and shook her finger at the mother she imagined in the second chair, "You are the one that's imperfect. I'm never good enough for you … but it is you who has a problem. You could never appreciate me."

Working with the third split

The self-created criticism of the saboteur begins as a three-part strategy:

- To deny the emotional impact of the actual criticism from others
- To remain unaware of the internal influence of the introjected criticism
- To ensure that the vital and vulnerable self remains protected, out of sight, and unexpressed.

The relational attachment pattern of the saboteur is disdainful. They undervalue relationships and inhibit sadness, fear, and intimacy while being full of rage. They have an implicit fear of vulnerability.

With several clients, I have discovered that their internal criticism is a secret, as though they are ashamed of it. The constant internal criticism may be traumatic because there has been no reparative relationship that served to neutralize the toxicity of the criticism. I invite the client to say the criticism out loud, so that I can hear and feel the impact of it.

Then, I encourage them to amplify the volume and intensity of the internal criticism, so as to externalize what has been internal. I want the client to be able to distinguish the difference between the self-created saboteur and the introjected voice. I may engage the saboteur in a dialogue about the origin and purpose of the criticism. The tendency for self-created criticism often begins in early adolescence, as a strategy to protect one's self from others' criticism, control, and rejection. I focus our therapeutic dialogue on the original purpose of the criticism and how that purpose no longer applies in the client's life today.

In the first year and a half of her psychotherapy, Maryann would allude to "an inner voice that controls all that I do." She was reluctant to give me any details about what the voice said. One day she uttered, "The voice always pressures me. I just want to escape into a good book." She then realized that she had two different sensations: the first was that she was ashamed of having the voice, and second, that she felt overwhelming shame with the criticisms that the voice was saying. She was confused: "Sometimes I think the voice is my own and sometimes it's similar to my mother's harangues."

Over the next several weeks, I devoted some time in each session to give Maryann an opportunity to express internal criticisms out loud so that both she and I could hear them in their full intensity. Eventually, she was able to voice several of her internal condemnations: "I'm a fake"; "I didn't do it good enough"; "I'll never make it"; "I look so awful that everyone will laugh at me."

As we explored the function of each of these self-created criticisms, Maryann became aware that she had created the voice, "to beat my mother at her own game! If I criticize myself, I don't have to remember her criticisms." This led to her having a series of memories—memories that she had not previously been conscious of. "My mother was constantly invasive. I had to find a way to drown out her controlling voice." In a later session, she discovered that a second function of her self-created criticism was:

> to make me do what I didn't want to do. All through my life these internal criticisms pushed me to stay awake and study, to work hard, to put on a good face for people. The criticisms have helped me to be successful at work and in all my social activities because I am always working hard to adapt to the critics. I hate my self-criticisms yet I am afraid that if I give them up, I'll never be good enough. This is a shitty situation. I want to be free to be me.

Working with the fourth split

The sequestered self is hiding, longing for security, quiet, and escape from painful interpersonal relationships. The attachment pattern of the sequestered self is *isolated*. Relational withdrawal is used to manage the client's intense affect and to escape from either internal criticism or possible external criticisms. Psychotherapeutic methods that are effective for other parts of the self may not be effective for the sequestered self. The client withdrawing from interpersonal contact requires a unique form of psychotherapy to help in healing from the hidden wounds of cumulative relational failures. For a detailed case presentation on working sensitively with a client's sequestered self, see the article entitled: "Relational withdrawal, attunement to silence: Psychotherapy of the schizoid process" (Erskine, 2020).

When working with the sequestered self, I focus on providing security within our therapeutic relationship. Once the client has some sense of security in our relationship, I proceed with helping the client to feel their physical sensations, affects, and memories. This is much deeper awareness work, often quiet and less conversational than when working with the loss of sensations in the first split. Although they do not show trust, they need a psychotherapist who is reliable, consistent, and dependable. In order to facilitate the client's internal sense of security, I sometimes invite them to withdraw while they are in our therapy sessions, to go to their "quiet place."

I recommend that they close their eyes and take a few minutes to feel the safety of being in their private place. I speak to them slowly and reassuringly with, "I'm staying right here" and "I'm listening to you, even when you are silent." I don't expect a response. I'm patient and provide time for the client to make internal contact with their body sensations, feelings, and memories—without talking. While they are in their quiet, private place, I may speak to them in short validating sentences:

- "It is important to have a quiet place."
- "It is necessary to feel safe inside."
- "There is no need to hurry." "I am right here watching over you."

I have learned that when a client is in their sequestered place, the best thing I can probably do is relax and not try to make something happen. I often do some deep, calming breathing myself, while staying focused on the client's nonverbal experience. I create the time and place for them to feel both the security of their "quiet place" and my quiet, undemanding presence.

When the client has a tendency to withdraw from interpersonal contact, phenomenological inquiry—effective with many other types of clients—may not be appropriate. They may become silent or provide only superficial responses because they have experienced inquiry as an invasion, or as a demand for the "correct answer." Instead of using phenomenological and historical inquiry, *therapeutic description* may be more effective.

Therapeutic description provides the client with validation of their often unspoken emotional and physical experiences. Therapeutic description is based on attunement to the client's rhythm, affect, archaic and current relational needs, and an understanding of their cognitive process. Therapeutic description provides a vocabulary for previously unspoken experiences to be acknowledged and eventually talked about.

It also facilitates an interpersonal connectedness between client and psychotherapist by providing the client with a sense that, "my therapist knows my internal experience, my fear of relationship, the safety in silence, the importance of hiding, and the depth of my loneliness."

Therapeutic description is not the same as explanations or interpretations that may be given to other clients to enhance their cognitive understanding of their psychological dynamics. It is about attuning our self to our client's nonverbalized sensations and experiences and helping the person form a language to talk about their physical and emotional sensations.

The effective use of therapeutic description requires that we use a tentative voice, not a voice of certainty, and pay very close attention to the client's physiological reactions of acknowledgment, disagreement, or nothing. Here are a few examples of translating phenomenological inquiry into therapeutic description. Rather than asking:

- "Why are you quiet?", a therapeutic description such as, "It must be important to be quiet," may be much easier for the client to accept.

- "What are you feeling?", it may be more effective to simply state a description, "It must be difficult to find words to describe what you are feeling."
- "What is happening in your body?", it may be more contactful with clients who tend to use relational withdrawal to say something like, "Your body must be tense holding all those feelings inside all the time," or "Being in a safe hiding place seems so necessary."

Throughout Maryann's time in psychotherapy there were many times when I witnessed her momentary withdrawal. I would inquire, "Where did you go?" In response, she would immediately answer, "I was just thinking." If I inquired further, she would give me a deflective answer about something happening in her social life, or about what she had just read. I sensed that she was not "thinking" but that she was retreating to some internal place.

If I inquired with, "What just happened? You seemed to go away," her face would form a scowl and she would turn away in silence. I surmised that she heard each inquiry as an accusation that she was doing something wrong. I began making comments instead of an inquiry: for example, "My questions must seem invasive"; she responded by giving a "Yes" nod of her head. Whenever I would notice a brief retreat to her internal place, I stopped inquiring. Instead, I described what I imagined her experience to be: "It must seem necessary to go into a private, quiet place." She again nodded a "Yes."

When I would see her withdrawing, I began making therapeutic descriptions such as, "It is important to have a safe place to rest," "It must be overwhelming listening to people," or, "I'm right here, even when you are quiet." My comments attempted to describe her internal process and what she might need; they were not as invasive as my questions, and she remained free to stay in her safe internal place.

Maryann began withdrawing more frequently in our sessions. I would like to think that her willingness to withdraw to her place of safety while being in my presence was now possible because of the non-judgmental, non-criticizing perspective that I brought to our psychotherapy relationship during the previous years. She now seemed to feel safe enough in our therapeutic relationship to allow me to witness her retreat to her "hiding place." People struggling with a schizoid process will withdraw when there is a threat of invasion, but they often try to keep their withdrawal a secret. Yet, when they feel secure in a therapeutic relationship, they will sometimes withdraw in search of healing—a healing that occurs through the psychotherapist's sustained attunement to the client's affect and rhythm.

So, I increasingly sat in silence and relaxed with my yoga breathing. I watched her intensely for any clues as to what she was experiencing and I periodically made comments like: "There is no rush. Take your time to be quiet"; "Having a safe place is so important"; or, "In a private place, no one can criticize or control." I watched her head and shoulders for the little nods of agreement; these were my guide to continue with my therapeutic descriptions. Sometimes, there would be no nod. Then I would patiently wait in silence and, some minutes later, I made a similar therapeutic description that I hoped would reflect her inner experience.

In each session, I would reserve time long before the end of the session for us to discuss what was occurring in the psychotherapy process. She repeatedly informed me that my quiet, patient way of being with her was "a salve, a soothing ointment." Following another session, she said, "I had to invent a quiet place. Growing up, I had no safe place in which to go. My mother was always hovering over me. But you are just there. You are not demanding anything of me. You are not actually with me, but you are out there, safe. Like you are watching over my welfare."

With this kind of therapeutically supported withdrawal, Maryann began having vivid memories; she would withdraw into her quiet place for about ten minutes, and then she would suddenly have a memory. As we continued the supported withdrawal, her internal images were of an increasingly younger age. Her memories were not explicit, rather they were composed of impressions, body sensations, and procedural reactions. Through therapeutic implications, we were able to compose a story about her deep sense of loneliness.

In my experience as a psychotherapist, there are many errors that I have made while working with several clients who use a schizoid process to stabilize their affect. I have been fortunate to have clients who have served as my teachers, who have helped me understand and appreciate the whole schizoid process and—in particular—what they need in a healing relationship. Their honesty and ways of being in our sessions have periodically exposed dimensions of my countertransference that were not obvious with other types of clients, such as, my desire to achieve a specific outcome and my urge to "do" the psychotherapy quickly. With such an internal urge, it is almost impossible to attune to the clients' sequestered rhythms and affects.

I have learned that it takes patience and long moments of silence to reach the client's sequestered self, and much longer to provide a consistently dependable healing relationship (Erskine, 2021). It is essential that we psychotherapists foster a sensitivity to the client's never-spoken, emotion-filled, internal story; adjust our psychotherapeutic involvement to the rhythms of a frightened child; and, attune to the client's deep sense of fear and loneliness.

References

Aiken, C. (1934). Silent snow, secret snow. In: *The Collected Short Stories of Conrad Aiken.* Cleveland, OH: World Publishing, 1960. (This story may be retrieved from https://fullreads.com/horror/silent-snow-secret-snow/)

Berne, E. (1961). *Transactional Analysis in Psychotherapy: A Systematic Individual and Social Psychiatry.* New York: Grove.

Bowlby, J. (1988). *A Secure Base.* New York: Basic Books.

Erskine, R. G. (1994). Shame and self-righteousness: Transactional analysis perspectives and clinical interventions. *Transactional Analysis, 24*(2).

Erskine, R. G. (1995). A Gestalt therapy approach to shame and self-righteousness: Theory and methods. *British Gestalt Journal, 4*(2): 107–117.

Erskine, R. G. (2003). Introjection, psychic presence and parent ego states: Considerations for psychotherapy. In: C. Sills & H. Hargaden (Eds.), *Ego States: Key Concepts in Transactional Analysis, Contemporary Views* (pp. 83–108). Duffield, UK: Worth.

Erskine, R. G. (2015). *Relational Patterns, Therapeutic Presence: Concepts and Practice of Integrative Psychotherapy.* London: Karnac.

Erskine, R. G. (2020). Relational withdrawal, attunement to silence: Psychotherapy of the schizoid process. *International Journal of Integrative Psychotherapy, 11*: 14–28.

Erskine, R. G. (2021). *A Healing Relationship: Commentary on Therapeutic Dialogues.* Bicester, UK: Phoenix.

Fairbairn, W. R. D. (1954). *Psychoanalytic Studies of the Personality.* New York: Basic Books.

Fraiberg, S. (1982). Pathological defenses in infancy. *Psychoanalytic Quarterly, 51*(4): 612–635. doi.org/10.1080/21674086.1982.11927012.

Galgut, D. (2010). *In a Strange Room.* Toronto, Canada: McClelland & Stewart.

Guntrip, H. (1961). *Personality Structure and Human Interaction.* London: Hogarth.

Guntrip, H. (1968). *Schizoid Phenomena, Object Relations and the Self.* Madison, CT: International Universities Press.

Guntrip, H. (1971). *Psychoanalytic Theory, Therapy, and the Self.* New York: Basic Books.

Hazell, J. (Ed.) (1994). *Personal Relations Therapy: The Collected Papers of H. J. S. Guntrip.* Northvale, NJ: Jason Aronson.

Hesse, H. (1927). *Steppenwolf.* New York: Modern Library, 1963.

Laing, R. D. (1960). *The Divided Self.* London: Tavistock.

O'Reilly-Knapp, M. (2001). Between two worlds: The encapsulated self. *Transactional Analysis, 31*: 44–54. doi.org/10.1177/036215370103100106.

Perls, F. S. (1969). *Gestalt Therapy Verbatim.* Lafayette, CA: Real People Press.

Perls, F. S. (1973). *The Gestalt Approach and Eyewitness to Therapy.* Palo Alto, CA: Science & Behavior.

Perls, F. S., & Baumgardner, P. (1975). *Legacy from Fritz: Gifts from Lake Cowichan.* Palo Alto, CA: Science & Behavior.

Rubens, R. L. (1996). The unique origins of Fairbairn's theories. *Psychoanalytic Dialogues: The International Journal of Relational Perspectives, 6*(3): 413–435.

Winnicott, D. W. (1960). Ego distortion in terms of true and false self. In: *The Maturational Processes and the Facilitating Environment: Studies in the Theory of Emotional Development* (pp. 140–157). New York: International Universities Press.

Winnicott, D. W. (1967). The concept of clinical regression compared with that of defense organisation. In: C. Winnicott, R. Shepherd, & M. Davis (Eds.), *D. W. Winnicott: Psycho-Analytic Explorations* (pp. 193–199). London: Karnac, 1989.

Winnicott, D. W. (1988). *Human Nature.* New York: Schocken.

CHAPTER 3

Relational withdrawal, attunement to silence: psychotherapy of the schizoid process

Richard G. Erskine

> *Here was a man capable of withdrawing into himself like a Russian doll.*
> —David Foenkinos, *The Mystery of Henri Pick* (2016)

Violet was a confusing and, at times, difficult client who taught me about relational withdrawal and the importance of attunement to silence in psychotherapy. Although I previously had clients who were afraid of making intimate connections and struggled to talk about their inner life, I did not appreciate the significance of their urge to withdraw from relationships.

Prior to working with Violet I practiced psychotherapy in an active and engaging way, particularly with depressed clients. I encouraged clients like Violet to make both internal and interpersonal contact by asking them to talk about their feelings in the first person, to look me in the eye when talking, and to engage in social activities that included participating in an ongoing therapy group. However, Violet's way of being with me challenged my therapeutic approach and stimulated me to think and transact differently. She was the first of several clients to teach me about the *schizoid process*.

Violet came to individual therapy with a variety of complaints. She was a fifty-two-year-old professional writer who was unproductive in writing a new novel, disappointed that her previous book had received only minimal praise, and was "disgusted with being fat." She was disheartened because her husband alternated between ignoring her and controlling her. The most revealing thing she said in our first session was that she binged on sweets to ease the feelings of loneliness and hopelessness that would sweep over her. Her stories included a number of self-condemning comments. I was surprised by her remark that she was "fat"; she did not appear as such to me. Violet was stylishly dressed and her conversation was extremely polite. My first impression of Violet was that she was depressed.

In our psychotherapy sessions Violet would go into detail about her current life, often reciting what she did day-by-day while avoiding talking about internal sensations or feelings. She did voice some disgruntlement about her family life and gave several examples of how she was compliant with whatever her husband or members of her extended family wanted. I was amazed that she could provide detailed information about various situations in her life but there was no revealing of herself. Instead of looking at me she looked at the carpet or over my shoulder. Often I experienced that Violet was talking *at me* rather than *to me.*

Throughout the first year of our psychotherapy sessions I responded empathetically to Violet's stories which to me sounded both aggravating and depressing. I actively listened even though I sometimes felt drowsy during her sessions. Perhaps my drowsiness was an integral part of her, as yet, untold story. I knew I was missing an emotional connection with her. It was up to me to remain attentive to my misattunements with Violet's rhythm, affect, and perhaps her developmental level of functioning and, importantly, to decipher what was occurring in our intersubjective process (Stolorow et al., 1987). Unlike my psychotherapy with other depressed clients, my sessions with Violet tended to have more focus on the current events and an emphasis on how Violet could change her behavior. For example, I talked to her much more than I usually would about a healthy diet, maintaining a consistent schedule for her writing, and how to have an intimate relationship with her husband. At the same time, I tried to neutralize her continued self-criticism by pointing out her accomplishments and encouraging her to think positively. Still, my interventions seemed to have limited impact.

I thought it would be beneficial to include in Violet's psychotherapy some expressive methods that had been effective with other clients who were living with compliance, self-criticism, and a reactive depression. On several occasions, in response to some aspect of her storytelling, I asked Violet to imagine her husband sitting on a chair in front of her and to express her anger at her husband's demands. She refused and became silent for the rest of the session. As an alternative I asked her on a few occasions to look at me and tell me about her anger. Each time she turned her head away and went silent. I was intrigued by how long she could remain silent.

I questioned myself. Was my use of cognitive behavioral and expressive methods a countertransference reaction? If so, to what was I reacting? I discussed my work with Violet in supervision. The supervisor only reinforced what I was already doing and addressed neither my lack of attunement to Violet nor her lapsing into long silences. So, in my introspection, I searched for what was missing in our therapeutic relationship.

I realized that I was not making full interpersonal contact with Violet. Just like Violet, I was not fully present. I was confused by her. I did not understand how she functioned. No wonder I periodically felt drowsy or found my mind wandering to other situations. It was evident to me that in the absence of any emotional connection between the two of us, I compensated by becoming more and more behavioral in my interventions. Eventually I became aware of a parallel process: my focus on behavior change mirrored both her mother's and husband's attempts to control her behavior. My countertransference was in my wanting something to happen … so I focused on expressive methods, cognitive understanding, and behavioral change to ward off my worry about not being an effective psychotherapist. It became clear that I was not providing the kind of psychotherapy that Violet needed.

I encouraged Violet to make more interpersonal contact with me, to see my face, and to talk directly to me. I talked about my feeling sad for her and irritated at her mother's behavior toward Violet. I used relationally connecting words such as we and us. I wanted her to experience my listening to her and taking her seriously. But looking me in the eye was particularly difficult for Violet. The more I encouraged her to be interpersonally contactful the more she responded with either self-criticism or silence. Whenever I made any inquiry of Violet—whether it was phenomenological, historical, or about how she coped with a situation—she would either respond superficially or turn her head in silence. Throughout the first year and a half of our work together I asked Violet many questions about her childhood and the nature of various interactions within her original family. I received abbreviated responses.

Our sessions continued to be filled with many stories of her current life. Session after session I listened intently to Violet's descriptions of what was happening to her two children, her discontent with her husband, and her difficulties with writing and food. Not only did she repeat stories but, as time went on, the stories became more elaborate. Sometimes Violet did not remember what we had previously spoken about; it was as if she had not been present. I was concerned about her continued self-criticism and spent time in each session challenging how she negatively defined herself. I questioned myself as to why she continued coming to our psychotherapy sessions. I told myself that she must be receiving some benefit; she never missed a session. And I wondered about Violet's unrequited relational needs and if she was unconsciously struggling to make an impact on me, or to define herself, or to find security.

When I asked Violet to evaluate her experience of our psychotherapy sessions she was pleased. She said that they were much more helpful than her previous two attempts at psychotherapy. I was amazed. What was helpful? When I asked for details she could not describe what she meant.

All my attempts to make this psychotherapy interpersonal seemed like a failure to me. I felt inadequate. Yet Violet continued to come to our sessions in spite of her husband's many attempts to stop the psychotherapy.

Useful metaphors

We continued in this same pattern for almost two years. At that time I was studying psychoanalysis, particularly the British object relations perspective (Greenberg & Mitchell, 1983; Kohon, 1986; Sutherland, 1980). I was impressed by the writings of Michel Balint (1968), Ronald Fairbairn (1952), Masud Khan (1963, 1974), Margret Little (1981), Ian Suttie (1988), and Donald Winnicott (1974).

I particularly admired the writings of Harry Guntrip (1968, 1971) and his descriptions of working with clients who withdrew from relationship in a "schizoid compromise" (1962, p. 277). Jeremy Hazell (1994) collected several journal articles by Guntrip that depict how he developed an understanding of the schizoid phenomena and suggested a relational orientation to psychoanalysis.

Donald Winnicott had used the terms "true self" and "false self" to describe the fragmentations in an individual's personality when there is an emotionally overloading disruption in the child's internal stability and sense of self (1965, p. 147). Winnicott depicted the "true self" as the source of needs, feelings, and spontaneous self-expressions that become split-off, disavowed, and desensitized—"the equivalence of complete psychic annihilation" (Greenberg & Mitchell, 1983, p. 194).

Winnicott delineates the "false self" as the type of person who hides behind an emotionless facade, who cannot allow themself to be either spontaneous or relaxed and quiet because they are constantly attending to the criticisms and demands of significant others. I realized that these theories were only an approximation of what happened within my clients when as a child they lived with constant misattunement, ridicule, and stress. However, the theory served as a useful metaphor in guiding my therapeutic involvement with my clients. The theory was also helpful because it stimulated my thinking about early relational disruptions, intrapsychic processes, and archaic forms of self-stabilization.

I was faced with a puzzle:

- Was Violet's polite and proper presentation her "true" or "false" self?
- Did Violet have a "true self"?
- If so, who was Violet's "true self"?
- What sort of neglect or trauma would force the "true self" into hiding?
- If there was a hidden "true self," how could I build a healing relationship with the emotionally authentic Violet?
- Did the so called "false self" serve necessary functions or was it pathological?
- What if the concept of "true self" and "false self" did not represent what was occurring inside my client? How could I then make sense of her superficial stories, the lack of interpersonal contact, and the absence of any vitality, emotions, or vulnerability?

Playing with this puzzle enabled me to expand my thinking. I explored the theory of "true self" and "false self" from a non-pathological perspective—a perspective that redirected attention to the concept of *self-in-relationship*. Who we are is always contingent on the other people with whom we have been in relationship, therefore our sense of self is always cocreated in each relationship. This concept of self-in-relationship inspired me to reexamine my attitude and way of working with Violet.

I was uncomfortable with the terms "true self" and "false self." They did not depict how I experience my client(s). The words "false self" imply deceit whereas "true self" implies something worthwhile. These terms seem to suggest that something was wrong with the person who had a "false self." Perhaps Winnicott's "false self" had some important homeostatic functions such as stabilization, regulation, continuity, or pseudo-attachment.

Keeping Winnicott's ideas about splitting in mind I thought about two aspects of Violet's sense of herself. She had a *social self* that achieved a semblance of relational attachment by accommodating to the requirements of significant others. And, she also had a *vital and vulnerable self* that subliminally experienced feelings, needs, and energy but remained protectively internal and isolated.

I began thinking of Violet (and, later, other clients like her) as someone who learned to hide her vitality and vulnerability. She created a social facade (i.e., "false self") in order to give the impression of some form of relational attachment—a persona that anxiously adapted to the expectations of others, while hiding her own sensitivity and vitality. Her attachment pattern was *isolated*, different from either an *anx*ious or *avoidant* attachment pattern because Violet longed for a comforting relationship (Ainsworth et al., 1978). Violet's *isolated attachment pattern* was the result of childhood attempts to self-stabilize and self-regulate her fear of being invaded and controlled (Erskine, 2009).

An essential psychotherapy

Were Donald Winnicott, Harry Guntrip, and the other writers describing my client Violet? I thought so. Even though these authors provided some general guidelines about psychotherapy for clients who managed their life via a schizoid process, I was left without a specific therapy plan. Guntrip (1968) described how a person is driven into hiding out of fear and then experiences a deep, sequestered loneliness that drives him or her out of hiding back into an adaptive interface with the world. Such a person is constantly caught in the struggle between hiding or connecting to others, but in an adaptive way.

Guntrip (cited in Hazell, 1994) defined the necessary psychotherapy of the schizoid process as:

> the provision of a reliable and understanding human relationship of a kind that makes contact with the deeply repressed traumatized child in a way that enables one to become steadily more able to live, in the security of a new, real relationship, with the traumatic legacy of the earliest formative years, as it seeps through or erupts into consciousness.... It is a process of interaction, the function of two variables, the personalities of two people working together towards free spontaneous growth. (p. 366)

Winnicott described the essential ingredients of an in-depth psychotherapy for clients who manifest a schizoid process as providing a respectful, understanding, reliable environment, one that the client never had and *needs if he or she is to redevelop out of inner conflict and inhibitions*. Such an environment allows the person to find out for their self what is natural for them. Both Guntrip and Winnicott encouraged a psychotherapy that focuses on the client's internal processes and not specifically on cognitive insight or behavioral outcome, a psychotherapy that provides a healing relationship to a traumatized and psychologically fragmented client (Hazell, 1994; Little, 1990; Winnicott, 1965).

I was impressed by the loving commitment that these psychotherapists had for their clients. I too felt a profound responsibility to Violet even though I was confused, felt drowsy, or searched for how I could help her change. What if I followed Guntrip's advice and made contact with the "deeply repressed" instead of focusing on interpersonal contact or change? I made a commitment to myself to respect her silences, to support her withdrawal, and to create a safe place for the "deeply repressed" to express herself. This required that I be consistent and dependable in providing a secure therapeutic relationship even though I did not understand her unexpressed affect or tendency to withdraw. Guntrip, Winnicott, and their colleagues were defining an essential psychotherapy that focused on the client's internal process—a psychotherapy that provided a healing relationship (Erskine, 2020).

Discovering a vital self

We were now near the end of our second year of psychotherapy. I had been puzzling for weeks over the questions of "false self" and "true self" that I outlined earlier. I wondered if the quality of my psychotherapy would be different if I thought of Violet's silence and withdrawal as her attempt to protect a vital and vulnerable aspect of herself. And, that her polite, proper, and superficial presentation as a social facade had at least two important functions: protection and attachment. I also gave considerable thought to the Gestalt therapy concept of contact and interruptions to contact (Perls et al., 1951). I particularly thought about the significance of internal contact and how intense focus on contact with an external world could possibly interrupt internal contact. Perhaps my therapeutic task was to facilitate her internal contact. Clearly there were many contact interruptions in our relationship: I did not feel a connection to the essence of her; she did not express emotions; and she most likely was not in contact with internal sensations. She told stories and I listened but we still had almost no interpersonal contact. I wondered what would happen if I encouraged Violet to focus on her internal experience instead of telling me her many stories.

When there was a pause in Violet's telling the details of her story I invited her to close her eyes and stay quiet for a few moments so that she could sense her internal experience. At first she was frightened by the prospect of doing this in front of me. Encouragingly, I again asked her to close her eyes, to be quiet, to feel her internal sensations, and to not speak for a while—to concentrate on the sensations that were happening inside. She appeared to withdraw into herself. I wasn't sure if she was turning inward to feel her internal sensations or just returning to a familiar hiding place?

I was concerned about the possibility that she was merely complying with my request as she had learned to do with her mother.

She remained quiet for a few minutes. She then opened her eyes to see if I was still present. I assured her that I would stay present as she went inside. We experimented with her closing her eyes and going to what she called her "quiet place." At first she was able to withdraw for only a minute. Then little by little we extended the time to several minutes. By the end of the session she said that it was a "quieting experience." I was not sure what her words meant but her body seemed softer, more relaxed.

The next session began with Violet again telling a detailed story of her family life. After a short time I interrupted by asking Violet about her experience in the previous session. She said that she was afraid to "go internal" in front of anyone because "What I have inside is private. No one can know it." I asked her about how she experienced me in the previous session when she was in her quiet place. She said that she was "scared, but it was OK because you did not try to control me."

It was evident to me that Violet's quiet place was her attempt to self-stabilize and create a place of security. I told Violet that I thought it was important she visit her quiet place and that we explore what she was experiencing. I also said that I was willing to accompany her and I promised that I would do my best to not invade her. I also talked about how we had been rehashing stories about her family and that in my evaluation not much had changed in the past two years. She disagreed with me and said, "You listen to me. You never criticize or define me. You are gentle with me. That is why I come back." We concluded this session by agreeing that we had seldom talked about her internal experiences and that in the previous session we had begun an important exploration.

In the next session I invited her to experiment with closing her eyes and attend to her internal sensations. I told her that I would remain physically still but that I would watch over her in a protective way. She then withdrew into her "quiet place" and remained in silence for fifteen minutes. When Violet opened her eyes she told me that I had discovered her secret, "my quiet hiding place. It has been my private place, all my life." In the next several months we often experimented with Violet withdrawing from external contact and making internal contact with her feelings, needs, and body experiences. In the beginning of our experimental work she was without any words. She had sensations in her body but she did not know how to speak about them.

Violet described her "quiet place" as being in her childhood bed with the covers and pillow pulled over her head. In one session she said, "There are a lot of things in there that I don't want to feel." As she said this I realized that I had been feeling increasingly protective of Violet; I could sense her intense vulnerability. I imagined myself sitting in her bedroom, vigilant, quiet, and ready. My imagination was essential in keeping me focused on Violet's vulnerability during our long periods of silence. Interestingly, I never felt drowsy or distracted when Violet was withdrawn into her "quiet place." I was always alert and interested in her internal experience. This was so different than the sleepiness I periodically felt when she previously told me detailed stories about her family conflicts.

Whenever Violet was telling me her current, day-by-day stories I watched for the little signs indicating that she was withdrawing, such as averting her eyes, leaving long pauses, or jumping from one story to another. She was telling me in a coded way about the attachment disruptions in her life and her desperate attempts to feel secure. Her stories were a metaphorical message to me about how she required my sensitivity to her unique rhythm and her need for security in our relationship.

Now, in most of our sessions, I reserved some time to invite Violet into her vulnerable place. My task was to be patient, to respect her silence, to provide time for Violet to make internal contact, to encourage her to feel both the internal safety of her "quiet place" and the safety of our relationship. I spoke to her in a soft, reassuring voice with statements such as: "It's important to have a quiet place"; "It's so necessary to feel safe inside"; "There is no need to hurry"; and, "I am right here watching over you." I talked slowly and with a voice tone I might use if I were talking to a frightened child. I provided long pauses between my statements to allow Violet time to experience and process any affect related to what I was saying.

As Violet withdrew into her imagined bed, "covered by blankets and pillows," I relaxed and did some deep yoga breathing to keep myself centered and fully present. I kept my eyes on her all the time and listened to her sighs and other soft sounds while I watched her physical movements. I did not try to make something specific happen. But I wanted to create the time and place for Violet to feel both the security of her "quiet place" and my non-intrusive, caring presence.

As the months progressed I discovered that her "quiet place" was not quiet. It was also a place of fear, sadness, and profound loneliness. In some sessions when Violet withdrew to her "bed and covers" she was "desperate to escape" her mother's control. She had many examples, at various ages, of how hurt she felt by her mother's criticism. From deep in her chest she would cry with spasms of heartbreak, sorrow, and loneliness. In the beginning of this therapeutically supported withdrawal her cry was without sound. In subsequent sessions her cry became a full vocal cry. I remained present, listening, and periodically responding with compassionate sounds and mirroring what she had been feeling. It then became apparent to me that her highly detailed stories, her quickly jumping from one story to another at a speed that did not allow for any dialogue, was an unconscious strategy to not feel her loneliness. She was unconsciously looking for interpersonal connection and simultaneously fearing any human closeness.

On some occasions after a long period of what she called "going internal," Violet would make sounds that were a combination of mournful crying and disgust. These sounds were accompanied by gestures of pushing with her hands. She was without words to express her diversity of feelings. She often emerged from her withdrawal in physical and emotional distress, struggling to tell me about the various incidents of neglect and the constant criticism from her mother. My task throughout all this therapeutically supported internal work—like the task of parents with young children—was to help her develop a language so that she could communicate her internal distress and needs, her vitality and vulnerability.

As our psychotherapy continued in the following months Violet actively expressed an array of feelings. In some sessions she would withdraw into the vulnerability of her internal world—a world in which she remembered being terrified of mother coming physically close to her. Violet described how she would try to escape both her mother's touch and "mean words" by imagining that she was in her bed with the covers pulled over her head. She was proud as she reported how she could "hide in bed" even when sitting at the family dinner table. Violet had changed. On some days she could now describe her personal experience; she could tell me about what had happened to her, describe some physical sensations, and express what she was feeling.

Learning from the client

When I first learned to support Violet's withdrawal into her quiet place I often made phenomenological inquiries such as "What are you feeling?" or "What do you need?" (Erskine & Moursund, 2022; Erskine et al., 1999). I discovered that my inquiries interrupted Violet's withdrawal. She would open her eyes and start to tell me some story about her current life rather than respond to my inquiry. Phenomenological inquiry was an essential form of connection with most of my clients (Erskine & Moursund, 2022; Erskine et al., 1999). I was curious as to why my phenomenological inquiries were not working with Violet.

I realized that there had been an important theme in the stories Violet had been telling me over the past two years: both her mother and husband constantly labeled her. They both defined who she was. As a child, and now as a wife, she struggled to conform to their definitions of what she should feel and how she should think and act. Violet described how the only freedom she had from their definitions was when she withdrew into her "quiet place," not having to accommodate herself to their definitions and expectations. I pointed out that the theme of being labeled and defined was present in many of her stories and that perhaps my inquiry was similar. She described how she experienced my inquiry as a definition of her, sometimes as "a demand that I be different."

Over the next few sessions we made some fascinating discoveries about our relationship. When I would ask Violet "What are you feeling?" she translated it to mean "What you are feeling is bad." When I inquired about what she needed she interpreted my question to mean that something was wrong with her for having needs. When I inquired about her physical sensations she tensed her body because she did not know how to act. Violet was constantly accommodating, altering herself to fit what she imagined were my expectations of her—a clear example of transferring old emotional memories into our relationship. At first, understanding the transference was difficult for Violet. She could not see her own accommodating reactions although she could experience the juxtaposition between my behavior and the criticizing, controlling, and judgmental behavior of her family. She began to be more relaxed with me and was more willing to spend time in her "quiet place."

I experimented with limiting the amount of phenomenological inquiry I was using with Violet. When she would withdraw into her quiet place I was silent, observant, present, and feeling protective. At first my not inquiring provided Violet with an opportunity to go deeper into her internal experience. She could feel her sadness and fear. When she was withdrawn—

imagining hiding in her childhood bed—she would alternate between being frightened about making any sound and then quietly crying. But eventually she became worried that my silence meant that I had "gone away." I was in a dilemma. If I inquired, I interrupted her internal experience. If I was silent, she would interrupt her withdrawal because she was worried that I was not present.

In another session I invited Violet to withdraw to her "safe bed." There was about fifteen minutes of silence wherein I caringly watched over her in the same way that I watched over my children as I sat by their bed at night when they were sick with a fever. I watched Violet's labored breathing and the tension in her clenched hands. I made a statement: "You must be so scared." Violet nodded her head to indicate agreement. I was surprised, since I realized that I had just defined her experience. A couple of minutes later I again said, "You must be so scared. It is important to have a safe hiding place." She again nodded her head. After another two minutes of silence I again said, "It is so important to hide in your quiet place, particularly when you are sad." She again nodded, her breathing returned to normal, she unclenched her hands.

When Violet opened her eyes she said my description of her internal experience was important because it meant that I understood her and that she was not all alone. I was surprised. We discussed how my description of her internal sensations was different from her mother's and husband's criticizing definitions of her. She described my voice as "tentative" and my tone soft, "not a definite, authoritarian voice" that she was used to in her family. Later, with other clients who used relational withdrawal to self-stabilize, I again discovered the effectiveness of using *therapeutic description* as I learned to do with Violet.

Therapeutic description provides the client with validation of their often unspoken emotional and physical experience. It is based on attuning ourselves to our client's nonverbalized sensations and experiences and helping the person form a language to talk about their physical and emotional sensations. It offers an understanding so that the client can further articulate their previously unspoken experiences and the profound effects of relational disruptions. It provides a vocabulary for previously unspoken experiences to be acknowledged and eventually talked about.

Therapeutic description provides an interpersonal connectedness from psychotherapist to client. It is not the same as interpretations or explanations that are given to other types of clients to enhance their cognitive understanding of psychological dynamics. Therapeutic description involves a sensitive attunement to the client's way of being that includes timing, tone of voice, and carefully observing the client's nonverbal responses to the descriptions. However, if therapeutic description is used too early it could be experienced as defining or invasive.

Violet provided the best definition of therapeutic description when later in the psychotherapy she told me how she experienced my comments:

> "It is as though you knew my internal experience, my fear of relationship, the safety in silence, the importance of hiding, and the depth of my loneliness. You helped me find the words to talk about my inner life. Now I am more alive most of the time."

In summary

Violet continued her psychotherapy for four years. We had many sessions where she would go to her "quiet place," sometimes for twenty to thirty minutes. During these long periods of silence I practiced how to be *therapeutically quiet*: to not intervene; to tolerate my uncertainty about what was happening within Violet. I periodically spoke, but only to reassure her that I was watching over her or provide some sparse therapeutic descriptions. Gradually I acquired an intense patience—a patience that is so necessary in working with clients who use relational withdrawal and silence to self-stabilize and self-regulate. I was watchful of every breath, sigh, and movement she made. I listened to her silence and compassionately worried about her speechless struggle. There were often times when there would be a long silence but she was eventually able to describe her body sensations, sob in her loneliness, and be angry at her mother, while still often being scared of "getting it wrong."

In several sessions where Violet imagined being in her "safe bed" she would sit up and tell me about the neglectful events in her childhood, the strict rules she lived with, and her mother's constant demands for "perfect behavior." I could observe the tension in her arms, neck, and legs as she talked about her mother. On some occasions when I pointed out that her body tension may indicate that she was angry she would begin by shrugging her shoulders and say, "I don't know." But, as we focused on the language of her body, she would recognize that she was angry.

In our fourth year of working together we were talking face-to-face. Most of my transactions with Violet were composed of phenomenological and historical inquiry—an inquiry that was designed to help Violet discover and put into language her emotion-filled, and never talked-about, childhood experiences of parental neglect and control. During this phase of our psychotherapy I did not use therapeutic description; that sensitive way of communicating was reserved for the times when Violet was silent and withdrawn into her hiding place.

Our psychotherapy was now focused on Violet's becoming aware of herself. We gave a lot of attention to her body sensations and her various emotions. I acknowledged her memories and validated her emotions. Many sessions included my helping her put her untold story into words. I prompted Violet in defining herself. I shared with her how she had influenced me and how I had to change the orientation of our psychotherapy. At first Violet did not believe me but she eventually said, "In the beginning you wanted me to do something different, something I didn't know how to do, just like the other therapists. But then you changed. You got softer and quieter. That helped me be me. Did you really change because of me?"

In response to my various inquiries she told me stories about her marriage relationship. I could hear Violet's anger at her husband's "criticism and control." She was still reluctant to do any active anger work but she was now able to say "I don't like it" and "I don't want it." She and her husband began to have arguments for the first time in their almost thirty years of marriage. She was now defining herself, refusing to comply with her husband's demands, and expressing what she wanted in her marriage. Violet's husband became enraged at the changes she exhibited at home. He demanded that she terminate therapy. He threatened divorce. She was terrified about being alone.

At the beginning of the next meeting she shook with fear as she announced that this was her last psychotherapy session. She said that her husband had intensified his demands that she stop the psychotherapy. A wave of sadness swept over me. Violet had made some significant growth in her ability to express both her vitality and vulnerability. At least in my presence she was neither putting on a social mask nor withdrawing. She had changed significantly. I did not know what to say to relieve her distress.

I was dismayed; our ending was so abrupt.

A few years later I met Violet on the street. She told me that she was living alone in her own apartment and that it was she who had initiated their pending divorce. Her husband was now opposed to the divorce but she was determined. She angrily said, "I've had it with his control. I'm now almost sixty and it's time I live my own life. I'm coming back to see you once this is all over. I have more work to do."

Although I never heard from Violet again I will always be grateful that she taught me about the schizoid process and the importance of the psychotherapist supporting the client in making internal contact with the *vital and vulnerable self*. I came to appreciate the therapeutic results when I am attuned to my client's silence. I rediscovered the profound effects of relating to my clients with a non-pathological perspective.

References

Ainsworth, M. D. S., Blehar, M. C., Waters, E., & Wall, S. (1978). *Patterns of Attachment: A Psychological Study of the Strange Situation*. Hillsdale, NJ: Lawrence Erlbaum.

Balint, M. (1968). *The Basic Fault*. London: Tavistock.

Erskine, R. G. (2009). Life scripts and attachment patterns: Theoretical integration and therapeutic involvement. *Transactional Analysis Journal*, 39: 207–218.

Erskine, R. G. (2020). Relational withdrawal, attunement to silence: Psychotherapy of the schizoid process. *International Journal of Integrative Psychotherapy*, 11: 14–28.

Erskine, R. G., & Moursund, J. P. (2022). *The Art and Science of Relationship: The Practice of Integrative Psychotherapy*. Bicester, UK: Phoenix.

Erskine, R. G., Moursund, J. P., & Trautmann, R. L. (1999). *Beyond Empathy: A Therapy of Contact-in-Relationship*. New York: Routledge, 2023.

Fairbairn, W. R. D. (1952). *Psychoanalytic Studies of the Personality*. London: Routledge.

Greenberg, J. R., & Mitchell, S. A. (1983). *Object Relations in Psychoanalytic Theory*. Cambridge, MA: Harvard University Press.

Guntrip, H. (1962). The schizoid compromise and psychotherapeutic stalemate. *British Journal of Medical Psychology*, 35: 273–287.

Guntrip, H. (1968). *Schizoid Phenomena, Object Relations and the Self*. Madison, CT: International Universities Press.

Guntrip, H. (1971). *Psychoanalytic Theory, Therapy, and the Self*. New York: Basic Books.

Hazell, J. (Ed.) (1994). *Personal Relations Therapy: The Collected Papers of H. J. S. Guntrip*. Northvale, NJ: Jason Aronson.

Khan, M. M. R. (1963). The concept of cumulative trauma. *Psychoanalytic Study of the Child*, *18*: 286–306.

Khan, M. M. R. (1974). *The Privacy of the Self*. London: Hogarth.

Kohon, G. (1986). *The British School of Psychoanalysis*. New Haven, CT: Yale University Press.

Little, M. I. (1981). *Transference Neurosis and Transference Psychosis*. New York: Jason Aronson.

Little, M. I. (1990). *Psychotic Anxieties and Containment: A Personal Record of an Analysis with Winnicott*. Northville, NJ: Jason Aronson.

Perls, F. S., Hefferline, R. F., & Goodman, P. (1951). *Gestalt Therapy: Excitement and Growth in the Human Personality*. New York: Julian.

Stolorow, R. D., Brandchaft, B., & Atwood, G. E. (1987). *Psychoanalytic Treatment: An Intersubjective Approach*. Hillsdale, NJ: The Analytic Press.

Sutherland, D. (1980). The British object relations theorists: Balint, Winnicott, Fairbairn, Guntrip. *Journal of the American Psychoanalytic Association*, *28*: 829–860.

Suttie, I. D. (1988). *The Origins of Love and Hate*. London: Free Association.

Winnicott, D. W. (1965). *The Maturational Processes and the Facilitating Environment: Studies in the Theory of Emotional Development*. New York: International Universities Press.

Winnicott, D. W. (1974). Fear of breakdown. *International Review of Psycho-Analysis*, *1*: 103–107.

CHAPTER 4

Engaging with the schizoid compromise

Ray Little

Richard Erskine (2020) recently invited me to respond to an article he has written about his treatment of a schizoid client. We were both on a panel twenty years ago at a transactional analysis conference in San Francisco, the theme of which was schizoid processes. The conference papers were published as a theme issue of the *Transactional Analysis Journal* (Daellenbach, 2001). It seems timely now to revisit some of those ideas, having worked extensively with them in the interim, and to share some current thoughts about schizoid processes.

In Erskine's (2020) paper, entitled "Relational Withdrawal, Attunement to Silence: Psychotherapy of the Schizoid Process," he presented the case of Violet and described how that work taught him the significance of relational withdrawal and the importance of attunement in psychotherapy. Erskine's article provoked me to focus particularly on the notions of the schizoid compromise, withdrawal, and treatment considerations. The schizoid person's behavior is marked by withdrawal and inability to form close relationships: "There is a consuming need for object dependence but attachment threatens the schizoid with the loss of self" (Seinfeld, 1991, p. 3). The person protects themself by withdrawing from social contact.

In my article "Schizoid Processes: Working with the Defenses of the Withdrawn Child Ego State" (Little, 2001), I examined several theoretical descriptions of schizoid processes. I pointed out how the term *schizoid* has been used to describe both a personality structure and psychological processes. Melanie Klein (1946) employed the term both to refer to a splitting mechanism and to describe a developmental position. In discussing the splitting of the self, she highlighted how the other is experienced as a persecutor. Fairbairn (1952) described three prominent characteristics of schizoid personalities: an attitude of omnipotence, detachment, and a preoccupation with fantasy and inner reality. He later described an intrapsychic structure that consisted of the splitting of the ego and repression as a defense. He pointed out that schizoid personalities may appear to fulfill a social role with others with what seems to be appropriate emotion and contact while actually remaining detached.

Before continuing here, I want to let readers know that I, as a white British male, will be drawing on my clinical experience to highlight some of the theory. The clients and supervisees' clients described here are largely white European and North American. I acknowledge this because we need to ask ourselves whether the theory is applicable across all races, ethnicities, and cultures given that there is little research into these aspects of personality disorders. However, some papers relevant to these issues have been published in the last decade, including Hossain et al. (2018), McGilloway et al. (2010), and Newhill et al. (2009).

Developmental theory

A variety of theoretical models can be drawn on to elucidate the developmental history involved in schizoid processes and personalities (Fairbairn, 1952; Guntrip, 1968; Kernberg, 1984; M. Klein, 1946; R. Klein, 1995; McWilliams, 1994). Some of them refer to schizoid mechanisms, whereas others refer to schizoid personality disorders. One perspective on understanding the etiology of schizoid phenomena is to consider how the individual negotiated relationships as an infant/child and then internalized those experiences. Ego state relational units (Little, 2006) and object relations (Fairbairn, 1952; Guntrip, 1968) both describe how relational experiences, and the child's perception of them, become organized and internalized as relational schemas (Little, 2013; Žvelc, 2010).

On examining these schemas, we can distinguish between tolerable experiences that were integrated and intolerable ones that remain unintegrated. Tolerable nondefensive experiences are an aspect of the integrating adult ego state and represent autonomous, here-and-now functioning from an open system (Little, 2006, 2011) with the capacity for assimilation and accommodation (Piaget, 1952; Žvelc, 2010). Intolerable experiences remain as a dissociated structure consisting of defensive or maladaptive schemas (Eagle, 2011; Žvelc, 2010). I describe these schemas as child–parent ego state relational units (Little, 2006), which are located in unconscious, implicit memory. These relational units make up the internal structure of the schizoid individual. (For a full discussion of the theory of relational schemas, see Eagle, 2011; Little, 2006, 2011; Piaget, 1952; Žvelc, 2010.)

The basic need for attachment and object relatedness and the desire to "discover one's reflection in the look of the other" (Seinfeld, 1991, p. 33) exists in the schizoid personality, as it does in everyone. It is intrinsic to who we are as a species. When we think of the adult person who presents with a schizoid characterological structure, we may wonder what the nature of the person's early experiences were, particularly with their primary caregivers, that led them to feel such hopelessness and fear in relation to being with others. Those early experiences led them to feel a tension between attaching and not attaching (or nonattachment). For Ralph Klein (1995), the question revolved around "what kind of deal does the schizoid negotiate in order to gain the benefits of attachment while avoiding the anxieties and dangers of nonattachment?" (p. 45).

Ralph Klein (1995, p. 51) described two positions—nonattachment and attachment—that the schizoid individual may occupy. The first consists of the schizoid's self-sufficiency and self-reliance. The second consists of being close and involved with another but runs the risk of being let down, rejected, or abandoned. As one client said to me, "Relying on people is seen as a bad idea as they will eventually let you down."

Guntrip (1968) and Ralph Klein (1995) agreed on the nature of the schizoid condition. They disagreed, however, as to the point during development at which the condition originates. Guntrip, following Fairbairn (1952), suggested that in response to the traumas of postnatal life, we develop a split structure that he described as the *schizoid position*. This refers to the primary structuring of the personality. If the schizoid position develops to an extreme extent (Gomez, 1997, p. 66), it may become the schizoid personality. For Klein (1995, pp. 40–41), the condition occurs during the rapprochement phase of development. He stated that schizoid personalities are aware of the two sides of their dilemma, thus indicating a certain degree of psychological separateness. They are also aware of the difference between external reality and their internal world, which, as Klein stated, reflects difficulties emanating from the rapprochement stage (Mahler et al., 1971). However, my experience is that more severely withdrawn and introverted schizoid personalities do not seem to experience the two sides of the dilemma as Klein described it. They seem to only occupy the nonattachment side. It is as though they have relinquished any desire for attachment. In this way, Klein's notion that the schizoid develops at the rapprochement phase does not account for my clinical experience of working with schizoid personalities with whom there seems to be evidence of earlier trauma and relationship failings.

I agree with Kernberg and his colleagues, who suggested that schizoid personalities, like other personality disorders (Clarkin et al., 2006), rely on more primitive defense mechanisms (e.g., projective identification), which suggests an early developmental struggle/failure. In light of this, it may be that Klein was describing more integrated personalities.

Structure of the mind

Many of my schizoid clients have felt safest when they are at home, with solid walls around them for protection. As children, they would frequently withdraw to their bedrooms, or somewhere similar, to feel safe, often playing on their own. For example, Nicola worked as a doctor and was proud of her care for her patients. This care was something that she did not receive from her parents when she was a child. Her mother was cruel, violent, and unpredictable. As an adult, Nicola was phobic about socializing with people. She also located the cruel object of her childhood in animals and was fearful of them. She hated dogs and would not go near them, particularly if they were not on a leash. She viewed them as unpredictable and vicious. As a result, she would not go into her local park unless she was accompanied by her husband. Nicola's withdrawn state of being in exile was linked to her experience of a cruel and unpredictable mother. My countertransference picture of Nicola's childhood was of her in a cot terrified of the world around her as represented by her mother.

Marye O'Reilly-Knapp (2001), who was also on the 2000 panel in San Francisco with me and Richard Erskine, described the schizoid individual as an encapsulated self "hidden from the world and even from himself or herself" (p. 44). She saw the schizoid's withdrawal as an "autistic encapsulation [that is] the psyche's most primitive form of organization and the earliest form of withdrawal" (p. 46).

If the person's experience as a child and the idea of closeness to others as an adult does not involve the internalization of a caring relationship, and instead is experienced as some kind of "master–slave" relationship (R. Klein, 1995), this often results in an internalization of a bad object relationship as described by Fairbairn (1952). He saw the good object internalized as memory, whereas the bad object relationship is internalized in a much more vital and fundamental sense than memory alone (as cited in Guntrip, 1968, pp. 21–22). Perhaps what Fairbairn was referring to was that a good object is experienced as benign, whereas a bad object is experienced more intensely and as profoundly charged with affect and frustrated needs.

Ralph Klein (1995) used the term schizoid from the perspective of Masterson (1988) to describe a further disorder of the self (in addition to borderline and narcissistic personality disorders). In taking an object relations view, Klein saw the schizoid as either in a self-object relational unit as a slave attached to a master or as a self-in-exile fearful of a sadistic object. This view of the person's internal world represents a split structure.

Some schizoid personalities may perceive the master/slave unit as more acceptable than being in exile and therefore attach to others at a cost to themselves; other schizoid personalities may prefer withdrawal and fantasies to that of being closer, which is felt as more threatening. For the withdrawn schizoid, fantasy serves to maintain some sort of link to the world of relationships when actual people and reality are intolerable. Fantasy can be fulfilled by novels, films, pornography, and gaming, all of which can stimulate fantasy relationships (Manfield, 1992).

As children, such individuals may live, through fantasy, in the world of the stories they read and may imagine themselves playing a part in the adventures of the characters. They come to inhabit their fantasies. This is a more extreme version of what most children do and serves the function, as previously mentioned, of maintaining some link to the world of relationships. The fear of being in exile, with its experience of isolation and nothingness, may be avoided by maintaining a "tie to the bad object" (Seinfeld, 1993, p. 65). Fairbairn (1952) described these ties as "the libidinal bonds whereby the patient is attached to these hitherto indispensable bad objects" (p. 74). Further, Grotstein (1994) depicted this as "the unwavering loyalty that schizoids maintain towards their objects" (p. 116). The schizoid personality's connection to the external world is usually superficial. They have withdrawn from the outer world and are living in an internal world of fantasy. However, by maintaining a relationship with the bad object, schizoid individuals keep in touch with the world, protecting themselves against a flight from reality and descent into nothingness. Guntrip (cited in Hazell, 1994) suggested that the individual preserves the ego by "taking refuge in internal bad-object phantasies of a persecutory or accusatory kind" (p. 164).

Considering all of this, Ralph Klein's (1995) description of the withdrawn position as nonattachment may not be strictly true. Withdrawal from the world of potential real-life attachments to an internal world may be a retreat to a position where attachments of a sort are maintained. The internal world of bad object relations consists of attachments, albeit to a bad object. This internal world is a world of attachments in a similar way that external relations constitute attachments. To live in this internal world is to occupy a world of relationships rather than an objectless/relationship-less world.

I am suggesting that the nonattachment position Ralph Klein described can also be seen as consisting of no external relationships but instead a retreat to an internal phantasy world of attachments that, to some extent, can be controlled.

Case study: *A Beautiful Mind*

This process of internal attachments was brought home to me dramatically by the film *A Beautiful Mind* (Howard, 2001), in which Russell Crowe plays the part of Nobel Prize winner and mathematician John Nash. I will use this film and the biography it is based on to illustrate the schizoid withdrawn state and the internal world with its relational schemas and its defenses against objectlessness and the black hole of nothingness.

In the film, Nash initially comes across as withdrawn and obsessed with patterns and numbers. He is seen as strange by his fellow doctoral students, from whom he is socially isolated. They describe him as aloof, without affect, detached, and isolated. "He's not one of us," one of them was reported to have said (Nasar, 1998, p. 13). In the film, Nash has an exuberant roommate, Charles, who appears to be everything Nash is not. Charles is heard to suggest that they get a pizza: "You know, food!" Charles appears outgoing and interested in alcohol and women. At one point, Charles asks Nash about friends. Nash replies, "I don't much like people, and they don't much like me." Nash fights with Charles in his room, pushing a table to and fro, which Charles pushes out of the window. In another scene, Nash is sitting on the roof of the building chatting to Charles and shouting at students below. There is a point later in the film when Nash is helping the military solve a code-breaking problem and catches sight of someone watching him from the balcony. He calls that person "Big Brother." The person later identifies himself as William and behaves with authority, telling Nash he will arrange for Nash to have top secret clearance to continue the work. Later in the film, when Nash tells William he needs to resign because his wife is pregnant, William responds by saying, "I told you attachments are dangerous."

What eventually becomes apparent is that Charles and William are visual and auditory hallucinations and part of Nash's internal world of attachments. Some of them are punitive and some more amiable. One of the things the film demonstrates is that Nash's life appears as an illusion with occasional excursions into reality. There seems to be a tension for Nash between rational and irrational thinking. Later in life, he considered that his "dream-like delusional hypotheses" (Nash, 1994, para. 27) had been irrational. He went on to say that "One aspect of this is that rationality of thought imposes a limit on a person's concept of his relation to the cosmos" (para. 29).

Nash, age thirty-one years, having worked for ten years as a brilliant theoretical mathematician, is diagnosed as suffering from paranoid schizophrenia after having a breakdown. Charles turns up again in the film, greeting Nash with a hug. Charles is accompanied by his niece, who expresses feelings with Nash, something he does not seem to experience a great deal. She seems to be the repository of Nash's unexpressed affect. As Nash later moves into remission, he realizes that, although he continues to see her over many years, she does not age. These characters are externalizations of Nash's internal world, his world of attachments and containers for his disavowed affect, attachments that, I suggest, are preferable to the black hole of nothingness. Nash's internal world is also a world of patterns and numbers, which is where he seems to feel safe and at home.

When Nash was a child, his parents were worried about him. He had a lack of childish pursuits and friends (Nasar, 1998, p. 32). According to his sister, he wanted to do things his own way. Other children thought him weird and bullied or just tolerated him (p. 36). It seems that he learned to "armor himself against rejection by adopting a hard shell of indifference and using his superior intelligence to strike back" (pp. 37–38). Nash used his superiority, standoffishness, and occasional cruelty to manage his loneliness, thus maintaining his self-esteem (p. 38).

Nasar, in her biography of Nash, described some of those schizoid personalities who are brilliant scientists and thinkers from whom society benefits but who are strange and solitary, such Albert Einstein, Isaac Newton, Immanuel Kant, Ludwig Wittgenstein, and René Descartes. She draws on the writing of Anthony Storr, a British psychiatrist and psychoanalyst, who wrote that the schizoid state is characterized by a sense of meaninglessness and futility. "Creative activity is a particularly apt way to express himself … the activity is solitary … [but] the ability to create and the productions which result from such ability are generally regarded as possessing value by our society" (Nasar, 1998, pp. 15–16).

The schizoid's experience

Schizoid personalities function at a borderline level of personality organization (Kernberg, 1984), a position between neurotic and psychotic. This level of functioning suggests that they have not managed to individuate and integrate sufficiently. These individuals often suffer as a result of poor interpersonal ego boundaries. Kernberg saw the schizoid personality disorder, with other personality disorders in this category, as having a poorly integrated sense of self and subsequent confusion about personal identity. These individuals have a predominance of and reliance on primary defenses (McWilliams, 1994), primitive object relations (Kernberg, 1984), and early persecutory anxieties associated with the paranoid–schizoid position (M. Klein, 1946).

On entering therapy, an individual with a schizoid presentation will probably feel anxious as a result of projecting either a sadistic object or the master-object representation onto the therapist. Alternatively, through projective identification, the person may locate the self in the therapist and inhabit the object aspect of the relational units.

The various theories just discussed and my description of schizoid processes and personalities emerge from clinical experience. What are being discussed here are those individuals who present for therapy with these characteristics and who are struggling in some way. Usually, they are seeking more contact and closeness but are fearful at the same time. There are also many people who could be described as having a schizoid personality who do not experience any tension and are content with their lives.

I think of the schizoid personality structure as having developed as a defense and as a means of managing early experiences of trauma or developmental deficit and rupture. I see their internal world as consisting of a split structure that has come about as a result of failures in bonding and attachment. The infant retreats inwardly, maintaining a more superficial relationship with attachment figures.

Seinfeld (1996, p. 78), citing R. D. Laing, wrote that in human development there is a polarity between separateness and relatedness, both of which represent profound human needs. The person with a schizoid personality experiences this process in a more extreme way. They are usually highly anxious, with the fear of closeness being experienced as a fear of dependency or a fear of merging with a subsequent loss of a sense of self. Separation may be experienced as isolation or being in exile. Both positions are experienced as frightening. Thus, nowhere feels safe for the schizoid individual. This is in contrast to the narcissist, who feels safe when merged with an idealized object, or the borderline, who feels safe when clinging and merging with a rewarding object.

Withdrawal: home base

Everything starts and ends at home

Any description of a schizoid presentation will include the characteristics of withdrawal, self-sufficiency, detachment, aloofness, and lack of affect. Withdrawal is often the home position of the schizoid individual. Ralph Klein (1995) described this as a nonattachment position and McWilliams (1994, p. 100) as a primitive defense. It is where schizoid personalities seem to spend most of their time and also how people often think of them.

Withdrawal into a different state of consciousness is an automatic, self-protective behavior that can be observed in infants. The same can be seen in adults who may retreat from others to their internal world of fantasy. Some infants' temperament may lead them be more inclined to withdraw, and there is some suggestion that they may be particularly sensitive (McWilliams, 1994, p. 100).

For example, I often see a certain man who lives in our locality walking around the streets. He wears the same clothes most of the year, and his unkempt beard gives him a medieval appearance. I have never seen him with anyone. We nod at each other as we pass, occasionally exchanging a polite greeting. I make a point of saying hello, but nothing more is said. He walks on, not really looking at people. He buys his lunch at a local shop and then eats it sitting on a park bench. He does not appear to work. My fantasy is this is the sum of his life, that this is how he spends his time. I cannot imagine that he has ever had a relationship in his adult life.

The appearance I am describing might be thought of as a more extreme withdrawn schizoid presentation. I doubt that he and others like him would seek out therapy. He may not even be uncomfortable with the way he is. His position may be a result of how he negotiated early life experiences and his relationship with his caretakers (R. Klein, 1995). His is a severe, introverted schizoid presentation, functioning in isolation, living in the citadel of his mind, perhaps living in imagination rather than in the external world with its possibility of relationships. The dread of relationships with the possibility of being smothered, suffocated, possessed, imprisoned, or absorbed (Guntrip, cited in Hazell, 1994, p. 166) feels claustrophobic. This extreme schizoid withdrawal was described by Guntrip (1968) as follows: "Womb fantasies and/or the passive wish to die represent the extreme schizoid reaction, the ultimate regression, and it is the more common, mild characteristics which show the extraordinary prevalence of schizoid, i.e. detached or withdrawn, states of mind" (p. 58).

In considering these disorders, the description and behavioral elements need to be combined with a phenomenological and intrapsychic analysis in order to fully understand and possibly diagnose a schizoid personality disorder.

Returning to Erskine's (2020) work with Violet, he initially focused on her withdrawal behavior, commonly exhibited by schizoid personalities. She was, for him, confusing and, at times, difficult. He described how in his work with her, he learned about relational withdrawal and the significance of attunement, particularly to silence, in psychotherapy (p. 14). Violet's internal world emerged early in her meetings with Erskine when she described how "her husband alternated between ignoring her and controlling her" (p. 15). This also echoed her relationship with her mother. Her comments about her husband were probably a transference projection of that internal world as well as the reality of her experience with her husband. That was a point at which her internal and external worlds came together. Her experience of her husband became a hook on which she could hang her projections and probably represented the object from which Violet withdrew.

In my 2001 article, I wrote about Sebastian, who usually started a session by saying something placatory that we could talk about but that did not reveal his vulnerability. Sessions seemed to be isolated experiences for him, without continuity. He often seemed to have forgotten the previous session, having wiped it out:

> Sebastian often withdraws and seems to be watching me. It is as if he is on the inside of his head looking out of his eyes watching my every move. He has described having retreated into a castle, staying in the dungeon where he feels safe. He leaves a guard on duty. The drawbridge is down but can be raised at any time. If I see an expression of emotion on his face and respond, he is moved at having been seen but feels he cannot call out.

He feels it would be dangerous and frightening to do so. Sebastian has retreated from the world and is detached from interpersonal relations. He has numbed his emotional responses to people and events. (Little, 2001, p. 35)

More extreme introverted schizoid personalities occupy what Ralph Klein (1995) described as "the safe place or haven, the impenetrable fortress, and the point of no return" (p. 55). The citadel is a womb-like state free from demands or attacks, with no need to adapt (Little, 2001, p. 38). The person is unlikely to experience any ambivalence about relationships. On the other hand, those schizoid persons with milder characteristics are more likely to want relationships with others. Perhaps there is a continuum for those with schizoid personality: at one end, more integrated individuals and, at the other, more severe presentations.

When thinking about schizoid individuals' ambivalence about attachment—craving closeness yet fearing engulfment, seeking distance but complaining of loneliness (McWilliams, 1994, p. 193)—I distinguish between these two aspects of ambivalence and the kind where withdrawal is more profound and individuals retreat into fantasy and their internal world. I refer to the latter as an "introverted regressed schizoid" (Guntrip, 1968, p. 42), someone who does without relationships.

Maintaining withdrawal: attacks on the link

Withdrawal is both a behavioral process and a psychological strategy of retreating into fantasy and imagination and detaching from external reality and relationships. This entails withdrawing into an internal closed system to escape the dangers of engaging with the external world. Over time, a schizoid client may establish a psychological and emotional link with a therapist, one that may be experienced as a threat or as dangerous. As a result, the person's internal bad object relationship may attack the links to the therapist because the clinician represents a threatening external reality. This defensive process reinforces the client's isolation. The closed psychic system, with its bad object, impedes the relational-seeking aspect of the personality. This is akin to Fairbairn's notion of the client remaining loyal to the bad object.

For his part, Bion (1967) described how the psychotic mind attacks the perceptual apparatus that links it to the object. I have experienced less severe attacks on the link between myself and a client as part of a schizoid defensive stance. For example, Justine, on leaving a session, would sometimes say things to herself such as, "Did you see how he took your money at the end of the session? He's so greedy. All he wants is your money. You're just a cash cow for him. You shouldn't trust him." This was an attack on her emerging link with me. This demonstrates how the desire to attach and connect may be prevented by the antirelational unit attacking the link between the client and the therapist as the needed object/other by devaluing and belittling the therapist. This kind of post-session attack usually occurred when Justine had shifted in her position, taken a risk, and revealed more of herself to me. The attack was typical of the nonattachment, antirelational side of her personality and her attitude of not relying on others.

The internal attacks would often leave her isolated and alone between sessions. At such times, she had destroyed the cocreated new relational unit.

After such self-talk, when Justine arrived at her next session, she was often wary of and less likely to trust me. I watched for this behavior and experienced it as "one step forward, two steps back." The antirelational self will attack the relational-seeking self's links to its attachment objects/others. These rejecting behaviors often echo the original caregiver's response toward the person's infantile dependency needs (Seinfeld, 1991, p. 73).

Enforced withdrawal during lockdown

Writing this article in May 2020 during the lockdown resulting from the Covid-19 pandemic highlights and affects my experience and understanding of these processes. When I venture out to the supermarket, I experience an increase in anxiety. I walk down the road wary of an unseen threat. Another person becomes a threatening enemy who may be carrying a deadly disease. Going around the supermarket picking up groceries I notice how watchful and anxious I am as other shoppers come close to me. There is an induced paranoia. It is not until I return home that I begin to relax.

I can imagine that this is not dissimilar to what less anxious schizoid personalities experience much of the time when they are out among people, anticipating an attack and withdrawing to protect themselves from danger. For some, the experience is even more extreme, and it is appropriate to talk of terrors and horrors and fear of mutilation: a world occupied by monsters. The difference for me during the pandemic is that my withdrawal is not something I chose but something that was imposed on me and is not my preference. Yet the danger is real. Needing to withdraw and isolate from face-to-face contact with clients, colleagues, and friends when personal contact involves the risk of catching a life-threatening virus has given me a perverted sort of empathy for the schizoid personality!

Listening to clients and talking to supervisees these days, I have realized that being in lockdown suits some people more than others, depending on their characterological structures. Another lockdown experience that spoke to the defense of withdrawal was something I noticed while working with clients remotely. Because of the isolation that I experienced, and the lack of contact with colleagues and friends, I had a growing desire to be friendlier with clients than I would be normally. I felt the impulse to reveal more personal circumstances and experiences that had nothing directly to do with the therapy. I would end the session by saying, "I'll see you next week," which is something I would not ordinarily say. What I understood was that my need for attachment, connection, and contact was emerging as a desire to self-disclose as a result of my disconnection from friends and colleagues. It was also triggered by the abrupt end to the session. The process highlighted for me that, in a nonattached state—in this case imposed by circumstances—the need to connect was emerging and fighting to be met. I was thereby running the risk of a boundary crossing (Little, 2020) and a loss of my therapeutic frame.

Countertransference reactions

Returning to Erskine (2020), he wondered whether he had been caught in a countertransference reaction with Violet through the methods he was using to treat her, which he appropriately discussed in supervision. The supervisor reiterated what Erskine had already been doing and did not address his lack of attunement to Violet, including during her long silences. Erskine began wondering what was missing in the therapeutic relationship (p. 16) and stated that he "felt inadequate" (p. 17).

One aspect of Erskine's countertransference was that he wanted something to happen in the therapy, so he focused on expressive methods, cognitive understanding, and behavior change. In my own work, sometimes my countertransference reaction to a schizoid client who has withdrawn has been that I want to "shake them up" and have them engage more with me. I can find it difficult to stay involved with someone who lacks affect and is self-sufficient and self-reliant. As therapists, with such individuals we can often feel useless or superfluous. Other therapists have described the experience of frustration or even abandonment in the face of the client's lack of lively emotional engagement in the work. On the other hand, I have clients for whom my aliveness can be threatening as if it were a prelude to danger, a sign that I will become an intrusive or dangerous other. One of the things that helps me stay engaged in such situations is understanding the nature of the client's early trauma.

With my client Sean, I recall wanting to disclose something of my poor, working-class background, which was very similar to his. I was fond of him and felt a desire to verbalize my warm feelings. It was difficult to sit with him session after session with his affectless presentation. At times I had the fantasy that expressing my feelings with him would somehow bring him alive, breathe life into his lungs. However, in fact, my presence was threatening to him.

As described earlier, countertransference reactions may include feeling tender while also struggling with how to connect and form a therapeutic alliance, as well as to understand the client's inner world without evoking too much anxiety or becoming too detached. The danger is in treating the client as an object of interest instead of as someone wrestling with a dilemma with its dual anxieties and helping them make meaning of their experience.

Schizoid dilemma

My clinical experience is that those schizoid personalities who present for therapy often experience a dilemma (Fairbairn, 1952; Guntrip, 1968) with which they are struggling. On the one hand, the person wants connection and closeness but fears feeling unsafe, even entrapped; on the other, they want to withdraw and retreat into exile to feel safe with the accompanying experience of isolation and aloneness.

Manfield (1992) movingly described this process as "too distant from people, he believes he will disintegrate, dissolve into oblivion, vaporize, be lost. [But] … too close to someone, he is afraid of being co-opted, used, swallowed up, devoured, totally appropriated" (p. 215).

This process also demonstrates a tension between the needed relationship—that is, the desire for closeness—and the repeated relationship (Little, 2011) with its fear of retraumatization. Working as I do in the here-and-now of the transference–countertransference relationship entails the therapist being both the longed for attachment object and the feared object. The more the therapist represents the longed for other, the more he or she will be feared as the process begins to trigger memories of early traumatic experience. As the client allows the need for contact to emerge, they may also experience the fear of retraumatization and the expectation that the therapist will let them down. Thus, the therapeutic paradox is that the more the needs emerge, the more the fear of retraumatization is stirred. In the initial stages of therapy, the client has no idea that the therapist is going to be any different from those who were previously retraumatizing for them. This represents a transference expectation.

The therapist's stance when working with these presentations should include an understanding of this dilemma and the associated relational impasse (Little, 2011). This understanding may be offered to the client as an interpretation. For example, the therapist might say, "On the one hand (you have an anxiety about getting close), and on the other ... (you are anxious about being isolated)."

Being close means the schizoid individual has to face the fact that they cannot control the other and that being involved in relationships runs the risk of being rejected, attacked, and/or experiencing pain. Some people prefer isolation rather than engaging with this process.

For example, as a child, Marcia retreated to her room to avoid the demands of her parents, whom she described as misattuned and not interested in her, only in her older sister. As an adult, Marcia preferred being on her own, but her job required her to do certain things for people. This meant she had to leave the safety of her womb-like state, which echoed her childhood bedroom. In doing so, she had to encounter the world that she hated. In her therapy, her infant needs emerged, and she wanted her therapist to be perfectly attuned to her. She unconsciously wanted to incorporate him into her safe, womb-like space and have him be devoted to her, thus protecting her from disappointment, pain, and separation.

For the schizoid individual, every place and every experience is fraught with anxiety, whether that is being with people or being alone. Being self-reliant avoids the problem of having to rely on or be dependent on another, but it can leave the individual having to do everything themselves and having no significant social contact. The dilemma can be described as an experience between an antirelational self and a relational-seeking self (Little, 2001; Seinfeld, 1991). Attending to the behavioral manifestations of the dilemma often highlights the person's own split internal personality structure, and the manner in which they experience others represents a transference projection.

Erskine (2020) described Violèt as "unconsciously looking for interpersonal connection and simultaneously fearing any human closeness" (p. 22). The relational-seeking self desires connection, whereas the antirelational self wants to prevent that from happening. He described how Violet's "social self" has achieved some relational security by accommodating to the requirements of significant others, whereas her "vital and vulnerable self" remains "protectively internal" (pp. 18–19). Erskine made a note to himself "to respect her silences, to support her withdrawal, and to create a safe place for the deeply repressed to express herself" (p. 20). He wondered if he "thought of Violet's silence and withdrawal as her attempt to protect a vital and vulnerable aspect of herself" (p. 20). He understood that her "polite, proper, and superficial presentation as a social facade had at least two important functions: protection and attachment" (p. 20).

Schizoid compromise

In common with Erskine, I (Little, 2012) admire the writings of Guntrip and his descriptions of working with clients who have withdrawn from relationship into a "schizoid compromise" (Guntrip, 1968, p. 58). That phrase describes what the client is trying to deal with psychologically, and the compromise indicates how they are managing the dilemma, that is, finding a middle ground between the two anxieties.

Erskine (2020) described wondering how he might make sense of his client's "superficial stories, the lack of interpersonal contact, and the absence of any vitality, emotions, or vulnerability" (p. 18). He saw Violet as "someone who learned to hide her vitality and vulnerability," who had "created a social facade (i.e., a false self) in order to maintain some form of relational attachment" (p. 19).

Previously, I (Little, 2001, p. 39) discussed how retreating from contact leaves the individual isolated, lonely, and in pain. Some schizoid personalities may attempt to avoid the pain through "workaholism, intellectualization and other distancing defenses" (Manfield, 1992, p. 205). In some cases, the longing for contact will reemerge, and the person may want to move toward others; however, such movement also brings with it the anxiety of being close with its sense of being entrapped. Guntrip (1968) described this as the "in and out program" (p. 36), an expression of the hunger for and terror of contact and closeness, caught between the need and fears of close personal connection. They are driven "in" by their needs and driven "out" by their fears. Some individuals manage this dilemma by establishing the schizoid "compromise in a half-way house position" (Guntrip, cited in Hazell, 1994, p. 166). This is a way of keeping others around but preventing them from getting too close or becoming endangered by them. This may, for example, be achieved by maintaining contact at an intellectual level or by being present physically but absent emotionally. More often than not, relationships are kept emotionally neutral, an approach that undermines the possibility of forming friendships and romantic relationships.

In the United Kingdom there is an attitude known as the "stiff upper lip," a cultural endorsement of the expression of the compromise that enables people to stay socially connected while hiding their emotions. Many "polite" behaviors in certain cultures are also an expression of the same compromise, one that is, in essence, a defensive position between the two fears of isolation, on the one hand, and enslavement or merging/fusing, on the other. The question for the individual is, "How do I keep people around without getting too close or being alone?"

The compromise is a remedy to the oscillation of the in-and-out program, but the individual does not give themselves to anyone or anything fully.

Therapy of the compromise: the therapist's stance

The initial therapeutic task with schizoid clients is to create sufficient safety (R. Klein, 1995; Little, 2001; O'Reilly-Knapp, 2001), including a containing, holding environment that is both non-wounding and unobtrusive and that creates an opportunity for the hidden, vulnerable, relational-seeking self to reemerge. The therapist needs to be curious regarding why the person went into hiding, what their terror is about, and the nature of the defenses involved. In addition, it is important to comprehend how attempts at contact by the therapist may be experienced by the client as intrusive and frightening. For example, in the work with Violet described by Erskine (2020), she was afraid to "go internal" in front of anyone because "what I have inside is private. No one can know it … my quiet hiding place. It has been my private place, all my life" (p. 21). The therapist needs to demonstrate an understanding of the schizoid dilemma and compromise and offer an attuned interpretation. In the inevitable push and pull of therapy, the therapist should try, as much as possible, not to behave as either a master or a sadistic object/other. Ware (1983) encouraged us to go slowly: "It must be remembered that the cure of schizoids is a slow, painstaking process, taking only small steps at a time" (p. 15). I believe that we need to wait outside the "cave" until the person appears or invites us in. What may help them emerge from their particular cave is maintaining the clinical frame and boundaries, which will enable them to begin to feel safe from engulfment or intrusion. Going in after them may repeat the experience of an intrusive caregiver/other.

To establish safety for the client, I occasionally agree to a schedule that begins with meeting every other week and then, after some time, moving to weekly. In my consulting room, I have three sofas, and the client can sit wherever they choose so they can feel safe enough. The therapist needs to attend to variations in the client's capacity to be present in whatever way they can manage. When a client does withdraw after having been more in contact, I wonder what went on that they became more withdrawn, which is often beneficial to interpret and discuss with them.

Schizoid clients generally begin treatment feeling anxious. During the therapy, this anxiety may be further triggered by moves toward the therapist and/or vice versa. These clients are sensitive to and impacted by changes in the therapist's mood, demeanor, and/or behavior. In fact, the client's withdrawal may well be triggered by the therapist's behavior.

For Ralph Klein (1995, p. 71), therapy is oriented toward reality, which thereby disrupts transference expectations. In my view, this disruption results from a cocreated relational experience. Erskine noted that both Guntrip and Winnicott encouraged a psychotherapy that focuses on the client's internal processes and not specifically on cognitive insight or behavioral outcome, "a psychotherapy that provides a healing relationship to a traumatized and fragmented client (Winnicott, 1965)" (Erskine, 2020, p. 19).

From a relational transactional analysis perspective, therapeutic action needs to entail working in the here-and-now of the therapeutic relationship in which the therapist is experienced as both an old object and a cocreated new object working directly with both relational units in the transference–countertransference relationship. The client's experience of the transference expectations reinforces their withdrawal from relationships. This is the nature of unconsciously engaging in psychological games and enactments.

As the therapist and client begin to develop a therapeutic alliance, the new cocreated self-other relational unit develops. For the client, this is a new lens through which to view and experience the world in contrast to their internal structure, which is projected onto the world of relationships. If the client begins to feel safe enough in the therapeutic relationship, they are more likely to experiment with taking risks with the therapist, such as sharing thoughts and feelings more freely. The nature of the client's compromise changes through their experiments.

For example, Lizzie, a woman in her late thirties who has always been independent and self-assured, came to see me because she felt there was something vaguely wrong. She did not trust anyone and could not recall ever doing so. But some things she had read recently led her to wonder if there was something wrong with that. The only contact she had with people was as the manager of an education service. From what she said, it seemed she could be helpful to those for whom she was responsible but without really feeling for them because she had no real emotional relationships. She found it difficult sitting with me because the familiar roles of helper and helped had been reversed, and she was the one requiring help. Her compromise position had always consisted of being helpful.

Any time I showed more than a bland presentation, Lizzie would complain of being intruded on. Over many years, in which I felt I had to sit patiently waiting for her to emerge, she began to tell me her early story of deprivation from an uncontained and intrusive caregiver. She gradually moved from her isolation, withdrawal, and a compromise position of being helpful and responsible for others to one in which I as her therapist became the one person who knew her story with its accompanying feelings. I felt that we had begun to cocreate a precious new narrative.

With another client who began expressing more of her feelings, fantasies, and inner world, it seemed she was experimenting with expressing previously repressed feelings and in so doing shifting her compromise position. She could justify her new behavior on the grounds that as a therapist, I was a professional and therefore different from others. This enabled her to change while remaining the same, thus maintaining her compromise of not revealing her emotions to the world. However, we could also see that she was nullifying me to some degree.

As therapists working with these presentations, we need to be wary of being excessively devoted to having our clients establish closeness, intimacy, and attachment to us or others in their lives, as if intimacy is a defining feature of psychological health and well-being. We might wonder if attachment is being fetishized, to quote a colleague, while acknowledging that to connect is a human need.

Dissociation

Dissociation is, in essence, disconnection from unintegrated states. One type of dissociation is depersonalization (a feeling that one is not in one's own body and is disconnected from one's sense of self), which Guntrip (1968, pp. 41–44) listed as a characteristic of the schizoid. Being disconnected from aspects of the self is a major defense of schizoid personalities. Living in their heads, with apparently little relationship with their emotions, is a common mode of being, as if there is a cutoff or blockage between their hearts and their heads that prevents any communication between the two. Dissociation is commonly used to protect the self from aspects that are felt to endanger existence or that are too painful to engage with. Dissociation maintains the split internal structure, and the therapeutic goal in such cases could be described as moving from segregation and disconnection to association and integration. O'Reilly-Knapp (2001) highlighted how schizoids use dissociation to "protect the continuity of existence" (p. 45).

Aloof from the crowd

Under stress, schizoid personalities may withdraw either temporarily or permanently from their own affect as well as from external stimulation (McWilliams, 1994, p. 192). Internal dissociation from affect can manifest behaviorally as aloofness, with the individual seeming to look down on others. These individuals appear to hold others in contempt and disdain, on occasions patronizing them while fearing being patronized. This is an expression of the internal saboteur (Fairbairn, 1952) who rejects the need of others. They appear to be proud of being independent and self-reliant (R. Klein, 1995, p. 57).

In such cases, the therapist's countertransference reactions may include feelings of inferiority because of having an emotional response to the client. The tendency of the client to behave in an aloof manner may have its origins in the relationship with primary caregivers who were overcontrolling or over-intrusive (McWilliams, 1994, p. 195), although usually the main fear driving their behavior is of engulfment rather than abandonment.

For example, many years ago I worked with a man who appeared quite aloof and superior. Initially I thought him quite engaging, but over time I began to feel a strong desire to attack him and penetrate his defenses, even to subjugate him in some way. I felt quite aggressive toward him and wanted to show him how he was making things worse for himself. I arrogantly felt I knew better than he did. After some time and reflection, I realized that he had disconnected from any intense feelings. He could talk politely with me about emotions, but he dissociated from his more intense feelings. In discussion with my supervisor, I came to see that, through projective identification, I was experiencing the intense feelings with which he could not allow himself to connect.

Therapist's defensive compromise

Lastly, I want to address a defensive position that therapists themselves may occupy: a schizoid compromise position, not a countertransference reaction. Schizoid individuals can be very sensitive to other people and often bury their aggression. As McWilliams (1994, p. 196) wrote, schizoid personalities are able to care about others while maintaining a protective stance (as was the case with Lizzie as described earlier), and some even pursue careers in psychotherapy. In citing Wheelis, McWilliams described how people with a "core conflict over closeness and distance" may take up the profession of psychotherapy because it "offers the opportunity to know others more intimately than anyone else ever will, while concealing the self" (p. 196).

For instance, therapy sessions are time limited. Therefore, at an emotional level, the therapist knows that whatever may go on and emerge in the session, it will end at a given time. Potentially, this time boundary permits the therapist to hide their own emotional response. In my experience as a supervisor, I have noticed that some therapists can avoid certain feelings or experiences by not commenting on them or by behaving in a particular manner that conveys the message that certain feelings do not have a place in therapy and therefore will not be addressed. An example would be the therapist who, every time sexual feelings enter the conversation, changes the subject. We all have our blind spots, but most of these are never examined. The therapist can "coast in the countertransference" (Hirsch, 2008) and thereby avoid disrupting the therapy, which would otherwise involve moving out of the safety zone of the "compromise" and disrupting the transference–countertransference relationship. It is as if the therapist's "[f]eelings can be identified and utilized interpersonally, although in a limited and circumscribed fashion" (R. Klein, 1995, p. 56).

Working as a psychotherapist can in itself be a compromise position for some. During the pandemic, working remotely has suited some therapists and clients. They feel more at ease. Hirsch (2008), citing Buechler, described how therapists with schizoid qualities may be inclined toward retreating emotionally, especially with clients who are also comfortable with emotional distance. The therapy may then become politely inactive. In my view, therapy should help the client enrich their lives and not be an alternative for life.

For some therapists, technique is often seen as the main method for facilitating the client's integration and growth. Thus, a further compromise for the therapist can be to use various techniques with the client while remaining affectively uninvolved. The therapist in a compromise position may not push themselves or the client beyond "states of comfortable equilibrium to states of disruption and surprise" (Hirsch, 2008, p. 65).

For some clinicians, the work of therapy provides some affective engagement in relationship while still maintaining emotional safety. In fact, schizoid personalities may "gravitate to careers in psychotherapy, where they put their exquisite sensitivity to use safely in the service of others" (McWilliams, 1994, p. 196).

Having said that, it is important to bear in mind that most therapists have a course of therapy during their training and will have engaged in reading, supervision, and self-analysis. As a result, they should have developed a narrative that explains what happened to them as a child. Managing to reconcile childhood experience in therapy and understanding the impact the past has on the present allows the possibility of developing an "earned secure" (Wallin, 2007, p. 87) attachment style.

If the therapist unconsciously retreats to a defensive withdrawal, or compromise position, this may be an indicator of them being under more extreme countertransference stress. Therefore, the concerns already expressed here regarding the therapist's compromise are a warning of the risks for the clinician.

Conclusion

It has been interesting to reread the literature from the past twenty-five years since I first read and engaged with it and particularly in light of the clinical experience I now have. Back twenty-five to thirty years ago, I had only limited clinical experience with schizoid processes. My first encounter with the literature was with Guntrip (in Hazell, 1994). As I reread him today, I continue to review my thinking and understanding and to examine my therapeutic approach. Guntrip still has a good deal to offer the practitioner who wishes to understand the inner world schizoid individuals occupy.

It is easy to overlook schizoid traits in clients, particularly when they are withdrawn, quiet, or enslaved and thus adapted to the other. They are not generally as disturbing to the therapist as borderline and narcissistic characterological presentations.

If I think of schizoid processes in contrast to schizoid personality disorder, I no longer see the dilemma as belonging only to the latter. In the twenty years since that conference in San Francisco where Erskine and I presented, I have come to believe, as some others do (Manfield, 1992, p. 204), that the schizoid presentation, with its flight from object relations and its subsequent compromise, is more prevalent and commonplace than we often recognize.

References

Bion, W. R. (1967). *Second Thoughts: Selected Papers on Psychoanalysis*. London: Karnac.

Clarkin, J. F., Yeoman, F. E., & Kernberg, O. F. (2006). *Psychotherapy for Borderline Personality: Focusing on Object Relations*. Washington, DC: American Psychiatric Publishing.

Daellenbach, C. (Ed.) (2001). The schizoid process [Theme issue]. *Transactional Analysis Journal, 31*(1). doi.org/10.1177/036215370103100102.

Eagle, M. (2011). *From Classical to Contemporary Psychoanalysis: A Critique and Integration*. New York: Routledge.

Erskine, R. G. (2020). Relational withdrawal, attunement to silence: Psychotherapy of the schizoid process. *International Journal of Integrative Psychotherapy, 11*: 14–29.

Fairbairn, W. R. D. (1952). *Psychoanalytic Studies of the Personality*. London: Routledge.

Gomez, L. (1997). *An Introduction to Object Relations*. New York: Free Association.

Grotstein, J. S. (1994). Notes on Fairbairn's metapsychology. In: J. S. Grotstein & D. B. Rinsley (Eds.), *Fairbairn and the Origins of Object Relations* (pp. 112–148). New York: Free Association.

Guntrip, H. (1968). *Schizoid Phenomena, Object Relations and the Self*. London: Hogarth.

Hazell, J. (Ed.) (1994). *Personal Relations Therapy: The Collected Papers of H. J. S. Guntrip*. Northvale, NJ: Jason Aronson.

Hirsch, I. (2008). *Coasting in the Countertransference: Conflicts of Self Interest between Analyst and Patient*. New York: Routledge.

Hossain, A., Malkov, M., Lee, T., & Bhui, K. (2018). Ethnic variation in personality disorder: Evaluation of 6 years of hospital admissions. *British Journal of Psychiatry Bulletin*, 42(4): 157–161. doi.org/10.1192/bjb.2018.31.

Howard, R. (Director) (2001). *A Beautiful Mind*. Glendale, CA: Dreamworks.

Kernberg, O. F. (1984). *Severe Personality Disorders: Psychotherapeutic Strategies*. New Haven, CT: Yale University Press.

Klein, M. (1946). Notes on some schizoid mechanisms. In: M. Klein, *Envy and Gratitude and Other Works* (R. E. Money-Kyrle, Ed.) (pp. 1–24). London: Hogarth, 1975.

Klein, R. (1995). The self-in-exile: A developmental, self, and object relations approach to the schizoid disorder of the self. In: J. F. Masterson & R. Klein (Eds.), *Disorders of the Self: New Therapeutic Horizons: The Masterson Approach* (Part 1, Ch. 1–7, pp. 3–142). New York: Brunner/Mazel.

Little, R. (2001). Schizoid processes: Working with the defenses of the withdrawn child ego state. *Transactional Analysis Journal*, 31(1): 33–43. doi.org/10.1177/036215370103100105.

Little, R. (2006). Ego state relational units and resistance to change. *Transactional Analysis Journal*, 36(1): 7–19. doi.org/10.1177/036215370603600103.

Little, R. (2011). Impasse clarification within the transference–countertransference matrix. *Transactional Analysis Journal*, 41(1): 23–28. doi.org/10.1177/036215371104100106.

Little, R. (2012). Love made hungry: The schizoid problem. *The Transactional Analyst*, Winter: 19–22.

Little, R. (2013). The new emerges out of the old. *Transactional Analysis Journal*, 43(2): 106–121. doi.org/10.1177/0362153713499541.

Little, R. (2020). Boundary applications and violations: Clinical interpretations in a transference–countertransference-focused psychotherapy. *Transactional Analysis Journal*, 50(3): 1–15. doi.org/10.1080/03621537.2020.1771031.

Mahler, M. S., Pine, F., & Bergman, A. (1971). *The Psychological Birth of the Human Infant: Symbiosis and Individuation*. New York: Basic Books, 1975

Manfield, P. (1992). *Split Self/Split Object: Understanding and Treating Borderline, Narcissistic, and Schizoid Disorders*. Northvale, NJ: Jason Aronson.

Masterson. J. F. (1988). *The Search for the Real Self: Unmasking the Personality Disorders of our Age*. New York: The Free Press.

McGilloway, A., Hall, R., Lee, T., & Bhui, K. (2010). A systematic review of personality disorder, race and ethnicity: Prevalence, aetiology and treatment. *BMC Psychiatry*, *10*(33). Retrieved from http://biomedcentral.com/1471-244X/10/33 RCH ARTICLE Open Access.

McWilliams, N. (1994). *Psychoanalytic Diagnosis: Understanding Personality Structure in the Clinical Process*. New York: Guilford.

Nasar, S. (1998). *A Beautiful Mind*. London: Faber and Faber.

Nash, J. F., Jr. (1994). John F. Nash, Jr. biographical. Retrieved from https://nobelprize.org/prizes/economic-sciences/1994/nash/biographical/.

Newhill, C., Shaun, M., & Conner, K. (2009). Racial differences between African and white Americans in the presentation of borderline personality disorder. *Race and Social Problems*, *1*:87–96. doi.org/10.1007/s12552-009-9006-2.

O'Reilly-Knapp, M. (2001). Between two worlds: The encapsulated self. *Transactional Analysis Journal*, *31*(1): 44–54. doi.org/10.1177/036215370103100106.

Piaget, J. (1952). *The Origins of Intelligence in Children*. New York: International Universities Press.

Seinfeld, J. (1991). *The Empty Core: An Object Relations Approach to Psychotherapy of the Schizoid Personality*. Northvale, NJ: Jason Aronson.

Seinfeld, J. (1993). *Interpreting and Holding: The Paternal and Maternal Functions of the Psychotherapist*. Northvale, NJ: Jason Aronson.

Seinfeld, J. (1996). *Containing Rage, Terror, and Despair: An Object Relations Approach to Psychotherapy*. Northvale, NJ: Jason Aronson.

Wallin, D. (2007). *Attachment in Psychotherapy*. New York: Guilford.

Ware, P. (1983). Personality adaptations (doors to therapy). *Transactional Analysis Journal*, *13*(1): 11–19. doi.org/10.1177/036215378301300104.

Žvelc, G. (2010). Relational schemas theory and transactional analysis. *Transactional Analysis Journal*, *40*(1): 8–22. doi.org/10.1177/036215371004000103.

CHAPTER 5

Silence, withdrawal, and contact in the schizoid process

Marye O'Reilly-Knapp

One of the most important questions a psychotherapist must consider is how to listen to a client's silence or maintain contact when the person withdraws. That became relevant to me early in my career and has continued to be of interest and relevance ever since. In an article I wrote more than twenty years ago entitled "Between Two Worlds: The Encapsulated Self" (O'Reilly-Knapp, 2001) I considered two questions: What is required in a therapeutic relationship so that the uncommunicable, walled-off parts can be spoken, heard, and understood? And at the same time, how can the integrity and stability of the client be maintained so that self-emergence is facilitated? Two new questions are at the center of this current paper: How can the therapist provide the space for silence to be supported? What is needed for the therapist to maximize her or his presence when a client withdraws?

Case vignette: Peggy

As a graduate student, I could select who I worked with in my clinical rotation. I noticed Peggy while talking with others on the unit. I would see her for a brief moment and then she would disappear. At the end of the morning, I decided that Peggy would be my very first client. I remember being excited to meet with her and get to know and hopefully to help her. Little did I know that my relationship with Peggy would begin my lifetime search for understanding the therapeutic process and the interventions needed to work with the sequestered part of the psyche.

In a journal I kept about our sessions together, I noted that the first time I spoke to Peggy I told her I would be on the unit three days a week and I would like to meet with her and talk. She did not say anything, so I hoped this was a yes rather than a no. The first session started the next day when I sat down in the dayroom and waited for Peggy to appear. I did this the same time each day I was on the unit. She did come. I greeted her and then we sat in silence for about ten minutes. The second week she told me to leave her alone. However, she continued to come and sit beside me. I sat in silence with her with an occasional comment about my thinking about her, checking about her eating and sleeping and activities on her unit. Most of the time she did not respond.

Over the next couple of weeks, our time together increased from ten to thirty minutes. Peggy tolerated sitting with me. In the eight months I worked with her, Peggy went from confinement on a closed unit to permission to go off the unit and onto the hospital grounds. She stopped using the bathroom floor as her escape and joined in some of the unit's activities.

I believe one of the pivotal points of our work together was in our third month. When Peggy did not turn up at our appointed time, I went looking for her. I was told by one of the clients that she was in the bathroom. I found her there lying on the floor. I told her I had been looking for her. I was upset and with raised voice told her that I did not want to see her on the floor, that she was better than that. I left telling her I would be waiting outside.

What worried me the most is that I could not think of any therapeutic approach that would validate my reaction. After all, I was a student, and I was concerned that my behavior may have been inappropriate and that there may be consequences. I was also concerned that Peggy might experience this as a rupture in our relationship. A few minutes later Peggy came out of the bathroom. She looked at me and then turned away. I told her I was glad to see her. I asked her if she heard me and she nodded her head, "Yes." I asked about her retreat to the bathroom but she did not respond. For the rest of our meetings, she never returned to the bathroom floor.

As I look back, I know my distress was appropriate and effective. As Bettelheim (1976) wrote: "The infant must first become important to a human being he can influence and who therefore becomes important to him" (p. 229). This quote resonated with me because Peggy certainly influenced me as she lay in the bathroom. I believe that with my response she saw me as genuinely caring about her. I became important to her. Over time she responded. Much of what I did with her was to be present and allow her to connect with me at her speed. We created a space relatively free of impingements. I made contact by sitting with her in silence. Although I did not have the theoretical basis I have now, I began developing a strong foundation for a therapeutic framework through reading the works by Erikson (1963), Bowlby (1969), Perls (1969), Balint (1968), Piaget (1971), May (1953), and Bruch (1969). In working with Peggy, I believe my naivety allowed me to be open with her and more accessible to new information. When I eventually said good-bye to Peggy, I was sad and had tears in my eyes. I gave her a small cake with a card to celebrate her birthday. She insisted on putting the cake in the locker by her bed. I often wonder where Peggy is today.

Case vignette: Sue

In my first year in private practice, I had a referral from the university where I consulted. Sue had been a student and was just released from the hospital, where she had been treated for a severe schizoid state. In her first session, Sue talked about her hospitalization and her fear of losing touch with reality. She was afraid that she would go so far away from reality that she would not be able to get back and would go insane. In her latest hospitalization, she tried to escape from the chaos created by her anxiety by retreating back inside, a schizoid flight to find a safe place. However, in the process she lost touch with her selfhood as well as the external world. I told her I could not ensure her that this would not occur again but I would be there for her, whatever happened.

To begin, Sue recounted her life before she went to college and how she had come from a highly dysfunctional family. To help her stay together as she talked, I "held" her by asking her to slow her speech, to take deep breaths, to be aware of sensations in her body. I tried to support her in her struggles and to signal that I was there with her, that she was not alone. These steps were important as she talked about the death of her mother when Sue was only twelve years old and the loss of two sisters and a brother when they departed the household. Being the youngest, she was left alone with her father, who was physically abusive. The main purpose of therapy at that point was to provide Sue with a reliable, secure relationship where contact with her essence as a full human being could be realized.

Sue spent the next year encountering her childhood memories of abuse and neglect. Diminishing some of the tension and conflict of her struggles helped lessen her anxiety. She began to integrate some of her thoughts and feelings and to develop a core of her personal self. After two years Sue left the area to live by the sea. Periodically I would receive a note from her until that stopped. Some time later she called to tell me she was back in town and asked if I would see her. When she arrived for the session, Sue said she had been hospitalized again and she wanted to work with me once more. I took this as her desire to have contact even though she was fearful. We made a contract to "discover more."

The next three years were the foundation for the work that we did. I listened to her, took her seriously, reassured her, comforted her. I was there for her in her silence and there when she returned from withdrawal. Little (1990) described this state as "consummate patience" (p. 19). I valued Sue's aliveness and her unique identity as a human being. I admired her strength as she opened herself to new possibilities. This period of her therapy prompted me to recall Guntrip's therapy where he spoke about his hidden self: "He remained alive and you have let him out" (Guntrip, 1968, as cited in Hazell, 1994, p. 25). Guntrip described that through his therapy with Winnicott he was able to reclaim the part of him that had been concealed and come out of hiding with his therapist's help. Now, a part of Sue that remained alive and hidden was beginning to come out in therapy. She continued working with me for five more years and in that time she was hospitalized once. She left therapy and has been living in a retirement community and is doing well, with support from friends and her church.

The encapsulated self

In the schizoid position, an organizing system is constructed in an attempt to gain some control by avoiding overwhelming thoughts and feelings. Within the pattern of an isolated attachment, a withdrawn, regressed part of the individual lies encapsulated, locked away in enclosed, protective fragments which serve as an armor of detachment. The mechanism of withdrawal provides the individual a place to hide, although it also inhibits activity and has a profound effect on mastery and self-efficacy. Orange et al. (1977) describe the experience of self-loss as an "intersubjective catastrophe" (p. 55). In my article "Between Two Worlds" (O'Reilly-Knapp, 2001) I described part of the turmoil in the loss of self as follows:

> Basic needs and wants become lost in a massive, psychic withdrawal and relationships are dismissed because what is most needed is also what is most feared. The person is left suspended between both internal and external encounters with no real relationship with either. The world consists of object relations filled with fantasies and dreams and a shell created by primitive isolation. (p. 47)

I also noted,

> There is not only a primitive withdrawal … there is also a dissociative defensive stance used to protect the continuity of existence. The ability to separate experiences from awareness allows the individual to escape from perceived danger. Withdrawal, as well as separation from internal and external experiences, becomes the shield against overpowering circumstances. (p. 45)

My premise here is that in the schizoid process the person: (1) lives in a world of isolation, (2) exists within the matrix of unintegrated life experiences, and (3) copes as best as one can in the real world. Guntrip (1968) writes that there are attempts to connect that are thwarted and end up in perpetual isolation—as a "detached spectator" (p. 18). He described mental activity as disappearing into an inner world where there is absolute withdrawal from life, "into the living death of oblivion, an escape into passivity and inactivity" (1968, p. 92).

Case vignette: Bill

Bill called for an appointment out of concern that he was going into a backward spiral. He came for psychotherapy because he felt like he was going back to his "old" days, when he lived for two years in the woods after his return from Vietnam. It reminded me of how Guntrip (1968) described a part of the ego

> which knows and accepts the fact that it is overwhelmed by fear and in a state of exhaustion, and that it will never be in any fit state to live unless it can, so to speak, escape into a mental convalescence where it can be quiet, protected, and given a chance to recuperate. (As cited in Hazell, 1994, p.178)

I viewed Bill's time spent in the war as an important source for his present concerns. In psychotherapy, he needed a chance to recuperate.

Part of the schizoid dilemma is that the person lives within a world of isolation and unintegrated experiences and constructs a system of organizing events to avoid feelings and memories. In this position, splitting pushes out of awareness the need for contact and connection. For a client with a schizoid process, "a therapeutic relationship allows each Child ego state to emerge and be met with a safe, attuned response" (Erskine, 2001, p. 4).

In Bill's therapy, we began with two areas that had not been dealt with in his previous therapies; only later did he examine his childhood experiences. The day before he and his friend were to leave Vietnam, a grenade was thrown into their encampment and his friend was mortally wounded. In a session, I had Bill close his eyes and go back to that encampment where Bill held his friend in his arms as he lay dying. Bill was silent, tears coming down his cheeks. To help him give words to that traumatic event, I asked Bill to talk to his friend, tell him what he meant to Bill and how he felt about him. Finally, I asked him to say good-bye and to tell his friend what he would remember about their friendship. We both then sat in silence. Later I told Bill how sad I was. I was also thankful that he was there and that his friend was not alone as he died. After the session I had a message from Bill thanking me for being there for him and how he recognized how important it was for him to be there with his friend.

A second area dealing with the war was raised in a weekend intensive workshop that I co-led. When Bill came home from the war, his plane was greeted at the airport by antiwar protestors. They spat at his troop and called them murderers and baby killers. In the group setting through reenactment, group members listened as Bill described his return from Vietnam. He talked about his arrival home and the response of protestors as he left the plane. When he finished, group members talked about their feelings. Then members welcomed Bill with respect and love. One member in the group had been an anti-war activist. Both cried as she went to him and asked his forgiveness. This is an example of how an intensive therapy is necessary to affect difficult, unintegrated remnants of a person's past. This group setting gave him a place to resolve a painful ordeal.

Most of Bill's psychotherapy focused on reorganizing his internal sense of being and emerging from isolation and historical detachment. He described how he felt alone and isolated from the world. He described living his whole life alone and afraid. In one session he started to talk about his time in the woods. I encouraged him to close his eyes and go to the woods. I told him I would go with him. Much of the time he was silent, and I sat with him and reminded him periodically that I was with him. In subsequent trips to the woods, he began to remember how as a young boy, around five or six years old, when his father would become violent and go after his mother and any of the other children who were present, Bill would go into hiding, first under the kitchen table and then deep into his mind where he could not hear, see, or feel anything. According to Bill, he was invisible. Later, in school he got into trouble by talking in the classroom and fighting in the school yard. In high school he began to drink. When he joined the Army, he did better because the structure helped him. Over time in therapy, Bill described the story of his life, including the years of isolation and withdrawal and his feelings of hopelessness and helplessness. His fear was realized, his rage and despair were heard, his excitement and joy were celebrated. Bill lived for fifteen years after he finished therapy; he got to see his daughter graduate from college and his son finish high school. I heard from his wife that they had good times together before he became ill and died of kidney failure which was attributed to a toxic herbicide used during the war.

The "between space"

Intensive psychotherapy is necessary to affect the core of an individual who manifests a schizoid defense structure. Effective therapy requires working with both the hidden, sequestered part of the psyche as well as historical events. With someone whose basic needs and desires become lost and relationships are dismissed, he or she is left suspended between both internal and external world encounters with no real relationship with either. The inner world consists of fantasies and dreams with a shell of primitive isolation. The external world is experienced as something with which the person is uninvolved, where he or she neither wants nor has expectations of help from another. Due to "sustained relations broken down at their most basic level," there is self-loss, no connection to either self or others (Orange et al., 1977, p. 55).

An understanding of emotional conflicts, unmet needs and the loss of relationship are all important in dealing with loss of self. Both here-and-now contact with the therapist and a return to states of fixation and dissociation provide the path for unfreezing of early ego formation and the unfolding of self. What was once constructed as protection and reinforced is now addressed in the therapeutic process. For both client and therapist, the process is unique to that particular relationship. Theory and technique are used as a guide with continual assessment by the therapist of the therapeutic process.

Case vignette: Sandy

After consultation with an expert in the field of dissociative identity disorder, I agreed to work with Sandy, whom I had met at one of the weekend workshops I did. Over a year, she attended several more. She had been seeing another therapist in the state where she lived 400 miles away. Although she had asked me to work with her, I did not want to interfere in her current therapy. However, when she became suicidal she called me; I would talk with her and then call her therapist to discuss her treatment. He told me he was going to terminate his work with her. I was conflicted and went for supervision. It was then, having the consultant's opinion and support, that I made the decision to accept Sandy as a client. After she terminated with her therapist, she and I began telephone sessions.

Readers may be wondering why I included Sandy as a case example in this chapter. The reason is that I have found several of my clients who had dissociative identity disorder (DID) also demonstrated a schizoid position. This was not evident in the beginning of therapy because the fragments that were presented masked the withdrawn, regressed self. In this chapter, most of the discussion will concern the schizoid condition.

In addition to weekly phone sessions, Sandy attended weekend workshops four times a year and a week-long residential treatment workshop in the summer. There were also occasional individual in-person sessions in my office when she was in the area. Because a strong therapeutic alliance had been established in our meetings over the first year and a half, her work moved rather quickly into the memories and feelings she had repressed.

During our telephone sessions, Sandy was often silent, and I would be with her, telling her I was there. She started sending me drawings in the mail after a session, and this helped her to find the words as we talked about the drawing in our subsequent session. She began to allow her hidden self to show in her drawings and to talk about her vulnerability. As she started to recall the reasons she had locked herself away, she began to work with the split-off and painful memories. She dealt with her fears by drawing pictures of anger with red and black circles, fear as balls of orange and yellow, and sadness as blue and white squares. She talked about being trapped in circles of anger, balls of fear, and squares of sadness. Each drawing had a feeling and a story, and I listened to them all. I sat with her as she went into the rage, or terror, and despair. Slowly, the drawings facilitated the emergence of her self. Later, she began drawing pictures in which she was no longer trapped. There was a flow to the brush strokes and a lightness to the colors. The supportive, safe environment of the sessions allowed her to deal with the intense affect. Time was provided for her to reenter the here-and-now and talk about her work with me. Because the work was exhausting, we allowed time for her to recuperate. Often a resting phase after the work helped her integrate new material. In the weekend workshops, she would go outside and sit under a tree after she had worked. She also used a journal to help her process additional information.

With Sandy, not only was a part of her withdrawn and hidden, she also held altered states of dissociated defensive structures. She had integrated several of her dissociated structures before coming to me, and for those that remained, I incorporated a method called "mapping" (Kluft & Fine, 1993). This type of recording represents a visual diagram where dissociated parts are identified and given a voice. It was like putting the pieces of a puzzle together. In this process Sandy had a visual representation of her narrative and the fragments that needed to be unified. As she filled in her "story lines" she was able to identify past experiences, form meaning out of events, and eventually develop an understanding of the past. This method was particularly effective for Sandy because she was an artist and had a deep appreciation for graphics. Being able to give meaning was an important step for Sandy in remembering and then appreciating the assets she possessed to help her survive.

The impact of impingements

Moving the body allows a person to shift in his or her surroundings as part of discovery and "sense of real being" (Clancier & Kalmanovitch, 1984, p. 84). Spontaneous movement is essential for exploring the environment without the sense of self being lost. Winnicott described the importance of someone being present and not making demands, which allows for establishing an "internal environment" in which the self can be alone in the presence of another. When there is impingement or interruption of continuity in the body, there is "restlessness of the environment" (Winnicott, 1988, p. 127).

With the schizoid condition, movement becomes impeded. Winnicott's theory (Newman, 1995) of impingements is useful in this regard, and his actual drawings illustrate the seclusion that occurs and how relationship patterns of isolation result. He used the analogy of a bubble wherein the baby is surrounded by the environment. When pressure on the outside is adapted to the pressure inside, there is a "continuity of existence" (Winnicott, 1988, pp. 127–128). In a state of being, before and after birth, movement is a way for the baby to discover the environment. This move out into the surroundings is a part of discovery and the sense of existence. When pressure outside is greater, there is impingement and disruption of continuity.

When impingement or encroachment is repeated, the individual returns to isolation. This isolation is different from loneliness in that it is a retreat from danger. In these cases, the person who withdraws from others "has experienced gross impingements from the beginning and has had to withdraw in order to preserve the core self from violation" (Abram, 1996, p. 35). The state of being for the baby and even later life experiences can trigger such withdrawal. A pattern of relationship develops whereby, even without restrictions or intrusion from the outside world, the feeling of being restrained may lead to seclusion of self from others. In the schizoid process, isolation into what Bettelheim (1976) called an "invisible fortress" severely restricts contact with others.

Case vignette: Jane

For the first month of her therapy, Jane directed me to "just listen." If I even nodded my head, she insisted that I was not listening. She told me my words got in the way. By attending to Jane with my presence, I joined her without intruding. At times I broke the silence to tell her I was listening, but I think this had to do more with my own comfort than hers. Most of the time I just listened. I questioned my effectiveness, even though I realized at the time my silence was vital to Jane's progress. I believe she needed what Little (1990) expressed as a "settled state, undisturbed by impingements" (p. 44) and Erskine et al. (1999) described as "therapeutic presence," a way of being there (p. 98). This attention was the entry into work about her mother, who was always telling Jane and her siblings what to do. Jane felt like she was being smothered. She could not tolerate any reaction from me, and she later talked about how important it was for me to hear her. She reported she could now breathe. Continually assessing my own responses to Jane and her process helped me to safeguard our therapeutic relationship.

The trauma existing in silence and withdrawal

Maintaining a connection with someone who is silent or goes into hiding requires the therapist's full attention. Silences can occur when there are no words or if the words are too difficult to say, so help is needed to find the words or to say the words out loud. The client may also be silent when his or her experience is preverbal. It is also important to notice sounds as well as physical movement and for me to monitor my own thoughts and feelings as I sit with a client.

What am I experiencing? Is the connection with the client maintained? If I lose contact, what does that mean? It is important to remain calm and to tolerate silences so that a stable, settled state is created in the therapeutic setting.

Case vignette: Linda

When we began group sessions, Linda would come into the office, sit in the corner, and remain silent most of the time. She had been referred by a colleague who thought a group setting might help her interact with others. After graduating from college Linda took a position as a receptionist in a law firm. She was single and lived alone. Her family constellation consisted of her parents, sister, brother, and aunt. She said she called periodically to talk to her parents and would learn about her siblings, and her aunt called to see how she was doing "once in a while." It appears most of her time was spent alone.

Linda appeared distant and uncomfortable when she was involved in conversations both before and during group, and she was the first one to leave after the group was over. She reported she would "go away mentally" when others were talking so that she could steady herself. The difficulty was that she lost connection with what was going on. Because she needed more time than the group could give her, I suggested she come into individual sessions to do the regressive work she needed. Her individual sessions were lengthened from fifty minutes to ninety minutes to give her time to settle in and fully experience my presence.

In the first individual session, Linda sat on a pillow in the corner and was quiet. I listened to her silence and sensed tightness in her body. When she started to speak, she would stop midsentence and become frustrated, saying she wanted to stop and go away. When I asked her about going away, she talked about hiding herself far away where no one could see or hear her. I asked her to close her eyes and go into her quiet place, and I focused on being a witness to her withdrawal. The first sessions she remained still and calm in the withdrawal for about ten minutes. She talked later about how she frequently went to that place when she was afraid. It was a place where she felt safe.

As the sessions progressed, Linda began to remember being afraid and alone. She had been shivering and said that she was cold, so I covered her with a blanket. This was a source of comfort as she began to remember her mother screaming and "doing crazy things." She started to remember the times her mother tied her to a chair because she was making too much noise or the time mother locked her out of the house for a whole night. Her father traveled for work and was not home most of the time. From the time she could walk until she left home to go to college, Linda's mother continued acting out while Linda took most of the abuse to protect her sisters. In her sessions, she began to deal with her feelings of terror because no one was there to help her. I reminded her that I was with her now. She wept with despair as she recognized her experience of not having a caring mother. I sat beside her and held her hand as she cried and screamed for help. And when she raged, I took her anger seriously about her mother's brutality by saying I was also angry at that behavior. One of the many times she went back to being tied up, I asked her to allow me to untie her. As she went through this she cried out "never again." Linda opened her eyes, she reached out to me and I took her in my arms.

Contact in silence and withdrawal

Interaction with another is central to the discovery of one's self. Fairbairn (1952) highlighted the hunger for contact and connection. From in utero through the life span, the individual is in continual interaction with others, and these exchanges become part of the sense of self. Mitchell (1988) considered the relational matrix as one in which "the establishment and maintenance of relatedness is fundamental, and the mutual exchange of intense pleasure and emotional responsiveness is perhaps the most powerful medium in which emotional connection and intimacy is sought, established, lost, and regained" (p. 107). The child learns a style of connection and these learned modes are maintained throughout life. It is in the relationship with the therapist that connection that was lost or never provided can be established and retained so that a new relational pattern can develop.

Guntrip (1968) described the ultimate problem in psychotherapy with a schizoid process as "the rebirth and regrowth of the lost, living heart of the personality" (p. 12). As described earlier, with Peggy, I spent a good deal of time in silence. I arrived at the same time and waited for her. My presence was an invitation to her: I am here for you, I am waiting for you. My presence also signaled: "I want to be with you." As I sat anticipating Peggy's arrival for a session, I thought about our last time together. I looked forward to spending time with her. I believed she was able to sense my desire to be with her.

Part of Sue's therapy involved her struggle to maintain her saneness, while at the same time deal with overwhelming feelings and memories. I arranged for her to hold my hand as she began regressive work. At times I would ask her to squeeze my hand to stabilize her and to be a link to me and hopefully to reality. Her clasp of my hand served as a reminder to her: You are here with me, you are not alone, I am not going away, and finally, I want you to stay with me.

With Jane, I was quieted by her, which allowed her to tell part of her story without interruption. Once she had a sense of me there with her, she then moved into interchanges with me. I envisioned her process as: I know you are here, I want you to know I am here, and then we can be here together.

In the work with Linda, I sat with her in silence honoring her withdrawal. She needed me to be there for her to acknowledge the existence of her withdrawal, and later, to validate and normalize her withdrawal. Being present in the moment is one of the most powerful positions we have as a therapist. It takes desire and concentration to stay in contact and to provide a space for the client's narrative to be recounted and understood. The position of witness provides an invitation to the client: I am here with you, I see you, I hear you, I am interested in you.

With Bill, I waited with him when he went into his hiding places. I sat with a little boy who desperately wanted to be out in the world and be safe. He needed a place where he could explore, which he did by taking me with him, in fantasy, to the woods and under the kitchen table. There he went further into his inner sanctuary, where I sat and waited for him to come back from the hiding place we shared under the table or in the woods. Along with dealing with his anguish, there were times when we played for that little boy's benefit. Sometimes there were songs, talks about baseball, laughter, and at times I even held him in my arms. My presence had the tone of "I encourage you to come out of hiding, I invite you to be in the world to explore and have fun. I know there are places in the world that are scary and there are also wonderful places for you to be. Let's find ways for you to be safe."

In Sandy's drawings, unconscious material was brought into awareness. Giving words to her sketches helped her construct her narrative. They provided a path by which to uncover and understand her withdrawal patterns. Appreciating how important graphics were to her, my remarks often included: "I see you, I picture you all alone in your hiding place, I see your struggle, I imagine you appreciating your strength."

With all the individuals described in this chapter, I considered silence and withdrawal because of the importance both occupy in the schizoid process, even though it sometimes limited the exploration of other forces at work. For a more detailed account of therapeutic interventions, the reader is directed to my article "Between Two Worlds" (O'Reilly-Knapp, 2001).

In the therapeutic relationship, the therapist joins with the client in experiencing the affective connection needed for oneness and for the emergence of self-states. Because of the extreme isolation and annihilation of self and others that characterize those with schizoid disorders, therapy needs to respectfully and consistently support the client's unique position, deal with the need for contact, and take into account intrapsychic processes. Providing a safe place for the emergence of the self and the establishment of a therapeutic bond is primary. The withdrawn space of encapsulation and the loss of relationship in the withdrawal need to be understood as attempts to survive. How the individual, with the therapist's support and encouragement, can move from a position of avoidance of contact becomes a major portion of the therapeutic work. Arieti (1974) wrote that the therapist needs perseverance in reaching such individuals. Tustin (1986) identified patience, tact, and skill as requisites for the therapist in working with a withdrawn person. Staying in contact takes effort for both the client and the therapist, effort well worth it in the end.

Conclusion

I hope this detailed discussion and the case vignettes will add to our knowledge about the importance of silence and withdrawal in working with schizoid processes. The ultimate purpose of therapy for clients with a schizoid condition is to provide a place for the reorganization of an internal sense of being and emergence from isolation. In this chapter, I have attempted to answer two fundamental questions: How can the therapist provide the space for silence to be supported? What is needed for the therapist to maximize her or his presence when a client withdraws? I have shown here how I used contact to maintain connection with each client during episodes of silence and withdrawal in the schizoid process. The stability and integrity of the therapeutic relationship allowed for the integration of a split self and ultimately an emergence from seclusion. Although the work was difficult, I never tired of it. In fact, I was honored by the trust given to me by these brave individuals.

References

Abram, J. (1996). *The Language of Winnicott: A Dictionary and Guide to Understanding His Work.* Northvale, NJ: Jason Aronson.

Arieti, S. (1974). *Interpretation of Schizophrenia.* New York: Basic Books.

Balint, M. (1968). *The Basic Fault: Therapeutic Aspects of Regression.* London: Tavistock.

Bettelheim, B. (1976). *The Empty Fortress: Infantile Autism and the Birth of Self.* New York: The Free Press.

Bowlby, J. (1969). *Attachment and Loss, Vol. 1: Attachment.* New York: Basic Books.

Bruch, H. (1969). *Psychoneurosis and Schizophrenia.* Philadelphia, PA: J. B. Lippincott.

Clancier, A., & Kalmanovitch, J. (1984). *Winnicott and Paradox: From Birth to Creation.* London: Tavistock.

Erikson, E. H. (1963*). Childhood and Society.* New York: W. W. Norton.

Erskine, R. G. (2001). The schizoid process. *Transactional Analysis Journal, 31*: 4–6.

Erskine, R. G., Moursund, J. P., & Trautmann, R. L. (1999). *Beyond Empathy: A Theory of Contact-in-Relationship.* London: Routledge, 2023.

Fairbairn, W. R. D. (1952). *Psychoanalytic Studies of the Personality.* London: Tavistock.

Guntrip, H. (1968). *Schizoid Phenomena, Object Relations and the Self.* New York: International Universities Press, 1995.

Hazell, J. (1994). *Personal Relations Therapy: The Collected Papers of H. J. S. Guntrip.* Northvale, NJ: Jason Aronson.

Kluft, R. P., & Fine, C. G. (1993). *Clinical Perspectives on Multiple Personality Disorder.* Washington, DC: American Psychiatric Press.

Little, M. (1990). *Psychotic Anxieties and Containment: A Personal Record of an Analysis with Winnicott.* Northvale, NJ: Jason Aronson.

May, R. (1953). *Man's Search for Himself.* New York: W. W. Norton.

Mitchell, S. A. (1988). *Relational Concepts in Psychoanalysis: An Integration.* Cambridge, MA: Harvard University Press.

Newman, A. (1995). *Non-compliance in Winnicott's Words: A Companion to the Writings and Work of D. W. Winnicott.* New York: Free Association.

Orange, D. M., Atwood, G. E., & Stolorow, R. D. (1977). *Working Intersubjectively: Contextualism in Psychoanalytic Practice.* Hillsdale, NJ: The Analytic Press.

O'Reilly-Knapp, M. (2001). Between two worlds: The encapsulated self. *Transactional Analysis Journal, 31*: 44–54. doi.org/10.1177/036215370103100106.

Perls, F. S. (1969). *Ego, Hunger and Aggression: The Gestalt Therapy of Sensory Awakening through Spontaneous Personal Encounter, Fantasy and Contemplation.* New York: Vintage.
Piaget, J. (1971). *The Construction of Reality in the Child.* New York: Ballantine.
Tustin, F. (1986). *Autistic Barriers in Neurotic Patients.* London: Karnac.
Winnicott, D. W. (1988). *Human Nature.* New York: Schocken.

CHAPTER 6

Relational needs and schizoid phenomena

Dan Eastop

Was Fairbairn (1952) being provocative when he wrote that "according to my way of thinking, everybody without exception must be regarded as a schizoid" (p. 7)? There appears to be a sense of mischief in his words, but it remains a wonderful starting point for a discussion on the schizoid process: the idea that on some level we all share the psychological ability to split off experiences, compartmentalize the self, and use withdrawal into inner reality as a means of organizing our relating and how we regulate being in contact with others. It also serves as a beginning to a discussion about how, as therapists, we might use our own experiences of schizoid phenomena to help our work with clients who rely on relational withdrawal to stabilize and regulate their affect. It may help us to remain present and in contact with such individuals, appreciating the creative, adaptive ways a schizoid person will regulate and control relational contact.

When we are with a schizoid individual and there seems to be little emotional contact, as therapists we need to find ways to maintain contact within ourselves, that is, to remain solid and present and at the same time to facilitate the client's reestablishing contact with their affect and physical sensations. When someone is "talking at me, rather than to me" (Erskine, 2020, p. 15), therapy becomes a performance, an acted-out interaction rather than an experience of authentic contact. Exploring how relational needs (Erskine et al., 1999) are experienced moment to moment, and how they are expressed by the client, offers structure to the therapeutic work.

We cannot know what is happening in the inner world of a client. We are always reaching for understanding: assimilating, noticing, and developing ideas and clues to a person's internal experience. Our experience of this reaching for (or waiting for) can often hold crucial information about how to be in contact with certain clients. We have to indwell, to put ourselves into the internal experience of the client who uses a schizoid process. In fact, I find it necessary to go searching for the person in their schizoid withdrawal. I search for a connection with the fragmented, split-off, or hidden parts of my client. When I sense that I do not know what my client may need from me, when I feel there is something lacking in our interpersonal contact, or when I do not know what we are doing, it is essential that I attend to these internal experiences and use them as guides. In attending to my countertransference, I am building a collection of impressionistic images, developmental and relational pictures, and a sense of what relational experiences were missing in my client's early life.

In this chapter, when discussing the schizoid process or a client who engages in schizoid phenomena, I am not referring to a person diagnosed with schizoid personality disorder. Johnson (1994) viewed character structure as existing on a continuum. At one end is the personality disorder and at the other is a higher level of functioning that he called a "character style" (p. 11). An individual with a schizoid personality is at the disorder end, and someone with an avoidant personality is at the style end (Little, 1999, p. 3). In defining an integrative psychotherapy perspective, Erskine (2011, p. 3) used a three-part continuum—schizoid style, schizoid pattern, and schizoid disorder—to distinguish the frequency, duration, and severity of the client's internal splitting and their use of archaic self-protective procedures.

Using the idea of a continuum, I experienced the client discussed here as having a unique way of relating that I describe as a schizoid pattern. We often speak of working with schizoid phenomena or with a schizoid process, but I think it is also helpful to talk about the psychotherapy we do as working within the schizoid process. This involves being prepared to work within the therapeutic transference (Little, 2011) alongside the theoretical belief that "the sense of self and self-esteem emerge out of contact-in-relationship" (Erskine & Trautmann, 1996, p. 317).

In making the concept of relational needs a cornerstone of the psychotherapy, I can remain within the client's unique process:

> Relational needs are the component parts of a universal human desire for intimate relationship and secure attachment. They include 1) the need for security, 2) validation, affirmation, and significance within a relationship, 3) acceptance by a stable, dependable, and protective other person, 4) the confirmation of personal experience, 5) self-definition, 6) having an impact on the other person, 7) having the other initiate, and 8) expressing love. (Erskine, 2011, para. 17)

Working closely with relational needs provides a way to understand and track the client's attachment style, relationship history of needs met and not met, and patterns of accommodation and coping while also providing a here-and-now guide to the client's current needs in the therapeutic relationship. I am attentive to these various expressions of transference, including various ways of relating to me, expressed and unexpressed emotions, and the qualities of our intersubjective dialogue. Each of these provides me with a unique lens to view what is happening within the person. As Erskine (2001) described,

> Transference is the active means whereby the client can communicate his or her past. This includes the neglects, traumas, and needs that were thwarted in the process of growing up, as well as the defenses that were created to compensate for the lack of need fulfillment. (p. 4)

In working with clients who exhibit a schizoid style or pattern, I find it crucial to find ways to anchor myself in the relating so I can remain fully present. Working closely with relational needs, I can better understand my clients' histories, the story being enacted in their transference, my own countertransference, and what they require from me in order to have a healing relationship. The concept of relational needs creates an anchoring in the relating and a structure to my understanding of which needs are emerging in the foreground of the relating and which are in the background, either disavowed or waiting to emerge.

Many clients who have either a schizoid style or schizoid pattern will enter therapy with little or no appreciation of their current or historical relational needs. A psychotherapy that is relationally focused involves creating an interpersonal environment in which the person's relational needs can freely emerge, be felt and known, and be responded to in active, contactful relating.

Case study: Helen

I will use a case study of psychotherapy with Helen to illustrate the concept of relational needs. I will show how different relational needs moved in and out of the foreground of our relating, including which needs were out of the client's awareness, yet to emerge. I will highlight the quality and nature of how relational needs were expressed or not expressed and describe how I used my countertransference to discover and attune to the relational needs of this withdrawn, hard-to-reach client. It is possible to see a cluster of relational needs unique to clients who have either a schizoid style or pattern, and this awareness can guide our work. Relational needs are often out of the client's awareness and may be disavowed, inverted, or blended together. In my experience, working with relational needs within the schizoid process facilitates the emergence of the true self (Winnicott, 1965), that is, an intrinsic sense of self that is "vital and vulnerable" (Erskine, 2020, p. 18).

Helen entered therapy with no awareness of her relational needs and appeared unconscious of having any needs at all in relation to others. Therapy involved her gradually seeing herself as having unique relational needs, understanding how these were neglected by significant others, and discovering how she created ways of coping. Her primary way of coping and adapting involved being a hardworking student and disavowing her feelings and needs. This continued into higher education, where she achieved several degrees in mathematics and science.

In Helen's early childhood, her mother focused her attention on Helen's two brothers. Significant memories for Helen included her father dying when she was seventeen and her leaving home for university. She took pride in being the "trailblazer" of the family and described how she went it alone as a "self-sufficient unit." When her mother moved the family to a new house, Helen no longer had a bedroom and so seldom returned home. She said, "I'm like a bad penny" to describe how she always seemed unwanted.

In our psychotherapy sessions, Helen behaved as a "good client," always arriving on time and rarely missing a session. She was the same way at work, a good employee who worked hard and waited for praise. As a result, she performed at a consistently high level in her work but was always exhausted and lonely. Her husband worked in the same company, and they had two children. Helen described herself as having a "breakdown" in which she felt emotionally and physically incapacitated. Her doctor diagnosed a major depression. I understood her breakdown to mean that Helen's sense of self, her internal structure, became so emotionally overwhelmed that it no longer provided the psychological functions of stabilization and regulation.

As I pieced together a picture of Helen's script system (Erskine, 2015a, 2015b), it became clear how her early experiences, her relationships with others, and her ways of coping matched the isolated attachment style (Erskine, 2011) people like her use to organize their relating with others. Her core script beliefs had shaped her career and approach to life. These included: "I am alone in the world," "Other people are scary," and "I must work hard for others." These and other behavioral patterns reinforced the necessity of finding ways to fit into the world.

Eventually, Helen's script system exerted such overwhelming pressure on her work persona that she was unable to interact and perform in the workplace. Under the pressure of her script beliefs, she could no longer integrate her affect, physiology, and cognition. The result was a breakdown in her sense of self—the capacity to integrate physiological sensations, various affects, and thought processes—and a retreat to a less demanding internal world. Deciding to come to therapy was difficult for Helen because it was an admission to herself that she could not cope and needed the support of a psychotherapist to reestablish a secure sense of self and to be able to work again. Her initial struggle in therapy was about the polarity between her childhood patterns of self-reliance and self-containment and the therapeutic opportunity to be vulnerable and receive support from someone else.

Prior to her breakdown, Helen's role at work had changed. Previously her tasks had been solitary, and the isolation from other people had become her "comfort zone." However, she had been made a project manager, which required her to interact with numerous workers as well as to rely on others. Helen described herself in this breakdown as if she were in a "mixing bowl with no ingredients, with an emptiness and loss of purpose." She told me she felt like a "jigsaw puzzle broken up and swept off the table" and described how her depressive phase felt as if the world had been turned on its head. Her usual ability to rationalize and order things had been taken away, and she felt stripped of her normal self. Helen experienced a great deal of shame in going through the breakdown and being off work. She talked about losing her role and purpose and being embarrassed about what others would think of her on her return.

In the beginning of our work together, I frequently asked Helen what she needed from her session that day in an attempt to give her a sense of choice and bring us into contact with what she needed. Over time, I discovered that my questions were misattuned to her patterns of being in relationship. The inquiry was too confusing and opaque for her; she was not in a place to communicate her needs or even to access what her needs were in the moment. I began to see her confusion as an important communication in itself. The "I don't know" to the question of "What do you need?" was an expression of her unmet relational needs, needs that were unknown to her. I wondered if her "I don't know" meant "I don't know who I am." In those early days, Helen was unable to define herself, particularly in relation to the "authority" of a psychotherapist. Instead, our work centered on Helen finding her own needs in relation to me rather than my explicitly inquiring about them. However, both Helen and I became increasingly aware of her relational needs as they emerged both in our person-to-person relating and through the transference.

Security

In the beginning, I did not yet know of Helen's rich, creative fantasies and ideas. I was preoccupied with the rigidity of how she presented herself, her routinized behaviors, and how she related to me. The more I tried to make contact, the more she pushed me away. I began to appreciate Helen's overwhelming need for safety in the therapy. This was not initially obvious because of the way she presented herself: she was not nervously quiet or shut down nor did she show a clear need for protection. As Erskine and Moursund (2022) described, "The need for relational security is most likely to be foreground at the outset of treatment" (p. 109). Helen strove to uphold a narrowed perspective on her life that discounted and avoided other aspects of who she was, particularly her relationships with others. Her life had involved carefully structured, controlled relations with people; she remarked that she was experienced by others as a loner, superior at times, not easy to interact with.

My experience of her relational need for safety in the therapy emerged in my countertransference. I felt controlled; the space, interactions, and rhythm of our work felt stifling. Early on I felt fixed, positioned, and unable to feel involved. I experienced Helen as needing to direct the dialogue. She ignored my questions and changed the subject so that our conversation remained superficial. She kept me at a distance, avoided interpersonal contact, and declined my invitations to explore her affect. She needed to feel safe: safe in herself, safe in relating with me, and safe in the parameters of what our psychotherapy was for her. Helen's relational need for security in relationship was masked by her various attempts to control the process of the therapy sessions. She was often highly descriptive in her language, using words or intellectualization to fill the space. It was as though she were saying: "If we stay over here talking about this stuff, we won't get near to the vulnerable me inside."

It eventually became apparent that Helen was withdrawing from interpersonal contact in the midst of our sessions. I suspected that she used this form of withdrawal in all her relationships. She appeared to have developed a carefully constructed social self, a part of her that was able to interact with others but in a rigid and narrowly prescribed way. She had a well-rehearsed social facade. Guntrip (as cited in Hazell, 1994) described this social self:

"This fundamental detachment is often masked and hidden under a facade of compulsive sociability, incessant talking and hectic activity. One gets the feeling that such people are acting a somewhat exhausting part" (p. 168).

The beginning phase of therapy with Helen could be seen almost entirely as a demonstration of the importance of the relational need for security in relationship. She observed me from the safety of emotional withdrawal and revealed little of her inner experience. I was unsettled and distracted by her repetitive, prepared, and superficial stories, which kept us in "safe" areas of discussion. I was perplexed: "Where am I going with this?"; "How come I can't seem to feel a relational connection with this person?"; and "How come I am left confused and cold, out of touch?"

As with many clients, Helen's relational need for safety in relationship was crucial for any psychotherapeutic work to take place. However, this need is often not conscious because the person, like Helen, may have prematurely, and without awareness, assumed the function of stabilizing and regulating themselves: a pseudo sense of security. Reliance on a social facade as a protective way of relating and maintaining control with others can mask the underlying need for a profound physical and emotional sense of security. O'Reilly-Knapp (2012) compassionately depicted this attempt at pseudo security, describing how "a social facade masks the pain and loneliness of an isolated existence" (p. 3).

Many individuals who rely on schizoid processes had early childhood caretakers who repeatedly overlooked and neglected the person's physical and relational needs while also being invasive and/or controlling. Such neglect or invasion/controlling resulted in the person accumulating physical and affective memories that are often disavowed and unconscious. This can result in them placing their personal needs secondary to the needs or even demands of their caregivers. They learned to hide what they needed—to split off from their own awareness—and to attend instead to the needs of their caretaker. This relational pattern is often reenacted in the therapeutic relationship, which is what Helen was doing by reenacting with me an early childhood pattern she had learned in order to cope with emotional neglect.

The schizoid individual may be extremely attuned to the therapist's needs, often appearing to be kind, thoughtful, compliant, and/or passive. As clinicians, we need to keep in mind the early experiences of the accommodating child, the adapted self that is skilled at meeting the needs of others and disavowing, splitting off, and/or detaching from their own. Stewart (2010) highlighted this: "If a therapist brings his/her archaic needs for security into session, then there's a likelihood he/she will communicate in covert ways messages such as 'I need to be taken care of' or 'I am overwhelmed by your needs'" (p. 43). The client's accommodating to the therapist is a form of withdrawal: "I sense you need caring for so I will go away" or "I sense you can see my vulnerability and I am scared."

The behaviors that emerge from a person's social self are centered upon conforming and accommodating to others. It is as though the client were saying, "I need you to accept me in my adaptation"; "Please accept this version of me"; or "I will be OK for you." They are displaying a social self that struggles to maintain a facade that provides an artificial sense of acceptance, validation, and security. With many schizoid individuals, there may be periods of therapy in which the person needs to maintain a sense of safety by repeating a familiar story. When Helen told me the same stories, I was initially frustrated. There was no real contact between us, no emotional connection, and I did not know how to be involved with her. My reactions reflected part of Helen's story. I was often emotionally distant and uninvolved. Eventually, I learned the importance of patience and staying present.

Initially, I became another person to whom Helen accommodated. I felt that she was not interested or, more importantly, did not want to see me as a relatable other. But she also needed me to be there every week, to be reliable and consistent, to be a mirror to her rigid and repetitive style of relating. It was a long time before she could allow herself to see me as a person separate from my professional status. It was a revelation for both of us when she began to allow herself to see that the psychotherapy offered much more than support for her job performance.

As our work shifted into a new phase, Helen needed to idealize me in order to create a new sense of safety, much like a child needs a stable adult who is predictable, consistent, dependable, and responsive to their emerging needs. With Helen's increased idealization of me, she perceived a new quality of safety in our therapeutic relationship. She described needing a safe space to speak her thoughts to a sensitive listener who would not criticize, overwhelm, or make demands of her. This new phase allowed Helen to become aware of needing safety in the relationship with me. She needed a therapist who was involved in her life, whom she could trust with her ideas, and who would foster her changing sense of herself.

Impact

In supervision I shared how I believed I was not making an impact on Helen's life and how uninvolved I felt I was in our work together. I was in deep countertransference, feeling I had so little influence and so little emotional connection with her. There was something happening between us that I needed to understand and resolve. I wondered if I was mirroring her experience of me. Did Helen sense that she had no impact on me or on anyone in her life? Was she living without any emotional connections? Her relational need to make an impact became apparent to me through my experience of how hard I was trying to relate to her.

Helen was skillful at making as little impact on others as possible. She painted a picture of herself as being on the outskirts of social groups all her life, fearful of others, wanting to fit in but not knowing how. She described "floating around cliques at school" and "nabbing people for chats." Her adolescent experience of being an outsider and finding social interaction scary had continued into her work life and was an ongoing source of anxiety. She described feeling "invisible" to others, "not having a place," and "not having an impact." I imagined how lonely she must have been, and yet the sadness I felt did not match the matter-of-fact way she spoke. Helen's interactions with others were mainly through maintaining a social facade characterized by passive accommodation and adherence to social rules and etiquette. Manfield (1992) suggested that there is often a "careful screening" going on with schizoid individuals that helps protect them from "anything that might expose them to attack or rejection or may be later used to pressure or coerce them" (p. 208). This seemed to be the case with Helen.

Clients who rely on a schizoid process to manage the affect inherent in relationships often experience an emptiness, a being "missed," and an unfulfilled "longing for something." At the same time, being in a contactful relationship is a huge risk for them, the risk of being known and therefore possibly invaded or controlled by the other. Some schizoid individuals express their internal confusion and hurt through script beliefs such as "No one is there for me," "I'm on my own," and "I'm not important." Erskine and Moursund (2022) wrote, "Relationships in which one does not experience having an impact on the other person are one-sided … just as with a thwarted need for self-definition, they foster the belief that one is unimportant and that others don't care" (p. 112).

Guntrip (as cited in Hazell, 1994) described this internal polarization of desire and fear as the schizoid compromise, that is, being half in a relationship while simultaneously being half out. This polarization then exacerbates an internal experience of loneliness. For instance, Helen described the tension she felt as a duality between "feeling alone and needing others." She noticed an uncertainty around depending on others and a "strange, uncomfortable" feeling when she felt others were dependent on her. Helen had not planned to have a family but had two children whom she described as "like accessories" and "little friends." Fairbairn (1952) reported how it becomes possible to recognize essentially schizoid phenomena in clients' experiences, such as

> full-fledged depersonalisation and derealisation, but also relatively minor or transient disturbances of the reality-sense, e.g. feelings of "artificiality" (referred to the self or the environment), experiences such as "the plate-glass feelings", feelings of unfamiliarity with familiar persons or environmental settings and feelings of familiarity with the unfamiliar. (p. 5)

It was heart-wrenching to hear about Helen's struggle to be in contact with her current family members. She reported feeling unfamiliar within her own family, a jarring confusion of "Who am I to these people? Who am I when I'm with these people?" These are the exhausting challenges faced by those living with schizoid processes who attempt to be parents and to be in intimate relationships.

This schizoid compromise results in the formation of a social self, a split-off part of the self that is adept at accommodating to different relational situations, including the relationship with a psychotherapist. This social self may dominate and distract from the person's attempts to express the vital aspects of themselves such as various affects, unique interests, pleasures, desires, dislikes, or any aspect of vulnerability.

Helen's strong need to remain safe within herself and to regulate the impact she had on the world around her meant she would repeatedly experience misattunement and misunderstanding from others. Although her affect was often hidden and her stories were distracting, I committed myself to doing my best not to disregard Helen's relational needs for security and self-definition or to make an impact on me. Although her needs were not obvious, I finally realized that they were being expressed in her stories and metaphors, enacted in her behavior, and engendered in my confusion and lack of involvement. (See Erskine, 2015a, for a description of how unconscious early attachment patterns are expressed in psychotherapy.) This helped me to think about Helen's experience in her day-to-day life. I imagined what it would be like for her to go to work and her emotional struggles with the people in her life. I found myself willing to vicariously experience what life was like for her. After I started to work with this introspection, I found ways to attune to Helen's rhythms and affects. I allowed myself to drift in and out of contact with her and to notice where I went in my sensations, thoughts, and awareness. I began to allow myself to go with the experience of being in relation with her rather than asserting my image of how a psychotherapist ought to be.

Helen had become accustomed to the repetitive pattern of our sessions. She would arrive exactly on time. She would appear small and young-looking at the door. She would move into the room, making as little noise or impact on her surroundings as possible. She would present me with her payment in the same way a child might present a ticket for a fairground ride: nervously and deliberately. She would then find her position on the couch, careful not to intrude on the space around her. Clients similar to Helen may be in psychotherapy for a long time without making an impact on the therapist. They adapt to what they imagine are the therapist's requirements and continue to hide their own needs. They rarely cause disruptions or act out. For instance, Helen was shocked when I asked her to message me to let me know how an important medical appointment went. It was difficult for her to comprehend that she had made an impact on me, that her health mattered to me.

Many people who use a schizoid process to manage their emotional and relational life actively regulate both the impact they make on others and the degree and type of impact others make on them. They move through life without impacting others, and so they are often not aware of the effect they have. In the family stories, such clients reveal that their childhood was marked by the impossibility of defining themselves or of making any significant impact within the family. They report that their need to make an impact was not enjoyed or welcomed. Growing up, they endured extensive disregard of their relational needs, so they stopped expressing their vital and vulnerable selves in favor of a version of themselves that worked for others. They were often without the experience of "making an impact" on others from an authentic part of them—the vital and vulnerable self, what Winnicott (1965) called the true self.

The relational need to make an impact becomes paradoxical for such individuals. The schizoid process often involves the individual working hard not to make an impact on the therapist, to control the space, to remain internally and relationally safe. With Helen, I felt the "impact" in my countertransference, my confusion, my sense of the lack of emotional vibrancy in the work, and the fatigue I often felt. Helen was making an impact on me; it was subtle but it was impactful. She was relating from her sequestered, vital, and vulnerable self.

If we are to be effective with such individuals, we must maintain a belief that we are gradually having an impact on them. This is where understanding the object relations theories of Fairbairn (1952), Guntrip (1969), and Winnicott (1965) can support practice so that we patiently trust what is going on behind the scenes, become aware of the phenomena emerging in the relating, and trust that the intrapsychic structure of the schizoid individual means that on some level we are becoming part of the person's internal landscape even though it may not appear so in our session-to-session relating. We must hold an appreciation of the level of stress and shame that these clients can have when a social facade is strong. Behind the scenes, the person may be observing words, responses, and expressions that can feed their fantasies about how they need to be in order to be acceptable to the therapist. Fairbairn (1952) described his schizoid clients' self-criticisms with the term "internal saboteur" (p. 101). The withdrawn self splits further to create the internal saboteur who turns against the vulnerable self. One of the functions of this saboteur is to anticipate criticism from others and regulate the person's behavior (Erskine, as cited in Zaletel, 2010). The internal saboteur serves to keep the vulnerable self hidden and repressed. It is the anti-wanting self that is contemptuous and despising of neediness and ensures the schizoid individual neither seeks nor obtains what they want (J. Klein, as cited in Little, 1999, p. 36).

Self-definition

In my work with Helen, I came to realize that her relational need to make an impact and for self-definition were simultaneous and interrelated, both part of her need for self-expression and validation. A person relying on a schizoid process struggles with a lack of self-definition and also to comprehend that they have an impact on others: "If I don't know me, how can I impact others?" Erskine et al. (1999) described how "children who grow up in an environment that demands conformity, unquestioning obedience to rules and norms, may never learn how to be themselves" (p. 137).

For example, when Helen was in school, the teachers and other students defined her by her academic ability. In her adult life she was defined by her position and status at work. Her sense of self seemed strongly anchored to her performance on the job and how others perceived her. Helen was frustrated with repeatedly seeking validation through her role at work, particularly because it was "behind the scenes." She often despaired and was confused about how all her efforts to "be good" and perform well were not acknowledged. One of the few times I saw her express anger was in response to the pressure she felt to perform a certain way at work. That anger led us to explore how she could get a satisfying response to her need for self-definition and to have a sense of making an impact on others.

As the therapy progressed, my appreciation deepened for Helen's strong attachment to her work life and how meaningful it was for her to retell stories about her work experiences. I began to see these as essential to her sense of self and self-identity. Her work life made her feel real and connected to something. It created structure, attachment, and fulfilled her needs according to her script beliefs of having to work hard and do well for others. All her energy would go into managing and surviving her week, although she was often exhausted by the weekend. She did not have friends she saw regularly and found it difficult to initiate and keep in touch with people (she spoke of people seeming to drift away). The effort she put into work, particularly interactions with others, meant she needed to withdraw internally on weekends in order to recuperate. For a long time, she viewed her therapy as supporting this process, a chance to verbalize her grievances so she could survive the next week at work.

Guntrip (as cited in Hazell, 1994) described how the schizoid individual:

> Without a satisfactory relationship with another person he cannot become a developing ego, he cannot find himself. That is why patients are so often found complaining "I don't know who or what I am, I don't seem to have a mind of my own, I don't feel to be a real person at all." Their early object-relationships were such that they were unable to "find themselves" in any definite way. (p. 129)

This reflects a core reason for the schizoid person to be in therapy: to find or reclaim their self-definition. I wondered how I could help Helen with this when she needed such self-protection. How could I find her without losing her again? I needed to continue carefully, always holding in mind her fears around interpersonal contact and her need to protect herself.

Further into our work together, Helen arrived excited to tell me about a work awayday she had helped to coordinate around the theme of pirates. She had dressed up and organized games and activities. The excitement and change in her energy amazed me. I knew Helen was showing me something new and different, a spark of vibrancy that I had been waiting patiently to see for a long time. This marked a turning point in her therapy as we began exploring her creativity and her enjoyment in planning creatively for others. Helen was starting to allow herself to express a different, emergent energy, away from the structure of her daily life toward something creative, playful, and fun. These moments of vitality were polar opposites to the repetitive staidness of her social facade. I was excited to finally see them and at the same time careful not to overwhelm her with my responses. I did not want to scare her away by expressing too much excitement or suddenly changing how I was with her.

As we explored fantasies about what she would do outside of her long-term workplace, she shared her dreams about wanting to teach. I encouraged that through my inquiry and involvement, and she eventually decided to volunteer as a classroom support at a secondary school. This was a hugely significant decision: to move out of her comfort zone based around work and home life and to work alongside children who needed individual support. I was deeply moved when she reported the connections and relationships she was forming with the children and how she was appreciating their particular needs in learning. Helen began to reflect on her childhood through the experiences with the children, which led to richer exploration of her emotional memories. In Greenberg's (2016) words:

> I tend to find these particular clients difficult to connect with because their real self is so hidden, even from themselves. … All of their aliveness goes into their fantasy life. I have

learned that if I am patient and those clients decide I am trustworthy, they will give me glimpses of the riches they have inside themselves. (p. 338)

Finding Helen's creativity came out of us exploring her inner world of metaphors and fantasies as well as from her experiencing me valuing and accepting the significance of those and letting her know about their impact on me. What had initially appeared as repetitive, superficial narratives around her work became a bridge to me appreciating how she made meaning within her world as well as glimpses of her vital and vulnerable self. Helen described herself at work as "a computer stuck and going round and round doing the same thing" and a "machine with grit in the machinery/cogs, grinding and missing connections." The more I attuned to and validated her wonderful metaphors and images, the more I heard faint expressions of unmet relational needs.

Such needs are often held within fantasy or "at a symbolic level" (Yontef, 2001, p. 8). They can be kept out of cognitive awareness or securely compartmentalized internally, away from contact with others. Within the safety of fantasy, an individual can imagine relational needs being satisfied but without genuine interpersonal contact with others. We can listen for and find these needs as our clients share subjects that feel safe to them. This interplay was described by Orcutt (2018) as follows:

> The therapist begins with showing interest in what is of interest to the patient. This may be as pertinent as the patient's intellectualized ideas about the presenting problem, or may diverge to topics of special interest to the patient such as books or computer games. This is to establish a mutual safe space with the patient, where verbal transaction can take place in an uncommitted way. This uses what Ralph Klein (1995) has called the schizoid patient's ability to form "relationships by proxy" and so defensively "act against the risks involved in connecting to, and sharing with the therapist" (p. 90). This ability can allow the patient to test out a harmless reciprocity in the sessions. Over time, the experience of this interplay may prove to feel safe enough so that the patient may begin to further test the possibility of a closer exchange. If all goes well, interchange becomes therapy as protective strategy transforms into relationship. (p. 44)

Instead of challenging or ignoring Helen's repetitive narratives around work, I moved into her work world with her. Through cognitive attunement, inquiry, and involvement in her retellings, I became deeply knowledgeable about her workplace: the people, the systems, how she worked, what she did. She was teaching me about her inner world, and the therapy began to deepen when I accepted what had initially appeared to be trivial. I began to understand through working with Helen how to be involved in whatever is of interest to my client.

Work was safety for Helen. It gave her an identity and provided for some of her relational needs. Nevertheless, she was gradually able to verbalize how her work did not provide the valuing she needed. She realized how little impact she was having in her work life, regardless of how hard she worked to adapt to its requirements. Our sessions became more about her making contact with herself in a reflective way rather than controlling the space with retellings of what had happened to her. She was able to speak more emotionally and vulnerably about her experience as a mother and her struggles in connecting with her son.

Forming an identity from a place of schizoid withdrawal or protection comes from acknowledging and accepting a relational need for self-definition. As a result, the "organization of a once-hidden self can now begin to form an identity" (O'Reilly-Knapp, 2012, p. 8). Through our work, I learned to appreciate my active part in facilitating Helen's growing awareness of a relational need for self-definition and how to move into the schizoid individual's world by working within the client's metaphors and fantasies, to sometimes share in her experience of a lack of self-definition. In doing this, it was important to remain present and in contact with myself, which requires a careful balance. My own sense of self-definition is often impacted when I cannot sense the other person's vitality, when my client is withdrawn and I cannot reach them. I am left to wonder about my own capacity to make an impact. With Helen, I learned to remain present as well as non-invasive and attuned to the nonverbal, the repetitions, and the clues that might be there in the person's social facade. I came to appreciate the experience of the schizoid phenomena and to notice the spaces between our interactions, to pick up on and use all the sensations available to me, and to be able to sometimes drift with the process while staying defined at the same time.

In my experience, there are observable phenomena that may signal the client's absence of self-definition; for example, the phenomenon of someone seemingly not arriving in a room and appearing to drift in and out of transactions. I observed that Helen lacked definition in terms of how she arrived in the therapy room. I understood this as a lack of aggress—a lack of initiative in both occupying the space and in relating—a passivity and an unclear definition in her physicality. Guntrip (as cited in Hazell, 1994) described how "the regressive urge to remain identified for the sake of comfort and security conflicts with the developmental need to dissolve identification and differentiate oneself as a separate personality" (p. 50).

Interrelating needs

Self-definition means an assertion of oneself, an expression of "me" in contrast to "you." Developmentally this is a huge task under any conditions. For the schizoid individual, maintaining the security of the hidden self takes precedence over the risks of differentiating. This is an example of how relational needs interrelate and interplay and how one need can be compromised by or contrasted with another: "It's not safe to define myself in contrast to others"; "I don't know myself enough to make an impact on you"; "When you initiate with me it feels unsafe."

I found that Helen's relational needs often fused together in clusters and appeared "theoretically interrelated" (Žvelc et al., 2020). I came to understand how the triad of relational needs to make an impact, for self-definition, and to have others initiate were all in the background of our relating. These were needs Helen was not aware of and did not outwardly express. I believe it aided Helen's therapy for me to hold the potential for them to emerge in our contact together, to be curious, and to watch for clues or expressions of them. These relational needs were thwarted at various points during Helen's life. She had given up expressing or seeking satisfaction of them and had found creative ways to compensate or adapt. Her therapy involved a slow growth in her awareness of her previously unmet, unknown relational needs.

Need to initiate

Helen's need for me to initiate contact was in the background of our relating during our early work. Her dominant need was to remain safe and in control of the space. My attempts to initiate beyond the safe parameters of what she was prepared for were brushed away. I could see from her physiology and her responses to inquiry how wary she was of initiations into relational contact. However, the more I stopped trying to do and the more I allowed myself to work within the schizoid process—to involve myself in whatever Helen was prepared to involve me in—the more I began to see the fragments of the need to initiate coming through, particularly in the form of developmental imagery.

As Helen trusted me enough to share more about her inner world, I was often reminded of how a young child might share ideas and thoughts. I imagined her not having the experience in childhood of a significant other alongside her at different ages, someone listening, involved, and impacted by her sharing ideas. It began to occur to me that Helen was, in her own way, initiating play in her therapy. She appeared to be enjoying my enjoyment of her sharing of ideas, concepts, and metaphors. If a child has not had others initiate with them, all their ideas for play stay internalized and in fantasy. In her workplace, I imagined Helen as a little girl trying to initiate and get on with the other kids, not understanding how they spoke and what they wanted from her. As Stewart (2010) suggested:

> It is important to be aware of the dynamics of initiating since sometimes it is clinically astute to wait until the client initiates reaching out to us. … The presence of the therapist's need to have the other initiate might be felt as a longing for the client to reach out to them, and a disappointment when they don't. … [Therapists should] be mindful of their own need in this regard and not make it an expectation of clients or withdraw when it's not met. (p. 48)

Again, the need to have others initiate may be bound up in the schizoid process and the unique style of relating that this involves: "I need you as a therapist to initiate contact but I need to regulate contact by withdrawing and presenting a social facade."

How do we as therapists hold on to the crucial need the client has when it is in the background of the relating? A schizoid person survives in relationships and interactions with others by relying on certain manners or creative personality adjustments, such as detachedness, robotic politeness, self-containment, or self-reliance. The underlying need for others to initiate is repeatedly missed as people relate to the social facade rather than the hidden self. This relational need remains out of awareness or hidden away, but it is there and will be within the field of relating in the psychotherapy. I imagined this confusion of unknown or hidden needs being expressed by Helen in statements such as "I need you as therapist to initiate contact with me but I am scared of what this is like" or "I need you to initiate but I can't tolerate this and need to regulate with withdrawal."

For such individuals, the idea of initiating with others, including the therapist, might be an unknown or frightening: "I didn't think it was OK to ask for what I need." Helen's relational need for the other to initiate was there, but it was a long time before I could initiate contact and move into a more relational style of inquiry. As with the relational need for self-definition and impact, her need for the other to initiate emerged into the foreground of our relating. These needs were there in the relating but often expressed inversely. She appeared to lack self-definition and instead relied on a social facade, a compromised version of her that hid away the vital and vulnerable self. Her efforts to minimize having an impact within the therapy conversely made an impact on me. Her need to have another initiate was experienced by her as threatening and emerged through careful attunement to metaphor and her intellectual playfulness. Could the out-of-awareness relational needs in the client relate to the ones the therapist picks up in the countertransference? I found how important it was to identify and track where Helen's relational needs were within our relating, that is, which needs were in the foreground, which could be noticed within my countertransference, and which were out of awareness or in the background.

Need for mutuality

Erskine and Moursund (2022) wrote, "The need for self-definition is the complement of the need for mutuality" (p. 112). For her part, Helen's relational need for mutuality was in the background of our relating until much later in our work together. Her predominant needs were to feel safe and to have her experiences and way of surviving validated and accepted. Any sense of mutuality between us would have been threatening and risky to her. Her loneliness and independence as a child did not include much companionship or many shared experiences with others. Her playfulness came through in her intellectual life and within fantasy. There was a gradual movement toward a more mutual relating as she grew in her self-definition and allowed me to be a more relatable presence. Zaletel (2010) described how with her client "[in] this therapy phase she expressed her needs of both mutuality and self-definition. Lara entered in contact with her real self and thus I, too, could become more of a 'real' person" (p. 23).

The more attuned I was with Helen, the more defended her vital and vulnerable self often became. I imagine the more we try to be in contact with the smoke and mirrors of the social facade, the more this increases a sense of unease or confusion for the client. However, as the person becomes more settled in the relating, the therapist can be as well. As Helen's therapy progressed, we were able to relate together in an increasingly equal, mutual way.

Working within a schizoid process, we might meet the social facade of the person who seems easy in conversation and willing to engage in therapeutic interactions. There may appear to be a need for a mutual or shared relating when, in fact, the hidden, vital, and vulnerable self does not need mutuality with the therapist at all. That part of the self needs the emergent process of self-definition, to move out from a cut-off, defended place to reclaim their voice and a sense of their uniqueness. There can be moments when it feels like the client is seeking some kind of mutuality or sharing of experience with the therapist when they are actually not ready to hear this and instead need the therapist to remain in an idealized position: bigger, protective, and an object onto whom they can project ideas from a younger, more vulnerable self. It might be like a scene in which a young child is sitting with adults at the dinner table attempting to join in grown-up conversation. This appears as a need for mutuality and shared experience when actually the stronger need is to have their own experiences responded to, validated, and accepted in an age-appropriate way (or even to get down from the table and go and play with the other kids!).

Need for survival

Reflecting on the therapy with Helen, I suggest that the relational need for survival describes the internal struggle for self-survival happening inside the world of the schizoid person and within the therapeutic relationship. As O'Reilly-Knapp (2001) reported in describing her work with a client's schizoid process,

> She used her withdrawal and dissociative states for protecting and sustaining her life" (p. 4). Defensive processes reflect the individual's need to survive in relationship. They are creative ways of maintaining safety in the maelstrom of relating with others. Beyond the need for safety is the need for the vital and vulnerable self to have survived as described in the "encapsulated self. (p. 12)

This is a process that goes on internally, privately, and silently. A client will show their struggle for self-survival through the transference.

The philosophical principles of integrative psychotherapy include the idea that "all human behavior has meaning in some context" (Erskine, 2013, p. 4). Taking this into account, I think the person who uses silence, withdrawal, or a social facade to cope with extreme distress or trauma needs to create an internal closed relational system in order to organize experience and keep the vital and vulnerable self alive. The therapist needs to appreciate and honor the function of this closed system and how the vital and vulnerable self has been in exile: deadened, put in a kind of deep freeze, the idea that to survive one must keep that part of the self "dead to the world." This becomes a need in itself. A client can show us in the therapeutic relating that "I need to be hidden," "I need to withdraw," or "To survive, I needed to seem dead in myself."

It is essential to acknowledge this need for solitary survival as part of a relational psychotherapy. Otherwise we may rush to offer the kind of contact and relating the individual may yearn for but also be highly fearful of. As Yontef (2001) outlined, from the perspective of the schizoid individual,

> It is dangerous to move into intimate connection if you cannot separate when needed. If you think you are going to be caught up, devoured, or captured in the connection, it is terrifying to move into intimate contact. On the other hand, if you do not feel connected with other people, especially if you do not believe you can intimately connect again, the separation or isolation is both painful and terrifying. (p. 9)

A relational need to survive involves the individual's fears around intimate contact and threat to existence. The vital and vulnerable self is locked in a closed internal system of survival. Guntrip (as cited in Hazell, 1994) described the internal tension with a metaphor: "a closed picture frame, the inside edge of which was an unbroken array of sharp teeth all pointing in at the patient" (p. 142). This precarious, fragile, self-contained inner world has to be acknowledged by the therapist as part of an in-contact integrative relational psychotherapy. Helen showed me that she needed to create a rigid structure of relating to others. Her way of regulating interpersonal contact was a tolerable compromise born out of necessity in order to survive early experiences in which her relational needs were not met.

Conclusion

To borrow Woodman's (cited in Kullander, 2008) phrase about dreams, I like to think of the schizoid individual as "like a deer at the edge of the forest" (p. 13). At first you may catch only a glimpse of her, and then she is gone in the blink of an eye. But this is enough to know she is there. Reflecting on the many hours I worked with Helen, patiently listening and attuning to her repetitious narratives, hoping to catch something of the vital and vulnerable self that she guarded so well, I found in myself a unique love and care for her in our struggles to find authentic contact with each other. This was someone who found intimate relating frightening and risky. Helen entered therapy not knowing what she needed or what possibilities lay ahead, but she followed a yearning inside herself for something different.

Therapy within a schizoid process is a like a slow rescue mission. It is our patient, caring and careful involvement with these clients that eventually allows someone to "unfold, like a flower" (Berne, 1961, p. 226) and emerge from the protected internal spaces in which they have hidden. Guntrip (as cited in Hazell, 1994) described therapy with these clients as being like "a steady recuperation from deep strain, diminishing of deep fears, revitalization of the personality and rebirth of an active ego that is spontaneous and does not have to be forced and driven" (p. 186). The therapeutic relationship is a place of growth and healing, a symbolic space of potential in which someone can begin to emerge and express their vital and vulnerable self. Within this growth, we must validate and accept the person's unique ways of surviving.

Helen and I worked together early in my practice, when I was inexperienced and did not appreciate what I now know about the schizoid process. I wonder if this not-knowing actually helped the initial phases of the therapy. I was not trying to impose myself too hard on the work or trying different strategies. I was prepared to work patiently and gently at the pace Helen needed in order for her to gain trust in the relating and to allow her true self and needs to emerge. When I first met Helen, I had no idea of the richness of her inner life or how creative she was in her fantasies, thoughts, and way of seeing the world. I was locked into relating with an adapted social facade that needed tight control over the therapy space in order to feel safe. The close consideration of how her relational needs shifted within the therapy offered anchoring in the often slow and repetitive early periods of our work. My attention to how her relational needs appeared out of awareness and yet longed to emerge gave me a guide to what could be happening in our relating.

Over the years we worked together, Helen taught me about what it means to be a therapist. Winnicott (1965) wrote of a "devotion" to the emergent self. This implies a commitment to cherishing the creative ways a person remains interpersonally safe, their styles of withdrawal, and the internal unknowns that epitomize the schizoid struggle to find contact with the external world, themselves, and others.

References

Berne, E. (1961). *Transactional Analysis in Psychotherapy: A Systematic Individual and Social Psychiatry*. New York: Grove.

Erskine, R. G. (2001). Psychological functions, relational needs, and transferential resolution: Psychotherapy of an obsession. *Transactional Analysis Journal*, *31*(4): 220–226. doi.org/10.1177/036215370103100403.

Erskine, R. G. (2011). Attachment, relational-needs, and psychotherapeutic presence [Keynote address]. International Integrative Psychotherapy Association Conference, Vichy, France, April 21. https://integrativetherapy.com/en/articles.php?id=73.

Erskine, R. G. (2013). Vulnerability, authenticity, and inter-subjective contact: Philosophical principles of integrative psychotherapy. *International Journal of Integrative Psychotherapy*, *4*(2): 1–9.

Erskine, R. G. (2015a). Life scripts: Unconscious relational patterns and psychotherapeutic involvement. In: R. G. Erskine, *Relational Patterns, Therapeutic Presence: Concepts and Practice of Integrative Psychotherapy* (pp. 91–112). London: Karnac.

Erskine, R. G. (2015b). Life scripts and attachment patterns: Theoretical integration and therapeutic involvement. In: R. G. Erskine, *Relational Patterns, Therapeutic Presence: Concepts and Practice of Integrative Psychotherapy* (pp. 73–90). London: Karnac.

Erskine, R. G. (2020). Relational withdrawal, attunement to silence: Psychotherapy of the schizoid process. *International Journal of Integrative Psychotherapy*, *11*: 14–28.

Erskine, R. G., & Moursund, J. P. (2022). *The Art and Science of Relationship: The Practice of Integrative Psychotherapy*. Bicester, UK: Phoenix.

Erskine, R. G., Moursund, J. P., & Trautmann, R. L. (1999). *Beyond Empathy: A Therapy of Contact-in-Relationship*. London: Routledge, 2023.

Erskine, R. G., & Trautmann, R. L. (1996). Methods of an integrative psychotherapy. *Transactional Analysis Journal*, 26(4): 316–328. doi.org/10.1177/036215379602600410.

Fairbairn, W. R. D. (1952). *Psychoanalytic Studies of the Personality*. London: Routledge.

Greenberg, E. (2016). *Borderline, Narcissistic and Schizoid Adaptations: The Pursuit of Love, Admiration and Safety*. New York: Greenbrooke.

Guntrip, H. (1969). *Schizoid Phenomena, Object Relations and the Self*. New York: International Universities Press.

Hazell, J. (Ed.) (1994). *Personal Relations Therapy: The Collected Papers of H. J. S. Guntrip*. Northvale, NJ: Jason Aronson.

Johnson, S. M. (1994). *Character Styles*. New York: W. W. Norton.

Klein, J. (1987). *Our Need for Others and Its Roots in Infancy*. London: Routledge.

Klein, R. (1995). The self-in-exile: A developmental, self, and object relations approach to the schizoid disorder of the self. In: J. F. Masterson & R. Klein (Eds.), *Disorders of the Self: New Therapeutic Horizons: The Masterson Approach* (Part 1, Ch. 1–7, pp. 3–142). New York: Brunner/Mazel.

Kullander, J. (2008). Men are from earth and so are women—Marion Woodman. *Awaken*. https://awaken.com/2018/03/men-are-from-earth-and-so-are-women.

Little, R. (1999). Schizoid processes: Working with the defenses of the withdrawn child ego state. *Transactional Analysis Journal*, 31(1): 33–43. doi.org/10.1177/036215370103100105.

Little, R. (2011). Impasse clarification within the transference–countertransference matrix. *Transactional Analysis Journal*, 41(1): 23–28. doi.org/10.1177/036215370103100105.

Manfield, P. (1992). *Split Self, Split Object: Understanding and Treating Borderline, Narcissistic and Schizoid Disorders*. Northvale, NJ: Jason Aronson.

Orcutt, C. (2018). Schizoid fantasy: Refuge or transitional location? *Clinical Social Work Journal*, 46(1): 42–47. doi.org/10.1007/s10615-017-0629-2.

O'Reilly-Knapp, M. (2001). Between two worlds: The encapsulated self. *Transactional Analysis Journal*, 31(1): 44–54. doi.org/10.1177/036215370103100106.

O'Reilly-Knapp, M. (2012). Organizing self-experiences. *International Journal of Integrative Psychotherapy*, 3(1): 1–14.

Stewart, A. L. (2010). Relational needs of the therapist: Countertransference, clinical work and supervision. Benefits and disruptions in psychotherapy. *International Journal of Integrative Psychotherapy*, 1(1): 41–50.

Winnicott, D. W. (1965). *The Maturational Processes and the Facilitating Environment: Studies in the Theory of Emotional Development*. Madison, CT: International Universities Press.

Yontef, G. (2001). Psychotherapy of schizoid process. *Transactional Analysis Journal*, 31(1): 7–23. doi.org/10.1177/036215370103100103.

Zaletel, M. (2010). Journey towards integration: The case of Lara. *International Journal of Integrative Psychotherapy*, 1(1): 11–24.

Žvelc, G., Jovanoska, K., & Žvelc, M. (2020). Development and validation of the relational needs satisfaction scale. *Frontiers in Psychology*. www.frontiersin.org/articles/10.3389/fpsyg.2020.00901/full. doi.org/10.3389/fpsyg.2020.00901.

Part II

A five-year case study and colleagues' reflections

CHAPTER 7

Allan: depression or isolated attachment?

Richard G. Erskine

> *In wildness is the preservation of the world,*
> *When we walk, we naturally go to the fields and woods:*
> *From the forest and wilderness come the tonics*
> *and barks which brace mankind.*
> —Henry David Thoreau, *Walking* (1862)

Allan's physician recommended that he call me for a series of psychotherapy sessions. In the initial phone contact, Allan said that he had been taking antidepressant medication for three years but without any noticeable results. He said that he always felt "low down" and did not have much energy, particularly when he was home. The doctor wanted Allan to try psychotherapy "to see if it will work." Allan and I agreed on three sessions to evaluate if psychotherapy was appropriate for him and whether we could work well together.

When Allan entered my office two days later, I saw a tall, thin man who was dressed like he was going hiking in the mountains. His attire and high boots were unusual for someone living in New York City. He spoke slowly and softly. When I inquired why he was seeking psychotherapy, all he could say was that he wanted his depression to stop. As I tried to establish a contract that would define the outcome of our work, Allan had difficulty stating any definable objective. I presumed that it was too soon to establish any goals; perhaps we needed to get to know each other first.

In the next two sessions, I learned that Allan was fifty years old, never married, and had lived in the same apartment since he was a young child. A bookkeeper in a large accounting firm, he was content with his job and liked the people at work, although he did not socialize with them because "I never go to bars." He said that he attended church almost every Sunday because he was in charge of the church's finances. Allan spent Saturdays and holidays hiking various portions of the Appalachian Trail and his four weeks of summer vacation camping in the wilderness where he could be "all alone with nature."

Allan's mother had died four and a half years earlier. As I inquired about Allan's possible grief, he was slow to respond. After shrugging his shoulders, he hesitantly told me about his mother's painful struggle with cancer. He claimed that he was not sad about her death but that he did miss her cooking. There was an absence of sensitivity in his response to my questions about his mother's death (Erskine, 2014a, 2014b, 2014c). I wondered if his flat affect indicated that he was not ready to talk about losing her or if it reflected a personality pattern. Allan had no memory of his father, who died when Allan was in kindergarten. Allan had a sister who was five years older, whom he had not spoken with since his mother's funeral. He sarcastically said, "I can't be in the same room with her. She's a know-it-all." Then he added, "Life is better all alone."

In our third session, Allan was contemptuous of his medical doctor's abrupt manner of speaking. At two different moments I inquired about his feelings of anger at his doctor's behavior, but Allan avoided my questions. The doctor had decided that Allan would slowly reduce and eventually stop the antidepressants. Allan said that he wanted to continue psychotherapy sessions with me "because it could help." He was not interested in forming an outcome-defining contract (Berne, 1966), but he volunteered that he would come for individual psychotherapy once a week for a year.

It was time for me to do some introspection, a sensorial search of my internal process: I found Allan pleasant, shy, and either withholding his responses or slow to respond to my questions. He was interesting when he talked eagerly about hiking and camping. At the end of this third session, I doubted whether I could help Allan resolve his depression. I still did not feel an affective connection with him. He was evasive whenever I asked him about his body sensations or other subjective experiences. Other clients had taught me that I need to maintain my own vitality and curiosity when I am working with someone who is depressed. With many such clients, I rely on phenomenological inquiry and carefully observe their style of answering my questions. That style is often more revealing of who they are than is the content of their answers. In the first three sessions with Allan, my phenomenological inquiry seemed to be more of a hindrance than a help. Unlike many other clients, Allan did not respond to phenomenological inquiry (Erskine et al., 1999).

Although his medical doctor described him as depressed, Allan did not manifest some of the symptoms of a depressive disorder. He had previously said that he lacked energy, yet he described himself as engaging in intense physical activities and being a "diligent worker" both on the job and in volunteering for his church. He said that he ate and slept well but was uninterested in social activities with people, even with the "nice people at church." In evenings after work, he was "plagued with miserable feelings." Allan defined himself at those times as "depressed" and added that in those moments he was compelled to "get out and walk … even if it is near midnight."

Was he depressed? Yes. But it did not appear appropriate to diagnose him as having a depressive disorder. It was clear to me that the various things he said about himself required careful attention. I did not understand his internal processes, but I listened for the covert meaning in his stories. I needed to be patient, attentive, and attune myself (the best I could) to his indistinct and subtle affects. I was reminded of Guntrip's writings in which he described several of his "schizoid" clients who entered psychotherapy because of depression (as described in Hazell, 1994).

I asked Allan if he had any thoughts of suicide. He described how he had always imagined escaping to "another world." As I inquired further, he said that he first thought about killing himself when he was thirteen years old and that throughout his life he had continued to think about dying and going to "a place of peace and quiet." I asked if he had ever attempted suicide, to which he answered "No." He lamented that he could not kill himself while his mother was alive because "I had to take care of her. I was all she had." While telling me this story, he used the word "despair," and the way he said it evoked concern in me. When I inquired further about what he was feeling, he dismissed my question with, "I'm fine." Each time I inquired about his affect he changed the subject.

I asked Allan how he imagined killing himself. With hesitation he described shooting himself in the head but quickly added that he did not now, nor had he ever, owned a gun. He described dying as going into a "peaceful, everlasting quiet." He was worried that suicide was a sin and that if he killed himself he would "not attain peace and quiet." By the end of that session, I was not worried that he was in imminent danger of suicide, but I was concerned that a long-term risk remained. His ideas about the quietness of death, the absence of close friends, the lack of energy when at home, and the death of his mother were some markers that could indicate a major depression, but he did not have many of the other characteristics (American Psychiatric Association, 2013). He ate well, walked extensively, and was able to concentrate on his work. He said that his apartment was neat and clean and that he was making plans for next summer's camping trip in northern Canada.

As I reflected on all that he had told me, I was certain that encoded in his self-descriptions and behaviors were unconscious relational patterns that were being lived out in his daily life (Erskine, 2010). If we were to continue with psychotherapy, I would have to explore several clues that he had given me: his sense of despair, his longing for peace and quiet, his excessive walking late at night, the family dynamics of his childhood, and various body sensations and tensions that indicated disavowed affect.

I only had a few minutes left in the third session. We had not formed a sufficiently close relationship such that a no-suicide contract would be effective. As we concluded the session, I felt that it was necessary for me to rely on his religious convictions and his statement that he did not possess a gun. And I had his word that he would come for psychotherapy each week for a year.

I sensed that something vital was missing in Allan's life. I was not sure what it was, but I kept thinking about how his life was devoid of any intimacy. Internally I made an emotional commitment. I wanted our psychotherapy to enhance the quality of his life and provide him with a desire to live. I walked home from the office that night questioning myself: "Was I wanting more for Allan than he wanted or was willing to do?" I knew what was possible in an in-depth psychotherapy, but I had no evidence that Allan knew the commitment, perseverance, and time that would be required to make some fundamental changes in his life.

The first year

The evening before our fourth meeting, as I contemplated Allan's agreeing to come to weekly psychotherapy, I was touched by how alone he seemed, how he preferred to be in nature and not with people, and how he had difficulty talking about feelings. I thought about his "depression" and wondered if he was describing the results of a prolonged schizoid withdrawal. One of the clues was that he did not respond well to my phenomenological inquiry. I was not sure if I could be effective in helping him achieve a satisfactory comfort in his life, but I was willing to invest myself in our therapeutic relationship. I was relying on my perception that Allan was serious about resolving his depression. He must have had some form of connection with me because he was willing to make a commitment for ongoing work.

In the first few weeks of sessions, I tried to inquire about the "low down feeling" and lack of energy that Allan had mentioned in our initial interview. He deflected my questions by talking about his work situation. He felt gratified by the "challenges of solving difficult tax problems" and "the freedom to do it on my own," but he disapproved of his coworkers' behavior because they were not as diligent as he was: "They waste a lot of time talking to each other." He chose not to include himself in their lunch or after-work activities. I asked about other friends; Allan was vague and eventually admitted that he had none.

As I raised my concern about how much time he spent by himself, Allan said, "Some nights after dinner I prefer to walk the neighborhood for a couple of hours. I watch people a lot, I often see faces I recognize." As I imagined myself in that situation, I felt an intense sadness. Yet Allan spoke of his situation matter of factly, with no emotion. He lapsed into long pauses, looking at the ceiling. In the next few sessions, Allan continued to describe his late-night walks through New York City and how he distracted himself from feeling "low down" by watching people. When I asked if he ever talked with anyone on his walks, he said, "I would never do that."

These stories caused me to wonder what he was not telling me. Did he have some secret that he was keeping private? I was curious about Allan, but my inquiries were only partially effective. He answered my questions but often with reticence. I wanted to know him, to know the depth and extent of what he felt, what he had lived as a boy, and how he managed his life. It was necessary to continually remind myself to be patient, to just let his story unfold.

Two months later, Allan again told me that he was "irritated" by his coworkers and wanted some changes in the office. There was a condemning tone to his voice. I wondered if his unhappy work situation was contributing to his low energy when he came home at night.

But when I implied that he could talk to his coworkers about his displeasure, Allan made it clear that he would never reveal his discomfort to anyone. His solution was to stay distant. Incidentally, from the moment I suggested that he could engage with his coworkers, he was distant with me. He averted his eyes and proceeded to talk about camping equipment that was currently on sale. It became evident that whenever I made a suggestion about changing his behavior, Allan would put an end to the discussion. Apparently he was closed to any therapeutic focus on his behavior just as he was closed to my inquiring about his affect.

In the next few sessions, rather than focusing on his behavior, I increased my use of phenomenological inquiry, particularly about his affect and body sensations. Although he was slow to answer, he usually identified tension in his neck and chest. Somehow that led us to talking about his difficulty in expressing emotion to people. He said, "I want to remain private. I don't want anyone poking their nose into my business." I asked if that included me. Allan answered, "Yeah, sometimes your questions are too damn invasive." I responded, "What happens inside you when I ask such questions?" Allan shrugged his shoulders and remained silent for the remainder of the session. During the next couple of sessions, he struggled to describe how he became physically tense, expecting me to criticize whatever he said, and how he quickly searched "for the right answer." I recognized that psychotherapy was not happening when he was giving me "the right answer."

I asked him to look me in the eye and tell me about his irritation, first with me and then with his coworkers. I wanted him to see my face and how I was impacted by what he did not like. It was difficult for him to voice his discontent, but after several sessions he was able to articulate some anger. I was not sure if these sessions were therapeutic or not. Allan's expression of anger may have been authentic or he may have been complying with my request or a bit of both. I was surprised when a few months later he said that he felt better after the sessions in which he expressed his anger.

I was curious about Allan's childhood, and over the next months I asked several questions about his early family life. Allan was physically tense whenever I did this and did not want to talk about his past. He often said, "I don't remember my childhood." I was curious about whether what I was observing with Allan pointed to his having an avoidant attachment style. That stimulated me to think about the formation of unconscious relational patterns in childhood—unconscious patterns that determine the quality of interpersonal relationships in later life (Erskine, 2008, 2010). It is evident from the child development literature that children who develop avoidant attachment patterns most likely had parents who were rejecting and punitive (Cozolino, 2006; Wallin, 2007) or at least predictably unresponsive to the child's needs and self-expressions (Erskine, 2009). Main's (1995) research indicated that mothers of infants with an avoidant attachment style were emotionally unavailable; they tended to be neglectful when the child was sad and were uncomfortable with physical touch.

It is now well recognized that, as an accommodating survival reaction to the caretaker's predictable unresponsiveness to their affects and relational needs, children learn to inhibit communicating emotions, needs, and internal experiences. As a result, they create an unconscious relational schema by which they inhibit emotional expression and undervalue the importance of relationship. They create an imago of interpersonal relationship where intimacy does not exist. Such children may form interpersonal relatedness strategies in which they do not express, or may not even be conscious of, their attachment-related feelings and needs. They may be disdainful of vulnerability and tender expressions of affection and/or prone to anger (Hesse, 1999; Kobak & Sceery, 1988; Main, 1990).

These ideas about unconscious relational patterns served to heighten my curiosity about Allan's childhood. I wanted to inquire about both his current life and his childhood, but he was not ready. Allan wanted to talk about the people at work and his activities at church. Each week he insisted on telling me about his experience hiking the previous Saturday. I began to form a developmental image of Allan as a six- to eight-year-old boy, a child without a father to take an interest in his adventures (Erskine, 2019).

This developmental image evoked feelings of compassion in me and increased my interest in his stories. I wanted to go hiking with him and see the woodland trail that he saw, to smell the same forest smells, to be a companion. I listened intently and asked factual questions about his hiking and work. Periodically, he allowed me to inquire about what he was feeling, imagining, or remembering. Then I was able to have a glimpse of his internal world, a private world he was reluctant to reveal. I felt an emptiness, like a vacuum, in my belly when I imagined that Allan's world was deprived of intimate contact with people.

When I listened quietly to his stories, I used my face and body gestures to indicate that I was present and attentive. I wanted to convey empathy even though he expressed little emotion. When I asked about his affect, he generally gave me vague answers and rapidly went into details about his current life. I stayed present and interested. We were developing an emotional connection but it was still fragile. I was perplexed and questioned myself: Was my wanting Allan to have contact and possible intimacy with people a countertransference reaction or was my desire responsive to his needs (Loewald, 1986)? Pondering this question allowed me to modulate making any comments, interpretations, or observations about his life. I knew that there was so much more to learn about Allan. Patience, observation, sensitivity, and curiosity were my therapeutic tools.

Our therapy proceeded in this way throughout the first year. I, in a countertransferential way, slipped into responding like a good father, curious and listening to his stories, which alternated between the events at work and what he did on his days off. Periodically, he talked about the people he saw on his evening walks. I still did not know much about what he was experiencing emotionally, such as when he was at home or when he walked the streets late at night "hoping for distraction from feeling empty." But I felt myself fully attentive and involved.

I was perplexed. I read some of the classic psychoanalytic literature about the transference–countertransference matrix (Brenner, 1979; Freud, 1920g; Greenson, 1967; Heinmann, 1950). Was I experiencing what Theodor Jacobs (1986) termed a "countertransference enactment"?

Were my behaviors concordant or complementary (Racker, 1968)? Over several months, my psychoanalytic peer group helped me to delve into my feelings and motivations. I took these conversations into account, formed impressions from what I was reading, and thought about several clients and the different forms of countertransference they stimulated in me (Novellino, 1984). I categorized my various internal experiences in three ways: reactive, responsive, and identifying (Erskine, 2012, 2013a, 2013b).

Sometimes my emotions and behaviors were reactive, a reliving of some unfinished emotionally charged experience in my own life. In these moments, I was self-centered and the client's therapy was disrupted. In many situations, I was responsive and attuned to the qualities of interpersonal contact that the client needed in order to heal from the wounds of neglect and trauma. In these instances, my affect, attitude, and behavior provided a "healing relationship" (Erskine, 2021). Often my affect, demeanor, and words reflected my identifying with the client's unspoken affect or visceral sensations. These various identifications guide me as to when to speak and when to be patiently quiet, in forming the phenomenological inquiry I might make, and in assessing the client's developmental level of functioning. I challenged myself with several questions:

- Were my various affects, urges, and caring behaviors a useful pathway to understanding Allan's inner experience? I was sensing the desire of a six- to eight-year-old boy to have an adult as his companion (identifying).
- Was I attuned to possible relational neglect that he might have experienced as a child? And would my compassionate responses actually be therapeutic (responsive)?
- Was the work with Allan reactivating unrequited relational needs from my own past (reactive)?
- Was my caring for him an unconscious identification with how Allan had prematurely cared for his mother (identifying)?
- Was I reacting to Allan's possible desire to be rescued by a good father (reactive)?
- Were we cocreating what he needed (responsive)?

I never found definitive answers to most of these questions. I was continually left to think about my motivations and to decipher the unconscious story enacted in his behavior, entrenched in his unrevealed affect, and envisioned in his fantasies about camping in the wilderness (Erskine, 2009).

Isolated attachment patterns

I kept thinking about unconscious relational patterns: those that can be described as "avoidant attachment" and those that take the form of "isolated attachment" (Erskine, 2009). Allan lived his day-to-day life in a more solitary way than individuals who manifest an avoidant attachment pattern. Although people with such a pattern often avoid expressing tenderness and empathy, they usually have a social life that includes group activities and superficial relationships. Perhaps Allan's unconscious relational pattern was more isolated; he was a loner. In this first year of psychotherapy, Allan did not talk about any interpersonal connection, and he avoided talking about his relationship with his mother. There was no indication of any emotionally close relationship in his current life and, I suspected, not in his childhood.

In drawing on my therapeutic work with other clients and discussions with members of an ongoing professional development seminar, it became apparent that a person may form an isolated attachment pattern as the result of a series of experiences in which caretakers were experienced as repeatedly unresponsive to the child's relational needs, untrustworthy, and/or criticizing and controlling of the child's emotional expressions (O'Reilly-Knapp, 2001). Because vulnerability was sensed by the child as dangerous, they succumbed to an implicit fear of control, criticism, and invasion. As a reaction to such non-contactful parenting, the child may develop patterns of withdrawal from interpersonal relationships, a social facade, intense internal criticism, and the absence of emotional expression (Erskine, 2001). On cursory observation, such people often appear to be emotionally reserved, quiet in the presence of others, and self-sufficient.

In looking back over the years of my psychotherapy practice, I often overlooked the significance of these subtle signs of the schizoid process. It has taken me a number of years to become sensitive to the unspoken story of such clients, a story replete with fear, shame, disavowed loneliness, self-criticism, and a compulsion to isolate. Allan was one of the clients who taught me to listen for the therapeutically significant story encoded in what such individuals do *not* say.

As Allan's first year of psychotherapy came to an end, I hypothesized that his pattern of attachment was isolated. He was a loner, had no meaningful relationships, and was reluctant to talk about feelings or his childhood experiences. In some sessions, he implied that he frequently criticized himself. Although I always inquired about his internal criticism, he would not reveal any content. During the second part of the year he had acknowledged and expressed some discontent with his coworkers, and on one occasion, with me. He still did not initiate conversations with anyone. When I encouraged him to reach out to people, he was annoyed with me, turned away, and quietly said, "You're bossing me." Yet he also said that he liked coming to our sessions, and he never missed one. I hoped he was forming some embryonic attachment to our relationship.

When we parted for summer vacation, I realized that Allan was teaching me how to relate to someone who was always suspicious of interpersonal contact, particularly if it was intimate in any way. I suspected that he was deeply afraid of what he called "invasion," but why? I was also curious about both his self-criticism, which seemed to lurk below the surface of our conversations, and the little criticisms he directed toward others. I looked forward to September when we could work together again. He was teaching me about relational isolation while I hoped that I was helping him with interpersonal contact.

References

American Psychiatric Association (2013). *Diagnostic and Statistical Manual of Mental Disorders* (5th edn.). Washington, DC: American Psychiatric Publishing. doi.org/10.1176/appi.books.9780890425596.

Berne, E. (1966). *Principles of Group Treatment*. New York: Oxford University Press.

Brenner, C. (1979). Working alliance, therapeutic alliance and transference. *Journal of the American Psychoanalytic Association, 27*: 137–158.

Cozolino, L. (2006). *The Neuroscience of Human Relationships: Attachment and the Developing Social Brain*. New York: W. W. Norton.

Erskine, R. G. (2001). The schizoid process. *Transactional Analysis Journal, 31*(1): 4–6. doi.org/10.1177/036215370103100102.

Erskine, R. G. (2008). Psychotherapy of unconscious experience. *Transactional Analysis Journal, 38*(2): 128–138. doi.org/10.1177/036215370803800206.

Erskine, R. G. (2009). Life scripts and attachment patterns: Theoretical integration and therapeutic involvement. *Transactional Analysis Journal, 39*(3): 207–218. doi.org/10.1177/036215370903900304.

Erskine, R. G. (2010). Life scripts: Unconscious relational patterns and psychotherapeutic involvement. In: R. G. Erskine (Ed.), *Life Scripts: A Transactional Analysis of Unconscious Relational Patterns* (pp. 1–28). London: Karnac.

Erskine, R. G. (2012). Early affect-confusion: The "borderline" between despair and rage. Part 1 of a case study trilogy. *International Journal of Integrative Psychotherapy, 3*(2): 3–14.

Erskine, R. G. (2013a). Balancing on the "borderline" of early affect-confusion. Part 2 of a case study trilogy. *International Journal of Integrative Psychotherapy, 4*(1): 3–9.

Erskine, R. G. (2013b). Relational healing of early affect-confusion: Part 3 of a case study trilogy. *International Journal of Integrative Psychotherapy, 4*(1): 31–40.

Erskine, R. G. (2014a). What do you say before you say good-bye? The psychotherapy of grief. *Transactional Analysis Journal, 44*(4): 279–290. doi.org/10.1177/0362153714556622.

Erskine, R. G. (2014b). The truth shall set you free: Saying an honest "goodbye" before a loved-one's death. *International Journal of Psychotherapy, 18*(2): 72–79.

Erskine, R. G. (2014c). Saying an honest "goodbye": Part 2: Three case examples. *International Journal of Psychotherapy, 18*(3): 52–62.

Erskine, R. G. (2019). Child development in integrative psychotherapy: Erik Erikson's first three stages. *International Journal of Integrative Psychotherapy, 10*: 11–34.

Erskine, R. G. (2021). *A Healing Relationship: Commentary on Therapeutic Dialogues*. Bicester, UK: Phoenix.

Erskine, R. G., Moursund, J. P., & Trautmann, R. L. (1999). *Beyond Empathy: A Therapy of Contact-in-Relationship*. London: Routledge, 2023.

Freud, S. (1920g). *Beyond the Pleasure Principle. S. E., 18*: 3–64. London: Hogarth.

Greenson, R. R. (1967). *The Technique and Practice of Psychoanalysis: Vol. 1*. New York: International Universities Press.

Hazell, J. (Ed.) (1994). *Personal Relations Therapy: The Collected Papers of H. J. S. Guntrip*. Northvale, NJ: Jason Aronson.

Heinmann, P. (1950). On counter-transference. *International Journal of Psycho-Analysis, 31*: 81–84.

Hesse, E. (1999). The adult attachment interview: Historical and current perspectives. In: J. Cassidy & P. Shaveer (Eds.), *Handbook of Attachment: Theory, Research, and Clinical Applications* (pp. 395–433). New York: Guilford.

Jacobs, T. J. (1986). On countertransference enactments. *Journal of the American Psychoanalytic Association, 34*(2): 289–307. doi.org/10.1177/000306518603400203. PMID: 3722698.

Kobak, R. R., & Sceery, A. (1988). Attachment in late adolescence: Working models, affect regulation, and representation of self and others. *Child Development, 59*(1): 135–146. doi.org/10.2307/1130395.

Loewald, H. W. (1986). Transference–countertransference. *Journal of the American Psychoanalytic Association, 34*(2): 275–287. doi.org/10.1177/000306518603400202. PMID: 3722697.

Main, M. (1990). Cross-cultural studies of attachment organization: Recent studies, changing methodologies, and the concept of conditional strategies. *Human Development, 33*(1): 48–61. doi.org/10.1159/000276502.

Main, M. (1995). Recent studies in attachment: Overview with selected implications for clinical work. In: S. Goldberg, R. Muir, & J. Kerr (Eds.), *Attachment Theory: Social, Development and Clinical Perspectives* (pp. 407–474). Hillsdale, NJ: The Analytic Press.

Novellino, M. (1984). Self-analysis of countertransference in integrative transactional analysis. *Transactional Analysis Journal, 14*(1): 63–67. doi.org/10.1177/036215378401400110.

O'Reilly-Knapp, M. (2001). Between two worlds: The encapsulated self. *Transactional Analysis Journal, 31*(1): 44–54. doi.org/10.1177/036215370103100106.

Racker, H. (1968). *Transference and Countertransference*. Madison, CT: International Universities Press.

Thoreau, H. D. (1862). *Walking*. In: R. Finch & J. Elder (Eds.), *The Norton Book of Nature Writing* (p. 192). New York: W. W. Norton, 2002. https://theatlantic.com/magazine/archive/1862/06/walking/304674/.

Wallin, D. J. (2007). *Attachment in Psychotherapy*. New York: Guilford.

CHAPTER 8

Allan: internal criticism and shame, physical sensations, and affect

Richard G. Erskine

> *It is joy to be hidden but disaster not to be found.*
> —D. W. Winnicott, *The Maturational Processes and the Facilitating Environment* (1965, p. 186)

During the summer recess, Allan was periodically in my thoughts. I was not certain that he would return to the psychotherapy sessions we had scheduled for the beginning of September because I had often sensed that we had a tenuous interpersonal connection. Allan was accustomed to doing things on his own. His quietness was illusive. He had occasionally commented about his internal criticism, and once in a while I heard a caustic remark about his coworkers or himself. I wondered about the extent of his criticisms, the history of his isolated attachment pattern, and the self-stabilizing functions of his relational withdrawal.

I was pleased when Allan returned. He was bustling with energy as he told me about his adventures in the Arctic wilderness. I was touched by the little snippets of connection between us that were interspersed with the stories of his adventures. I still had a developmental image of Allan as a lonely boy, hungry to be listened to and understood and at the same time deeply afraid of interpersonal contact (Erskine, 2019, p. 14). In the midst of one of his stories, he made a tangential comment: "There were no women to look at." I did not know what this meant, but I suspected that it was significant. It seemed important that I not comment on this remark while he was telling me lively stories about hiking and camping.

When Allan said, "There were no women to look at," my first thought was, "Of course there were no women to look at when camping alone in the wilderness." I pondered what his words might mean. Did I misperceive what he said? Although I was a bit confused, I thought it wise to wait to raise the question until I sensed he was receptive to discussing it. Among the important things that I learned from the writings of Eric Berne was to listen to every word the client says, particularly their parenthetical and tangential comments. It is in these utterances that the client reveals their unconscious organizing principles, which Berne (1972) called *script*. I was confident that Allan had inadvertently revealed something significant and made a note to investigate his comment once we had established a more trusting bond.

During September, I continued to listen to Allan's stories about his camping adventures. I looked at his professional-quality photos of wild animals and waited for opportunities to inquire about his internal experiences. He seemed a bit more tolerant of my questions than he had been the previous winter and spring, but frequently there were long silent pauses or no answer. He remained reluctant to talk about his affect or family history. When I asked about possible sadness, fear, or shame, he seemed unable to relate it to himself. He understood the sensations of anger but said, "I do my best to purge my anger."

After a few sessions that seemed unproductive to me, I was frustrated with Allan's apparent lack of emotion and superficial conversation. I had been waiting for an authentic expression of his inner life. Who was he under his social facade? What was the essence of Allan? Was his true self the man whose life was limited to work and hiking? Was he hiding his vulnerability or some big secret? I discussed my confusion with a valued colleague who raised even more questions, and over the next several days I remained perplexed as I pondered them:

- Was Allan actively avoiding letting me know about his inner process? If so, what was I doing wrong or failing to do? Was I too focused on his accomplishing something in therapy? Or would it be beneficial if I attended to the Allan who learned to hide his vulnerability?
- Was he so physically numb that he could not sense his affect? If so, it would be necessary for me to focus the therapy on his body and inchoate affect. Was his noncommunication an expression of shame?
- Was he one of those children who had no one to help them identify internal sensations and provide a way to talk about subjective experience? If so, my task was to help him identify internal sensations and develop a vocabulary for talking about his affect. This approach included constructing a narrative about his life.

I hypothesized that the direction I was looking for was embedded in the answers to these questions. It was clear to me that Allan needed a good deal of security and sensitive guidance in order to become aware of his inner process. Now it was necessary for me to address Allan differently.

I spent some time in each session bringing Allan's focus to the physical tensions in his body. I drew his attention to his tight chest and neck muscles and related the tensions to possible affect. At my initiation, we also spent a bit of time in each session talking about his "privacy." He described how he had always been private, even in his earliest memories. I suspected that when he spoke of depression he was talking about the sensations of shame (Erskine, 1994, 1995). He remained reluctant to talk about shame, but I returned to the topic for a few minutes in each session. He said that his depression (meaning shame) was "a great silencer."

I inquired about the nature of conversations he might have had with his mother when he was a young child. Each time his immediate answer was "I don't remember." I pointed out that he knew his mother's personality and that he could imagine the quality of their communication. In response, Allan sarcastically said, "My mother knew nothing about me or my feelings." In the next sessions, I tried to return to this topic, but Allan responded, "I've said enough about her." His reticence to talk about his relationship with his mother spoke louder than words. His pain and anger were palpable, even though he tried to keep them out of our conversation. I was willing to be patient, but I was also persistent in my focus on his feelings. I made a few inquiries about his relationship with his mother in each session.

A revealing dream

Two months into our second year, Allan asked if we could talk about the following dream: "I am trying to get to the Yukon. I rushed to the train station but the train to Montreal was canceled. I kept looking for another train to take me to the wilderness, but none of the trains were running. I don't want to stay in the city with annoying people." I asked Allan to tell the dream again, slowly, and add the following phrase to the end of each sentence: "and this is my life." As he retold the dream and added "this is my life," we paused after each sentence for Allan to sense the meaning of what he was saying.

Then I encouraged him to elaborate on each statement. With the first sentence of the dream he added, "I have no relationships. I am bothered, sad, and lonely, trying to go where there are no people to interfere with me. I am looking for quiet. … And this is my life." He was then silent for several minutes. I watched the tension in his shoulders carefully even though he made no eye contact or acknowledgment that I was in the room. I remained observant and breathed deeply in order to remain present. I knew something important was happening within Allan.

After several minutes of silence, we continued exploring the meaning of the dream. His comment on the second sentence of the dream was, "I have no people in my life because I was just trying to survive, be safe, and wanting no one to bother me." His voice became harsh: "Relationships are a problem. I don't need people. I get tired of people. And this is my life." As he continued, he added, "Something is missing in my life. I am empty. I don't know what it is, but I can't be with people." I was amazed that he was telling me such a personally revealing dream. This was the first time he had spoken so pointedly about his internal experience.

I asked him why he was telling me the dream that day. He said, "Most of the time I don't trust you, but today I wanted you to know my dream." Near the end of the session, I inquired about how he experienced me in that session. He said that he was relieved that I guided him to talk and added, "You didn't make any interpretation. You allowed it to be my dream, my meaning." I still did not have enough information about Allan's intrapsychic life to make a specific interpretation of his dream. Yet, in asking Allan to add "and this is my life," I was making a subtle interpretation about how the dream represented the ways in which Allan was living his life. I periodically use interpretation if I can sense the client's developmental level of functioning and have an understanding of how they think and feel. If I do make an interpretation, it is usually about a child's physical and relational needs and what quality of interpersonal contact may have been missing in the client's significant relationships. Often it is effective if I invite the client to decipher their own meaning.

Allan and I spent the next few weeks discussing the significance of the various elements in his dream, such as his yearning to be in the wilderness with "no one to interfere." When I asked what he experienced when he said "no one to interfere," Allan had two memories of his mother "interrupting me when I was playing" and his older sister "bossing and controlling me." I was elated because this was the first time in a psychotherapy session that he had divulged an explicit childhood memory.

In the next session I began by quoting Allan's statement that "I can't be with people." I asked him to explore what those words meant. I was again surprised when he offered a series of memories from when he was nine, eleven, and fifteen years old and wanted to be with friends. But he ended up disappointed and discouraged because they would tell him what to do. He said, "I hate people telling me what to do." This was the first time since the previous spring that he provided an opening to talk about his anger. However, he said that he did not feel any anger and dismissed my inquiry with a scathing voice: "I just can't be with people." His self-criticism was evident. I knew that we would soon have to address his self-critical comments because they were becoming more prominent in his conversations with me.

I kept thinking about his statement the day we explored the meaning of his dream: "Something is missing in my life." I waited for some clue to investigate with Allan what that meant and how it affected his life. I intuitively knew that the phrase was significant. I made a few inquiries, but Allan deflected my questions. I asked Allan what he was feeling during his late night walks around the city. He had great difficulty describing his sensations, and I introduced the word "lonely." At first he did not comprehend that there was such a feeling. He described it as "feeling empty." In subsequent sessions, we used the words "empty" and "lonely" interchangeably to talk about what he was feeling during his nighttime excursions. I often thought that his lonely feelings might have been even more significant than what we were discussing. I made a note to come back to loneliness in future sessions. But for now, we were dealing with several entwined issues that had to be put to rest before we did any in-depth work on his unconscious pattern of isolated attachment.

During this phase of the therapy, I periodically asked how Allan perceived my behavior and my effect on him. He was usually slow to answer, as though he was struggling to comprehend something. For example, in one session he said that I was "kind" to him and that I did not "interfere" with what he was thinking. I asked him if my behavior was similar or different from his mother's. With strain in his face he described the contrast between my "acceptance" of him and his mother's "constant disapproval." Over the next few weeks I inquired more about his mother's behavior, particularly his experience of her when he was young. He gave me little fragments of stories, and piece by piece the various stories began to form a picture of his mother dominating Allan's feelings and behavior.

On some occasions when I inquired about Allan's mother's behavior toward him, he gave his usual response: "I don't remember." I described how significant memories are stored in our body tissues and our emotional reactions and how unconscious relational expectations are formed in early childhood. Whenever I talked about how people function, Allan seemed captivated, like a little boy listening to an adult telling an exciting story. As we talked about ways of being in relationship, he said, "You don't act like I expect. You're interested in me." I acknowledged his comment with a historical inquiry: "Was anyone not respectful and not interested in you?" In the long silence that followed, I could see that he was struggling to answer. Eventually he said, "She was unrelenting in her criticism." Then he looked away and was silent for the last few minutes of the session. Although he said nothing, he looked sad. I wondered if he was trying to "purge" his anger.

The flow of psychotherapy

As I studied my notes to write this story of Allan's psychotherapy, I was aware that our therapy work progressed in a nonlinear way. I wish I could tell his story as a simple progression from one insight to the next, from one self-expression to the next, and how each phase of our work led directly to the resolution of another issue. But that is not the way it happened. Rather, we recycled various issues several times. In writing this case study, I am organizing the story chronologically, but readers should keep in mind that what we discussed in one session was often not mentioned again until much later. Some of what I am reporting here may appear repetitive because, indeed, that is often how the rhythm and pattern of psychotherapy goes.

Usually, in each of Allan's sessions, we addressed a variety of topics, such as his walking the streets at night, hiking on the weekends, his internal criticisms, estrangement from his sister, his physiological reactions and feelings, and our relationship. Early in our work I was quiet, attentively listening and acknowledging the significance of what Allan was saying. As this second year progressed, I became more proactive and often made links to what we had discussed in previous sessions. I inquired much more about his phenomenological experience and his childhood. One of my therapeutic tasks was to gather and hold the diverse elements of Allan's story in order to help him construct a coherent narrative about his life.

Self-criticism and shame

During the next few sessions, I made several other inquiries about Allan's mother's disdainful attitudes toward him, how he coped with her criticisms, and how he perceived our interactions. By periodically focusing on the characteristics of our relationship, the juxtaposition of my behavior and his mother's, stimulated Allan to recall several disheartening memories of how she had treated him (Erskine, 2015, p. 17). Over the next months, he had a number of additional memories of his mother finding fault with him. Often they were only fragments of a memory: an image, a body reaction, or the sense of repulsion that left him "feeling low down" and "empty." These bits of memory provided an opportunity for me to engage further in both historical and phenomenological inquiry. We were slowly assembling various pieces of a puzzle about a little boy who learned to hide his loneliness and show the world that he was self-sufficient.

Our therapeutic dialogue now provided more openings for me to bring Allan's focus to his physiological reactions and what was happening in his muscles. We began to form a vocabulary to describe both the muscle tension in his back and some of his affects. In the first year and a half, he had been unable to talk about his feelings. Now when he was occasionally feeling vulnerable, he made several attempts to verbalize his internal distress. My comments were aimed at increasing his awareness of physiological sensations and integrating his body reactions with his various affects. Then the focus was on integrating his affect with understanding his motivations and behavior. This reflected a goal of integrative psychotherapy, which is the integration of the client's physiology, affect, and cognition so that behavior is, by choice, in the current context and not activated by fear, compulsion, or conditioning.

In some sessions, Allan was now able to talk about being angry at his mother's treatment of him. Usually I encouraged him to look directly at me as he told me about his anger at her criticism and control. I wanted him to see my face and that I was taking his anger seriously. I also wanted him to see my sorrow about the way his mother had treated him. Eventually, I asked him to close his eyes and talk to the image of the young woman who "criticized, manipulated, and controlled" him. At first, voicing his anger to an image of his mother was difficult, but after a couple of sessions he was able to vehemently express it.

I pointed out how sad, even painfully lonely, it must be for a child to be constantly criticized. In one session, Allan seemed amazed as I explained that it was emotionally confusing when a child was sad, angry, and scared at the same time, particularly if there is no adult to help them understand and express what they are feeling. He responded ironically, "My feelings did not matter to her." I blurted out, "They matter to me!" He was quiet and his eyes were moist. In a soft voice he said, "Thank you."

It was late November, time for the Thanksgiving holiday, and Allan had a week off from work. He went winter camping in the mountains. When he returned to therapy he surprised me by talking about how he missed me. I asked what he missed. He answered that I was "quiet, patient, not demanding like my mother. You never criticize me. I like coming here … some of the time." I was amazed at what seemed like a transformative opening in our relationship. We went on to talk about other issues, and by the end of the session Allan appeared to be withdrawn again. Just as the session was finishing, I asked what he was thinking. He slowly answered, "I'm a fool for telling you. Now you won't want to work with me." His self-criticism had superseded all that we had talked about.

I was reminded how people who use a schizoid process to manage their affect may feel a sense of attachment and affection with another person when they are physically distant but that they fearfully withdraw into hiding when in close proximity (Galgut, 2010; Yontef, 2001). After some sessions with Allan, I reflected on the similarities between Allan and Harry Heller, the schizoid protagonist in Hermann Hesse's (1927) novel *Steppenwolf*. Hess artfully described the schizoid processes in his central character, who spends most of his time in an internal world of fantasized relationships while his actual life is devoid of interpersonal contact. Guntrip (1968) referred to this as life half in relationship and half out—a stranger to intimate relationships except those that exist in the person's mind.

During these couple of months, I began to notice a new pattern with Allan. In the previous year, he had made several passing references to how he criticized himself after each therapy session. At that time I primarily listened rather than probed with questions. It seemed important that I observe his process and attend to resonating with Allan's affect or unarticulated relational needs. Now some of our sessions began with Allan describing how he had chastised himself during the previous week. At first I assumed that he was replaying his mother's criticisms, but I was surprised when he described the criticism as being his own voice. I wanted to know about the intensity and vehemence of his self-criticism.

Over the next few sessions, I encouraged him to let me hear what was happening inside him, even to shout the criticisms out loud. When he finally spoke, the forcefulness of his words was lethal: "I'm useless," "I'm a weakling," "No one's interested in me." My encouragement for Allan to say the self-criticisms aloud was based on a fundamental Gestalt therapy concept: intrapsychic conflict is diminished when it is externalized (Baumgardner & Perls, 1975; Perls, 1973). I was certain that each criticism added to Allan's sense of feeling "low down" and "empty." While Allan shouted his self-criticisms, I responded with empathy to the vulnerable part of him that was receiving the criticisms.

I made sure that in each session I took some time to address these various self-criticisms. It became clear to me that although Allan wanted to talk to me each week, he was also disdainful of that wish. He rebuked himself for being "self-centered" and for "talking about feelings." He criticized himself and me for "talking about my mother and the past." He was again retreating from contact with me. It took weeks of tentative inquiry and much encouragement for Allan to tell me more of what was happening on the inside: "I'm a fool for going to therapy," "I don't have any needs," and "I'm worthless."

Eventually, I discovered that as he walked home from our sessions, he repeatedly told himself, "Feelings waste mental energy." We learned that he was most critical of himself when we had attended to his emotions or when I made reference to what children need from a sensitive parent. These brief moments of intimacy were discomforting for Allan. He had no memory of anyone else being attentive to what he needed or felt. One day, as Allan was leaving a session, he said, "When you are nice to me, the criticism begins."

As we addressed his internal criticism, it began to subside. Allan was able to talk about his childhood, how his mother was "cold and rigid," and that he sometimes felt "lost and low down." When I periodically described what every child needs in a healthy child/parent relationship, he was astonished. In the next few sessions, he was vulnerable and described being sad about what was missing between him and his mother. I was feeling good about our work together because Allan's awareness of his body, affect, and anticipations seemed to be increasing.

In each session, we were now talking about his continuing sense of shame and relating it to what he termed "turning inward." With tears in his eyes, he described a deep sadness because he was not accepted by his mother and sister for "who I am." He was afraid to express his uniqueness because "I know they will reject me." We also talked about the necessity of hiding his anger "because they will overpower me with their nasty comments. Mother was a controlling bitch." He described how he would hide in his bedroom for several hours each day and watch nature shows on TV. He told me how he could hide even when he was at the breakfast or dinner table with his mother and sister: "It is simple. I just remain private, and they're never curious about who I am. They tell me who they think I am and how I should be. But they don't know the real me."

To trust or not to trust

I was surprised when Allan began a session by saying, "I know you criticize me when you go home. You're nice to me in the office because I pay you. But you really don't like who I am." He was doubtful about staying in therapy. After listening to Allan's uncertainty for half an hour, I talked to him about how he had allowed himself to be vulnerable in my presence and how he had been sharing his emotional experiences with me. I suggested that sharing his internal processes may have disrupted how he had learned to manage his life and that terminating our psychotherapy sessions might restore an old perception of himself. Although he did not immediately respond, Allan seemed pensive. When the session ended, I assumed that my hypothesis had stimulated him to think about how he had been frightened of his increased awareness of his fear, sadness, and shame.

Early in the next session, Allan said that when he was at home, he thought that he could trust me, but when he was walking to our sessions he was certain that I was not trustworthy, that I would eventually criticize him and he would have to quit the therapy. Allan was actively transferring his emotional memories of his relationship with his mother into our relationship. I realized that it was his unconscious attempt to demonstrate his childhood relationship with his mother, the relational needs that were thwarted, and how he compensated for the damaging effects of his mother's criticisms by imagining my potential criticisms (Erskine, 1991). My task was to decode the unconscious childhood stories that were encoded in his transferential transactions, which were entrenched in his self-contained affect and embedded in his lack of relationships (Erskine, 2009). This was a ripe opportunity for more inquiry about the internal effects of his mother's criticisms and the various ways in which he could not rely on her. Although some of the theme was the same, the details of his life kept unfolding.

In the next session, I began by asking if Allan had any memory of my criticizing him. He answered, "No. Maybe you do it silently." Then, after several minutes, he said, "I'll eventually hear some negative comment about me." After a pause, "But you never do." Again we focused on the juxtaposition between my attitude and behavior toward him and what he had experienced with his mother. The contrast stimulated additional memories of his mother's "despising behavior" toward him. Now I was able to appreciate and modulate the responsive countertransference that had been engendered within me: I wanted to be a companion to him in the way that a five- to seven-year-old boy needs a father who listens, understands, and guides without any ridicule.

In one of the sessions during which he was imagining that I would reject him, I added my subjective experience by commenting, "I feel privileged to work with you. And your uncertainty about our relationships is central in the story of how you lived your early life." After a pause in which we were both quiet, I added, "You needed security in your relationship with your mother and her criticisms interfered with that security." His eyes teared up. He responded with, "My security was in my own room with my little TV. I watched the nature shows, over and over. They were my escape."

Self-criticism: a distraction from criticism

One day when he was paying for his therapy sessions, I was startled by his sarcasm directed toward me. When walking home, I recalled several occasions when Allan had criticized his coworkers. His criticisms were often slight or parenthetical, but I now realized that his negative remarks were frequent. I was disappointed in myself because I had missed the significance of his various criticizing comments. But, unlike Allan, I did not chastise myself. Instead, I wondered what was happening within Allan, what was unexpressed, and the functions of his criticisms of others.

In looking over my notes for the first year of Allan's psychotherapy, I discovered that I had made only one notation regarding his derogatory comments about other people. I had presumed that his disparaging remarks were his attempt to express controlled anger. As I reflected on other snide comments that Allan had made, I realized that I had disregarded my discomfort. Clients' sarcasm and ridicule usually put me on high alert because they may provide a momentary glimpse of the person's internal organization. I was concerned: Were his criticisms of people a projection and therefore a momentary relief from his own self-criticism? Were the belittling comments an active expression of what he had introjected from his mother and sister? Or did the criticisms he absorbed as a child activate his self-criticism of others?

I began our next session with a relational inquiry about how he experienced our interpersonal contact. A relational inquiry encompasses a series of questions about how the client perceives the psychotherapist and the quality of the mutual relationship, particularly what may be missing (Erskine, 2021). Relational inquiry is effective if the psychotherapist remains empathetic and is open to learning from the client's perspective. At first Allan did not recall his sarcastic comment. Then he defended it as "normal" and said, "That's just the way I talk." I asked him to think about the effect his criticisms might have on both me and other people.

He was pensive and then described how his mother's remarks always left him feeling shame for being who he was. He realized that he was inflicting shame on others. We wondered together if this is how he avoided his own feelings of shame.

It was evident that Allan had a pattern of criticizing. In the following session I made an interpretation composed of three points: that he had been sarcastic with me, that he frequently criticized others, and that he criticized himself just like his mother had treated him. He immediately tried to apologize to me, but I suggested that there was something more important than an apology. What was most important was that he understood the functions of his criticism as the first step in changing what he had been doing. In that same session, I took the opportunity to talk to him about the concept of introjection and explained how children will unconsciously identify with the detrimental behavior of their parents as a way to not feel rejection, hurt, or shame. As a result, later in life they treat either themselves or others in the same way they were treated. Allan grasped the concept quickly and told me some stories about how he acted with coworkers just as his mother had treated him. He was embarrassed by his behavior. I responded that I was more concerned about all the shame he had experienced over so many years because of his mother's disdainful comments.

In several sessions, I noticed that Allan would sometimes hold his breath and then sigh. When I first asked about that pattern, he said, "It's nothing, just the way I breathe." However, I suspected that each sigh was a signal of some internal experience. I continued to inquire about his body sensations, and it became evident that each time he held his breath for a moment and then sighed that he had heard an internal criticism such as "You can't do that" or "People don't want you bothering them." With several phenomenological inquiries, Allan was able to tell me that it sounded just like his mother's disapproving voice. We talked about how discouraging it was to constantly relive his mother's criticism. I asked him to make those comments again and loudly, like he was talking to little Allan. He repeatedly yelled his mother's words, then he lowered his head and was silent for several minutes. When he again looked at me he had tears in his eyes.

As our next session began, Allan said that he had a profound insight. He was "not sure how it works," but he was certain that his self-criticisms were his way of not remembering his mother's criticisms. All week long he was able to remember his mother's harsh tone. He said, "If I criticize myself, I don't hear her." He added, "Now I realize that she ridiculed me all the time, even before I went to school." We talked about how his self-criticism became more prevalent and vociferous than his mother's and a distraction from the emotional pain of his mother's words. His posture changed, and the tension in his face and shoulders relaxed as he cried.

We spent the next couple of sessions talking about his childhood and the effects of his mother's criticisms and disapproval on him at each developmental age. He again cried about how he had "always tried to hide from her." Over the next few weeks, he reported that he "stopped criticizing myself" and added "I criticized myself to stop her from controlling me, but what I say to myself is much worse and more frequent. I feel a lot of what you call 'shame.'

Then I go to my private inner room." I was curious about Allan's "private inner room" but I did not inquire. Spring was in full bloom, and we had many loose ends of the work to deal with before the summer break.

That spring we spent a good deal of time talking about Allan's shame and how shame was the result of both his internal criticism and the criticism he received in his family. Back in September, when I had first used the word "shame," he did not understand. Later he realized that his feeling "low down" and "depressed" were the symptoms of shame. He said that when he was "low down" he had always known that "something is wrong with me." He was now able to recall several incidents of his mother saying "What's wrong with you, boy?" whenever he was playful or loud. He described how throughout his life he had held himself back in any situation in which someone might tell him he was wrong. He added, "I always go to my private inner room." As he recalled these memories, he had an "empty feeling" in his belly and tension in his back. I had compassion for the loneliness of the boy who had such a mother.

As we discussed his body sensations, he was able to talk about being sad for not being accepted for how he was and his fear of rejection if he said what he thought or felt. He talked about how he believed his mother and began to say to himself "something is wrong with me. I have to hide." To protect himself from his mother's ridicule, he spent most of his time in his room. I reminded Allan that he had previously said that he "purged" himself of anger. We spent several sessions talking about how he worked to "keep silent," "hide in my room," and told himself "something's wrong with me" every time he felt angry. "I refused to be angry like her. I purged myself of anger, but I was depressed instead."

Allan was now actively telling me about his anger at his mother. On three occasions he grabbed a pillow and shook it with anger. He imagined it was his mother and that he was holding her by the neck. He shouted at her, "Nothing is wrong with me. I am a normal boy!" During those sessions, I encouraged him to physically express what he was feeling. I acknowledged his need to protest and validated the significance of both his anger and his sadness.

It was again time for summer recess. He agreed to return to psychotherapy the first week of September. He was looking forward to two summer events: walking the Appalachian Trail with the hiking club he had recently joined and taking a month-long camping trip in the Arctic. At the last session before the break, he expressed "a bit of worry" because last year he had felt "empty" when he was in the Arctic. He did not want to feel that way again. I again translated Allan's word "empty" and offered the word "lonely" as a description of his visceral/affect experience. I knew we had more to discover when he returned in September.

References

Berne, E. (1972). *What Do You Say After You Say Hello? The Psychology of Human Destiny*. New York: Grove.

Baumgardner, P., & Perls, F. (1975). *Gifts from Lake Cowichan: Legacy from Fritz*. Palo Alto, CA: Science and Behavior Books.

Erskine, R. G. (1991). Transference and transactions: Critique from an intrapsychic and integrative perspective. *Transactional Analysis Journal, 21*(2): 63–76. doi.org/10.1177/036215379102100202.

Erskine, R. G. (1994). Shame and self-righteousness: Transactional analysis perspectives and clinical interventions. *Transactional Analysis Journal, 24*(2): 86–102. doi.org/10.1177/036215379402400204.

Erskine, R. G. (1995). A Gestalt therapy approach to shame and self-righteousness: Theory and methods. *British Gestalt Journal, 4*(2): 107–117.

Erskine, R. G. (2009). Life scripts and attachment patterns: Theoretical integration and therapeutic involvement. *Transactional Analysis Journal, 39*(3): 207–218. doi.org/10.1177/036215370903900304.

Erskine, R. G. (2015). *Relational Patterns, Therapeutic Presence: Concepts and Practice of Integrative Psychotherapy*. London: Karnac.

Erskine, R. G. (2019). Child development in integrative psychotherapy: Erik Erikson's first three stages. *International Journal of Integrative Psychotherapy, 10*: 11–34.

Erskine, R. G. (2021). *A Healing Relationship: Commentary on Therapeutic Dialogues*. Bicester, UK: Phoenix.

Galgut, D. (2010). *In a Strange Room*. Toronto, Canada: McClelland & Stewart.

Guntrip, H. (1968). *Schizoid Phenomena, Object Relations and the Self*. Madison, CT: International Universities Press.

Hesse, H. (1927). *Steppenwolf*. New York: Henry Holt, 1929.

Perls, F. (1973). *The Gestalt Approach and Eye Witness to Therapy*. Palo Alto, CA: Science and Behavior Books.

Winnicott, D. W. (1965). *The Maturational Processes and the Facilitating Environment: Studies in the Theory of Emotional Development*. Madison, CT: International Universities Press.

Yontef, G. (2001). Psychotherapy of schizoid process. *Transactional Analysis Journal, 31*(1): 7–23. doi.org/10.1177/036215370103100103.

CHAPTER 9

Allan: isolation, loneliness, and a need to be loved

Richard G. Erskine

The third year of Allan's psychotherapy began with him telling me the details of his summer vacation, complete with exquisite photos of Arctic foxes and polar bears. He was always excited when he talked about his photography. After the first twenty minutes, I inquired about his internal criticism, something we had been working on a good deal in his psychotherapy the previous spring. He said that he was "less tense because there was almost no self-criticism." I made several inquiries about Allan's internal experience, and he described his sense of comfort when camping alone. He looked down and was silent for a couple of minutes. Then he added, "I felt empty, what you call lonely." With my continued inquiry, Allan talked about his mixed feelings of enjoying the solitary experience of the wilderness and, at the same time, realizing that something was missing that felt like "an emptiness in my stomach."

I surprised myself when I blurted out, "Were there any women to look at?" I remembered the tangential comment Allan had made the previous September when he said, "There were no women to look at." He turned his head away and was silent. I immediately knew that my remark was disturbing to him.

I was embarrassed by my indiscreet comment. My remark was not empathic with Allan's telling me about his empty, lonely feelings. I searched internally for what had prompted my inappropriate question. Usually it is easy for me to be empathic with clients' feelings of loneliness. I was perplexed. Was my countertransference a reaction, an expression of some unresolved aspect of myself, or was I identifying with some unspoken characteristic of Allan? I did not know, and I did not know what else to say so I remained quiet. I needed time to consider how to repair the rupture in our relationship. After some minutes, Allan returned to telling me about his vacation, but his facial expression had changed; his enthusiasm was gone.

Although he was talking, it seemed to me that he was putting on a social facade composed of pleasant but non-meaningful conversation. Throughout most of the previous spring, Allan's social facade had disappeared after a number of sessions in which we attended to his internal criticism and particularly after Allan realized that his self-criticism distracted him from remembering his mother's harsh criticisms of him.

At the end of the summer, when I thought about Allan returning to psychotherapy, I began to formulate a treatment plan. If he was no longer suffering from internal criticism, I planned to invite him into a series of therapeutically supported withdrawals into his "private inner room." I could observe how he often relied on relational withdrawal to stabilize and regulate himself, but I surmised that he was alone in his "private room." I firmly believe that the healing of cumulative neglect and trauma occurs through a contactful therapeutic relationship (Erskine, 2015). So, if we did engage in a therapeutically supported withdrawal, it would mean that I would have to be fully present with him, to listen to him if he spoke and even to his silences, to be an external guardian of his quiet and private place, and to help him process his affect and implicit memories. I had learned from other clients who used relational withdrawal to self-stabilize and ward off anticipated emotional invasion that a supported withdrawal provided the space and opportunity for them to feel viscerally more secure and validated. It was an opportunity to identify their own, often nonverbal, experience (Erskine, 2020). However, my plan was suddenly placed on hold. We had an urgent situation that required a different therapeutic posture.

Throughout the week, I was worried about the effects of my behavior. It was clear to me that my error had triggered a breach in our therapeutic relationship. Prior to that session, I had decided to take direct responsibility by opening the next session with, "I want to apologize for my lack of sensitivity to you when you told me about feeling empty. My question was inconsiderate. What happened between us when I asked about 'women to look at'?" When Allan heard those words, he hung his head in silence. I assumed that I had again caused him to feel a sense of shame. He looked away, his face was tense, and he remained silent for the next several minutes.

Allan eventually looked at me and said, "I guess I had better tell you the truth." There was another long pause and he added, "I'm so tense. You'll think I'm demented." There were a few minutes of silence, during which I remembered the previous year when we had spent many sessions talking about the various dimensions of his sense of shame: hiding his shame by avoiding people, the sadness in his conviction that he was not worthy of anyone's attention, his fear of ridicule and rejection, and his core belief that "something is wrong with me." He had just said, "You will think I'm demented." Was he again recoiling from internal criticism? Was he making a confession?

I honored Allan's silence but continued looking at him. I tried to communicate acceptance through my facial expressions. He then said, "That's what I do at night." I was not certain what he meant, but I knew that it was important to wait in silence while something churned inside Allan. After another long pause he said, "I have never told anyone … when I go walking at night, I am looking for a woman." With a nod I acknowledged what he had just said but made no direct comment. I knew that my patience was a valuable form of interpersonal contact, and it seemed important that I go at his pace. He was quiet for a couple of minutes and then added, "There are several women that I watch. I know what time they get off work and I follow them home." Allan was again silent. While he hung his head I thought about how painful shame can be: the intense sadness at not being accepted as one is and the fear of rejection for who one is.

After a few more minutes of quiet, I made what I hoped would be a normalizing comment: "There must be some important reason you are looking at them." He was again silent for several minutes. I repeated my comment. He looked at me and with tears in his eyes said, "I'm lonely." Slowly, bit by bit, we talked about the empty feeling inside his stomach and how he had some relief when he followed a woman and wondered what it would be like to be with her in her home.

In response to my gentle inquiry, he talked about the pain of loneliness. He described how he always felt "low down" when he finally returned to his apartment. Throughout that session, Allan was physically tense, caught between wanting to reveal his story and his reluctance to say anything. I decided to reassure Allan that he was not "demented," and I explained that his watching the women had some important psychological functions. I promised him that in our coming sessions we would explore his desire to watch them and, importantly, what he was needing as he searched for a woman.

Although I tried to reassure Allan, I ended the session with an intense mixture of thoughts and emotions. I felt compassion for Allan; he was lonely and depressed. Simultaneously, I was alarmed. I had a fantasy of Allan stalking the women, of his being a sexual predator, or worse. I had a duty to uncover Allan's intentions, to discover if he was "demented," to determine if he was dangerous to the women, and, if necessary, to protect them by reporting him to the authorities. I suddenly felt overwhelmed with responsibility. As Allan was leaving my office, I ran after him and invited him to return the next day for another session. He was reluctant. But later he called me to say that he was willing to come at lunchtime for an additional session because he had more to tell me.

When Allan arrived for that next session, he was physically tense. He made no eye contact and seemed to be withdrawn to some internal hiding place. I waited patiently, mostly in silence. I interspersed the silence with a few comments such as "I'm here for you," "There is no need to rush," "There must be a lot of feelings going on inside." After about twenty minutes, he looked at me and said, "What am I going to do?" At that moment, I sensed a little boy, lonely, depressed, and not knowing how to feel better. I was in a dilemma about whether to address the troubled child in Allan or to alleviate my internal tension and worry. I had spent part of the previous night distressed about Allan's behavior and the possibility that he was a potential danger to women. I spontaneously decided to use this session to directly address my worries. I asked him, "Do you have any sexual fantasies about these women?" Allan immediately responded with "Oh, no! I never do that." I continued with, "Do you ever want to hurt them?" At first he was appalled that I asked such questions, and then with tears in his eyes he said, "I only want them to be with me."

During the next several sessions, Allan described the stories he had invented regarding the women he followed at night. I consistently and continuously inquired about these various fantasies and particularly about his body sensations, affects, and hopes. A theme in Allan's stories included his imagining that the various women would be happy to be with him. As I learned more about Allan's imagined encounters, we identified that the most important themes included his fantasy that the women were kind to him, wanted to tell him stories about their lives, and were delighted to listen to his stories. Allan's imaginings were full of details about his hoped-for relationship with the women, such as their pleasure in having dinner together, discovering their joy in hiking with Allan, and the excitement of doing photography together. In each of his stories there was an imagined joyous connection between Allan and a woman. Near the end of one of our sessions, he confessed that, while following the women, he would repeatedly say to himself, "Can you love me?" However, by the time he returned home he was depressed.

I continued to wonder if sexual activity had any place in his fantasy. During our therapeutic dialogue, I interspersed some questions about his sexuality. From the various things Allan said I had the impression that he was not imagining anything sexual with the women. I asked some direct questions about his sexual history. Allan told me that he had a girlfriend when he was fourteen, they had kissed a lot, but he had felt guilty because he had touched her breasts. His mother had become enraged when she discovered that he was spending time after school with the girl and forbade him to see her again. He never had another girlfriend, never dated, and avoided any conversations with women. His life was sexless. I asked if he masturbated, looked at pornography magazines, or watched erotic videos. Allan was surprised by my questions and answered "No" to each of them. But in responding to my questions about masturbation, he described how his mother "was furious with me when she saw stains on my bed sheets. So, I stopped touching myself."

In between our sessions, I thought about the possible homeostatic functions that might be involved in Allan's silent quest for a woman, such as:

- Emotional regulation of his loneliness and depression
- An identity and sense of value in "who I am"
- An orientation of himself in relationship with women
- Compensation for unsatisfied relational needs
- Self-protection against the memory of the pain and fear of loss of interpersonal connection with his mother.

My heart went out to Allan when I realized that we had a great deal of work ahead.

We spent time talking about his "empty, lonely feelings." I validated the significance of his internal question, "Can you love me?" Now Allan repeatedly talked about being an "unloved child." Together we interpreted his mantra, "Can you love me?" as the lament of a neglected yet controlled child who yearned to be loved. During some of these conversations,

Allan cried. I watched for signs of anger but his sadness predominated. I focused on responding empathically and helped him to identify his current relational needs for validation, companionship, and self-definition. Periodically, he would slip into a withdrawn place. He would become silent, hunch his shoulders, and not respond to any of my inquiries. Sometimes it seemed that these reactions stimulated Allan to shrink even more into himself.

In another session I asked if he had ever spoken to any of the women. His body seemed strained as he answered, "I would never do that." As we talked more he said, "Then it will all go bad. She won't want me." I explored with Allan what he imagined would happen if one of the women wanted a relationship with him. He answered, "They will try to control me. They will criticize me." He pulled into himself and was quiet. Throughout this period of time I sensed that my inquiry and comments had to be delicate, and I was sensitive to how quickly Allan could slip into silence. I began to encourage him to take time to withdraw into his private place, to feel whatever he felt, to experience a sense of quietness or any memories. During these prolonged moments, I would quietly watch over him, just as though I were watching over a sick child.

In another session, Allan was "deeply discouraged." He had discovered that a waitress whom he frequently followed had a husband and two children. He was distraught: "I lost my dream." I responded to his sadness as though he had actually been betrayed by a partner. I talked to him about grief as he told me how he had longed to be with her. He was angry that she was married and not available. He then spontaneously talked about his mother: "She was never there for me. I was always alone. I am still alone." He then wept in childlike grief for the betrayal of a real person, his mother.

In each of the next few sessions I made historical inquiries about Allan's relationship with his mother during the years he was five to fifteen, after his father died. Allan increasingly had memories of how he responded to the "criticisms heaped on me" by both his mother and sister: "When they weren't hassling me they ignored me. But that was fine with me because I could be alone in my room." As I inquired about what he was experiencing internally when he was in his room, he replied, "I closed up inside. I guess I was protecting something. I told myself 'nothing matters.'" I inquired about what he was protecting, and he described the tensions in his stomach and chest. I suggested that the tension in his body was loneliness.

I could see that periodically Allan was briefly looking away and/or tensing his jaw muscles. I took advantage of those moments to invite him to close his eyes and go to his "private room." I promised him that I would neither come near nor would I go away but that I would stay present. At first he withdrew for only a couple of minutes, and then he would open his eyes to see if I was still attentive. Over the next many sessions, he was able to withdraw to his private place for longer periods of time. I sat quietly, observing each breath and the little gestures that he made.

After one session when Allan was in his private place for about twenty minutes, he described it as "cool and quiet and that's the way I like it." I offered that perhaps that was why he liked camping in the Arctic. He seemed to enjoy that comment and ironically said, "My mother was hot tempered and noisy … the farther from her the better. That's why I like it cold and quiet." We made an interesting discovery. Following withdrawals to his private place (usually for about ten to fifteen minutes), he was more relationally contactful and somewhat playful. It was as though his energy had been replenished with spontaneity and vitality.

A few weeks later, Allan was disturbed by a dream. He said that he knew the dream was significant. He was conflicted because he did not want to think about it, but he wanted to know what it meant. We talked about his ambivalence around knowing and not knowing before we attended to the content of the dream. Almost inaudibly he uttered, "I want to hide from the painful truth." He described the dream: "I am the age I am now but I am carrying a heavy backpack, a big weight, so I feel small. I'm trying to get on an old-style train to go to a faraway camping place. The steam locomotive could not move because a large woman was blocking the track. The woman began to stare at me but she had no face. I noticed that she had large pendulous breasts, but I knew that there was no warmth in them." Allan described how he woke up frightened by the faceless woman. After about an hour, he fell back to sleep, and just before morning he had another short dream: "The same large woman had her back turned to me and was directing a crowd of people, telling them what to do. She and the crowd of her faceless admirers continued to block the track. I was stuck on a cold train platform. I woke up with a low-down feeling, what you call depressed." Allan then said, "Last time you asked me to analyze the dream, but now I want you to tell me what it means." I was momentarily stymied; dream analysis is always idiosyncratic, visionary, and relational. Allan was directly requesting my involvement in his understanding of his dream experience. This alone was a significant change in his demeanor. To me he seemed like a young boy asking his father, "What does it mean?" I needed a few moments to think. I wanted to speak to him heart to heart. It seemed imperative that my words provide some healing understanding. Eric Berne (1961) described the therapist's use of a duplex transaction wherein the psychotherapist talks simultaneously to both the client's adult and child ego states. That was my challenge.

I quickly reviewed all that Allan had told me and realized how this dream captured some of the themes of his life script: being blocked in self-expression and choice, his mother's failure to acknowledge his vulnerability, observing people but without any face-to-face communication, and the absence of human warmth. I had a developmental image of Allan as a five- to six-year-old boy. I decided to tell him a story about how I understood the dream. I talked as though I were speaking to both the young boy and the mature man. I wanted his active involvement in deciphering the meaning of the dream so I decided to interpret the dream in small segments. I began with, "The boy is on the track of life; a boy full of steam and energy." I paused for Allan's reflection. He said nothing but nodded in agreement.

I went on, "He has a heavy weight on his back. It is such a big weight, like a pack full of commands and insults. It is such a big weight, perhaps even painful." Allan appeared to be emotionally moved, his eyes moistened, he swallowed hard but this time he did not turn away. After a few minutes he then said, "Before you, no one has ever understood." Allan motioned me to continue. I added, "He wants to go to a cool and quiet place to camp because the camp is his own private place." Allan answered, "I take that camp with me all day, every day. It is my refuge." I was feeling gratified because Allan was actively cooperating in our co-analysis of his dream, but then we were out of time. Neither Allan nor I wanted to stop. He asked if he could come later in the week for an additional session because he wanted to hear the rest of the story. After he left I rushed to my desk to write the details of his dream before I lost any of it.

Just before Allan arrived for an early Thursday morning appointment, I reread my notes about his dream. I was glad that we had had a two-day break because I could now focus on what I considered the most important element of the dream: the faceless woman. Allan began our session with a new curiosity about how the dream represented his life. As we reviewed what we had talked about on Tuesday, Allan added, "I have always had the weight of her negativity and criticism on my back. I wonder if that is why I can carry a heavy backpack when I go camping. I am used to her weight." After a pause he added, "I am tired of carrying her criticisms. They are not about me. She was unhappy with life. Perhaps she was always irritated with me because I was curious and full of life … until she forced me into hiding."

Allan asked me to continue analyzing his dream. In previous sessions, I had made my interpretation in a metaphorical way by talking about "the boy." As I thought about how well Allan had processed our previous conversations about his dream, I now assumed that he was ready for me to make my interpretation directly about him. I changed my language from "the boy" and "he" to "you." I looked him in the eye as I said, "It must have been impossible for you as a young boy to have a real face-to-face contact with your mother, particularly if she was criticizing and misdefining you. It seems that your mother could not face your uniqueness and vitality. Nor was she sensitive to your vulnerability … but she was able to stop your locomotion. Just like in the dream where the faceless woman stopped the steam locomotive." He said, "Yes, that's it." Allan was silent for a few minutes, but he was not withdrawn. He then looked me in the eyes and keep repeating, "That's it." We spent the rest of the session talking about the loneliness in being constantly criticized. Allan described an almost impossible struggle to define himself in the presence of a domineering mother. He said, "My only option was to withdraw to my private place, and when I got too lonely, I imagined being in the wilderness."

In the next session, Allan was eager to have me continue talking about his dream. I returned to the beginning of the dream with, "In the dream you were trying to go to a faraway camping place; even as a small child you needed to find some place of quiet." After talking a while about my interpretation, Allan exclaimed, "That is how I have always lived, searching for the quiet. I am getting on the train to get away from her but she is always stopping me." We continued with what I thought the dream meant, and then I asked a question: "Allan, you described the woman as 'faceless' and having 'no warmth or sympathy.' That is exactly how you have often described your mother's behavior to you. What do you think it means when you described the faceless woman in the dream as having 'large pendulous breasts?'" Allan quickly answered, "She was always disgusted with her breasts. She blamed me for destroying her figure. She was disgusted with me. That's what stops me in my tracks. There was no warmth or caring in that woman." In the next few sessions Allan had a number of memories about his mother's and sister's treatment of him, and he was angry.

As Christmas approached, Allan said that he was no longer depressed. Since October he had not followed any women. Instead, he spent his evenings working on his photography projects and planning his hiking and camping adventures. He confided that when he saw "a kind-faced woman" he would internally say, "Can you love me?" In several sessions he clearly stated, "My search for women is my longing to have my mother be kind and love me. I know that I will never get my mother to love me." His sadness was intense but he was present.

In the next session, Allan suggested that it might be time to terminate our work together. He talked about how he had changed and was no longer depressed. He wanted to move out of New York City but did not know where: "Some place with rugged mountains, a place for my photography." Although I celebrated the changes he was making, I was bothered by his suggestion of termination. I did not know what else might emerge if we continued to address his internal process. I lacked assurance that we had come to a good conclusion. I was aware that we had not addressed his early childhood, before the age of five when his father died. I talked to Allan about engaging in an investigation of the unknown, what might be unresolved. Out of curiosity he reluctantly agreed to continue until June.

References

Berne, E. (1961). *Transactional Analysis in Psychotherapy: A Systematic Individual and Social Psychiatry*. New York: Grove.

Erskine, R. G. (2015). *Relational Patterns, Therapeutic Presence: Concepts and Practices of Integrative Psychotherapy*. London: Karnac.

Erskine, R. G. (2020). Relational withdrawal, attunement to silence: Psychotherapy of the schizoid process. *International Journal of Integrative Psychotherapy*, *11*: 14–28.

CHAPTER 10

Allan: therapeutic withdrawal and painful memories

Richard G. Erskine

> *The real voyage of discovery consists
> not in seeing new landscapes,
> but in having new eyes.*
> —Marcel Proust, *Remembrance of Things Past* (1929)

After the Christmas holidays, Allan and I resumed our work. Allan usually talked about the events of his past week, his travel and hiking, and what he was doing with his photography. As soon as I had the opportunity, I shifted our conversation to discussing his self-criticism and how it served as a deflection from all the memories of his mother's criticisms. I encouraged Allan to speak his self-criticisms aloud, and we compared those to the degrading comments his mother and sister had actually said to and about him. Allan could see how he was criticizing himself just as his mother had criticized him, but he described his self-criticism as more frequent and harsher than what he remembered from his mother.

Allan was now aware that, since his mother's death about seven years earlier, the self-criticisms had increased. We discussed how the self-criticism served two functions: to distract him from the emotional distress caused by her criticisms and, at the same time, to remain emotionally attached to her by imitating her caustic remarks. These discussions about Allan's self-criticism and how it served to deny the actual criticism from his mother reiterated what we had previously discussed: they strengthened Allan's understanding of his internal conflict, which was composed of wanting a deep emotional connection with his mother and the fear of her constant negation of him.

During some of these conversations, Allan would hold his breath for several seconds and then sigh. I worked with another client who used a schizoid process to manage her relational distress, and it finally dawned on me that, like her, Allan's breathing pattern was his subtle sign of relational withdrawal. Although I had noticed Allan's breathing pattern for a couple of years, I had not attended to its significance. I now realized that Allan was withdrawing right in front of me whenever his affect was aroused. I had planned to initiate supporting Allan in a therapeutic withdrawal the previous September, but I inadvertently made a comment that took us to another important issue. I now decided to attend to Allan's pattern of sighing and to perhaps use it as an opportunity to support him in an ameliorative retreat.

In the next session, when we were talking about Allan's reactions to his mother's stern behavior, I noticed that he was again holding his breath. It was clear that this was an emotion-filled moment. I asked him to close his eyes and go to the security of his private place. I assured him that I would remain present and, importantly, not invade that special space. In the past, I had facilitated some therapeutically supported withdrawal, usually for just a few minutes, to help Allan manage distress. Now I thought that it might be useful if I encouraged and supported his relational disengagement both more frequently and for longer periods of time. I wanted to create a safe place for Allan in which he could experience a caring relationship but on his own terms and at his own pace—a place, perhaps, where he could discover even more of himself.

In response to my suggestion, Allan closed his eyes and silently curled forward with his chest to his legs. Two minutes later, I noticed that he momentarily looked at me. I responded with "I'm right here. I'm relaxed and staying with you." He closed his eyes again. After another couple of minutes I said, "I'm right with you. It is so important to have a quiet place." A few minutes later I added, "It's so necessary to have a safe and quiet place." Allan said nothing, his eyes were still closed, but his head nodded in agreement. He remained withdrawn for another five minutes. I softly reassured him that I was present. When he straightened up and opened his eyes, he looked more relaxed and said that it felt good to "just be quiet."

Halfway through the next session, when I could see Allan looking away, I again asked him to close his eyes and go to his private place. There were several minutes of silence except for my making a few reassuring comments such as, "I'm still here. I'm not going to move closer and I am not going away"; a minute later, "It's so necessary to feel safe"; two minutes later, "Being quiet and safe is so important." This pattern continued for fifteen minutes. With each of these comments, Allan remained silent but slightly nodded his head. When he opened his eyes he said, "The only quiet place I had was when I was watching TV in my room. And even then my mother would shout commands at me. My sister would come in and torment me." He spontaneously closed his eyes and withdrew for several more minutes. When he opened his eyes, he stared at me for a few silent moments and then said, "I wish you could have been with me in my room. You would have made it quiet."

For the next several weeks, in most of our sessions, I continued to suggest that Allan retreat to his safe inner place. He no longer leaned forward with his chest on his knees; now he curled up on the couch. He was able to remain in his internal private place for longer and longer, sometimes for thirty minutes. I continued to make descriptive comments every two to three minutes just to let him know that I was fully present and attentive. I was physically still but attentive to Allan's breathing and gestures.

I had learned from other clients who used a schizoid process to maintain emotional stabilization and regulation that inquiry or questions are disruptive. As one client said, "Questions are an invasive demand." Instead of any inquiry, I made resonating comments every few minutes that indicated my attunement with Allan's inner processes. Some examples were: "It feels so good to be quiet"; "No one is invading your safe place"; "I'm watching over you"; "It is so important to be at rest"; and eventually, "Sometimes it's so lonely inside." I always watched for the agreeing or disagreeing movements of his head. He never said a word when withdrawn, but I had the sense that we were establishing a growing connection between us.

Following twenty minutes of being in his private place, Allan said at one point, "I wanted to be alive but not in my family." Two other notable comments were:

- "In withdrawal I feel peace, a deep sense of quietness and relaxation in all my muscles until the loneliness sets in. It begins in my stomach and climbs up to my chest, and it may jump to the back of my neck; it gives me a dull headache."
- "I have a big pain when I am depending on my mother, wanting her, and knowing that she could never be in touch with me. I needed her but she was only there in her cold body, always wanting me to be a perfect child. I feel so alone because I need her so much, so much that I don't want her anymore. I just want to be alone so that my body is not tense all over."

With each supported withdrawal, an important therapeutic action occurred. Allan was increasingly having vivid memories of specific childhood events. He was often surprised and made comments such as, "I haven't remembered that for years," "I remember how I was trying to hide even before I went to school," "I forgot all about how miserable I felt each night when we were having dinner." He was telling me specific memories that documented what he had previously expressed in general terms. I made sure that we had sufficient time after each supported withdrawal to talk about his emerging memories. The beginnings of our sessions were no longer consumed by a review of his activities; instead, he told me about the childhood memories that he was having during the week. Allan was sad, and, although he did not talk about it, his anger was evident in the tone of his voice and his use of foul language.

In a session that began with Allan describing how he was now "taking photos of urban life," he became abruptly quiet, sighed, and looked away. I asked him to take a moment to go to his private place. After only a few minutes he recalled being about eight years old and how he would make funny faces and dance to try to please his mother. He described how he acted like a clown to get her to play with him. He said, "I remember that I would do anything to amuse her, to make her happy with me. I repeated my little performances many times until she would just walk out of the room. One time stands out in my mind. I remember my stomach aching and running after her. I don't remember her words, but the look on her face made me want to hide. I didn't know the word then, but today I would say she was disgusted with me. I was full of confusion. Today, as I think back, I would say that she was always disgusted with me."

In three different sessions, Allan told me a variation of that story. Each time I felt my stomach churning as I identified with the young boy's desire to be accepted as well as the painful sense of being rejected for doing what seemed so right. My countertransference had two forms: identifying and responsive. Stimulated by my identifying countertransference, I validated the boy's need to be accepted "just as I am." And, stimulated by my responsive countertransference, I talked about a child's joy of playing with an interested and involved adult. Allan cried as I described to him what a child of that age needed in companionship from an adult.

One day Allan was disturbed by a vivid memory from when he was seven years old. His teacher had been screaming at another boy and dragging him out of the classroom by his ear. Allan was terrified. While the teacher was busy he snuck out of the classroom and ran home. He could not get in the house, so the neighbors called his mother at work. When she arrived home, she was furious with Allan. She slapped him across the face and then marched him back to school. Allan had an intense body reaction, horror, and an overwhelming realization that he could never trust his mother or the teacher again. He remembered saying to himself over and over, "I'm all alone, no one will be there for me, I have to do what they say." He repeated those words to himself over the years, particularly when his mother made demands or when teachers gave assignments. Allan learned to anticipate what any adult might say to him and then circumvented their possible criticisms by criticizing himself.

In the remainder of that session, and in the ensuing weeks, I allotted some time to attend to Allan's emotional pain and fear, betrayal and distrust. Although what he had told me was a specific story of an actual event, I often thought of it as a metaphor for many other memories that remained nondescript. They were similar but lacked pictures or language because they were implicit and procedural. We investigated how Allan disengaged from people by transferring his experience of mistrust and betrayal into every relationship. We explored his three script beliefs ("I'm all alone," "No one will be there for me," and "I have to do what they say"), how they manifested in his current life, and how he collected evidence to reinforce each belief. We talked about how each fantasy, when contrasted with reality, served to confirm his various script beliefs (see Erskine, 2015, chapter 7, for a detailed explanation.)

In this same series of sessions, I allocated time to hear about Allan's life, provided time for supported withdrawal, attuned to his affects and rhythm, and took his memories seriously. As with most clients, there were many facets to our therapeutic work. As I studied my notes and reflected on the details of Allan's psychotherapy, I was challenged to write this case study in a logical and understandable sequence because psychotherapy is multidimensional, with many elements requiring deliberation. I often experience myself as working within a many-sided hologram in which every dimension is in some aspect interrelated with several others: body tensions, inchoate affect, self-soothing behaviors, unarticulated stories, and stylized procedures in relating. As I attend to one set of facets, I overlook others. Often, I am attending to two, three, or more psychological issues in one session. Or, I many not attend to some facet for a few weeks and then give it intense attention for a couple more. So please bear with me as I report the story of Allan and the many dimensions of our psychotherapy.

Each week, as we continued the supported withdrawal, Allan's memories were increasingly of a younger age. Never previously talked-about memories seemed to emerge in response to my careful listening and empathic acknowledgment and validation. I repeatedly brought his attention to his body sensations and previously nondescript affect. I talked about what a young child needs from an attuned parent while also creating enough silence for his internal process to gestate.

After Allan withdrew into several minutes of silence, he described his experience at a preschool age: "I always remained quiet when my mother said something because I knew that I must do what she said. It feels like I knew how to be quiet since I was a baby." As our weekly sessions continued, Allan's time in withdrawal was not always calm and secure. He was having body memories, painful physical sensations, and an "intense emptiness in my stomach." When he was withdrawn, I continued making resonating comments.

Allan told me about waking up one morning with a choking sensation in his throat. As we explored his body reaction, he had the impression that someone was forcing a spoon into his mouth. He was bothered because he had no visual image, "no real memory," only a choking reflex. Allan described his choking as a reaction to being force-fed. As I asked about how he was fed as a toddler, Allan replied, "I can't remember that far back." I responded, "You know your mother's personality, how would she have fed you when you were first learning to eat solid food?" He immediately responded, "She would force me to eat. She certainly forced me when I was nine or ten and did not like the food." Allan had no explicit memory of being a toddler, but his body was revealing a story.

I watched for the nonverbal signs that I was resonating with his experience. I did not want to make suggestions about what he was feeling or remembering, but I did want to reflect what I thought he might be experiencing, to provide words for his silent, wordless experiences. Each time I made a resonating comment, I made sure that I said it in a tentative voice, almost like a question. I wanted to avoid sounding like I was making a defining statement. I said, "Perhaps, even as a toddler, you were forced to comply." He responded angrily with, "Comply, shut up, and be good. That was my childhood. There was no place to be me. Except I had my private place."

Whenever we had a session during which Allan went into his private place, I often saved the last twenty minutes to cognitively discuss with him what he experienced during his withdrawal. During that time, he talked about school-age memories, how strict his mother was about rules and school work, and the uncomfortable sensations in his body. On some days, it seemed like we had to mutually create a language that described his inner sensations, various affects, and the memories that he had never spoken about. I periodically used the last few minutes of our sessions to make a relational inquiry about how he experienced my transactions with him. These relational inquiries were a safety net in our therapeutic contact because they provided me with the information I needed to adjust the therapy according to what Allan could assimilate.

A few times, although there were no words, Allan cried from inside his hiding place. Whenever Allan withdrew into his lonely sensations, he talked afterward about envisioning himself as a baby, left alone to cry. We had several sessions in which Allan was both withdrawn and regressed to the age of an infant or toddler. He curled into a ball and whimpered like a baby. He had a visceral sense of neglect, but he was not sure if it was an actual memory or just his imagination. We talked about the significance of implicit and procedural memory and how such memories are experienced as body sensations and undefined affect. During our post-withdrawal reviews, he was not only "sad for the little boy" but also said, "I am furious at how she neglected me, how she demeaned me. I feel like I could rip her hair out … like she did to me once. I could just break her face. I'm so angry."

About this time, Allan began his sessions by telling me, "The internal criticism is increasing." But the criticism was no longer in his own voice but in his mother's voice. He could remember her bitter sound and chastising words. He described the difference: "When I criticize myself, the words come very fast, almost in a code, more like a pressure in my head: 'I don't belong'; 'I'm worthless'; 'There's no use in talking.' But now I clearly hear my mother's voice. I can hear her awful sound when she says things like, 'What's wrong with you?'; 'You are useless'; 'No one wants to hear you'; 'You're a bother.' Those are her real words. They are in my head but now I can remember exactly when and where she said some of those things. I am not making his up. She actually said those things."

I was pleased with the flow of the therapy because Allan had been processing many memories. He seemed to be integrating body sensations and affect with clear cognitive understandings. Allan was currently involved with a group of avid hikers. He was amazed: "I even talk to a couple of them because we like the same things. They want to talk to me about the Arctic and places I discovered. Do you think I can show them my photos?" We often reviewed what we had previously discussed, but each reiteration seemed like an important building block establishing inner security. Allan was changing. He seemed to be present much of the time, with far less self-criticism. He had clear memories of his emotional turmoil with his mother and sister, and he had stopped following women at night. When I carefully inquired, he talked about his continued loneliness.

But I was concerned about another recent change: Allan was periodically hearing his mother's voice criticizing him. When I inquired about the internal voice, he said, "It's my mother's voice. I don't always hear all her words, mostly I hear her despising tone. She is always an influence in me, particularly when I am around people. She interferes and says, 'People don't want to be with you,' and 'You should be ashamed of yourself.' I don't like what I hear but I can't stop her voice. When I hear her voice I can't talk to anyone."

I was uncertain once again about where to place the emphasis in our psychotherapy. We were accomplishing much, but Allan's description of his "mother's voice" added a new aspect to our work. I was stymied by the multiple dimensions of Allan's psychological processes and what was unfolding. Between our sessions, I mulled over the options. I pondered four possible therapeutic directions: we could continue with the supported therapeutic withdrawal that we had been doing for the past couple of months; we could stop the withdrawal work and celebrate the progress he had made; we could coalesce his emerging memories into a cohesive narrative; or I could redirect the psychotherapy and focus on the possible introjection of his mother's affect, attitudes, and behavior.

It was now well into spring. We would soon have to consolidate the work we had accomplished. Metaphorically, I did not want to open a new chapter, and I also did not want to close the book. At this point, it would be respectful and wise to involve Allan in any decisions about his psychotherapy. After all, at Christmas he considered terminating, but I encouraged him to remain in therapy. That seemed to have been a fruitful decision. I thought about how Allan's relationship with his mother left him with few opportunities for choice, so I wanted to provide him with a chance to influence how we proceeded.

I interwove a discussion of the various alternatives I had been considering into our therapeutic dialogue. We talked about how the supported withdrawal sometimes gave Allan the space to relax and feel protected and how at other times going into his private place stimulated intense emotion-filled memories. From these emerging memories he was forming a consistent and coherent personal story about his life. He no longer had the urge to walk the streets at night looking for someone to love him because he had an acute awareness that he had been searching for the love he had been missing in his relationship with his mother. He realized, "My retreat to the wilderness was always an attempt to escape my mother's control. It worked for a little while, but then her voice always snuck up on me."

We discussed the advantages and disadvantages of Allan terminating at this point in the psychotherapy. He agreed to continue in September. If he returned, we would actively attend to his "mother's voice," how she had a profound influence on his life, his "empty" feelings, and any other obstacle that interfered with Allan being all that he could be. These couple of sessions were interspersed with Allan wanting to talk about his forthcoming camping trip, this time in a different part of the Arctic. He was keenly interested in the possibility of creating new wildlife photographs and curious about how he would interact with people on the ten-day excursion he would take with the hiking club. The next week I left for Europe, and he left for the north in time to catch the midnight sun.

References

Erskine, R. G. (2015). *Relational Patterns, Therapeutic Presence: Concepts and Practices of Integrative Psychotherapy*. London: Karnac.

Proust, M. (1929). La prisonnière [The prisoner] (Vol. 5 of *Remembrance of Things Past*). https://clearingcustoms.net/2013/12/17/what-marcel-proust-really-said-about-seeing-with-new-eyes/.

CHAPTER 11

Allan: my mother's voice—psychotherapy of introjection

Richard G. Erskine

When Allan returned in September to begin his fourth year of our work together, I wanted to make sure that he was in agreement with changing the focus of our psychotherapy over the next few months to attend to the introjection of his mother's personality. I intended to begin by talking about how the therapy would be different and getting a clear agreement about the purpose and direction of the work. However, my plan was temporarily diverted by Allan's enthusiasm. Like a young boy, he was excited to show me his photos. He talked about discovering a new camping area and his excursion with the hiking club. He appeared to need both my interest and patience and seemed almost joyful when I responded with curiosity about his adventures.

In response to several inquiries about his inner experience, Allan described being lonely at night when he was with his hiking group. He realized that he often withdrew when the others were sharing personal stories. He recounted, "I felt stuck. I didn't know how to join in the conversation, and then I was empty in my stomach. I wanted to join in but I could hear my mother's voice saying 'No one wants to hear you,' and 'You are a bother.'" He described how on most of the trip, "I just felt useless as a person. Oh, I could be a part of the group by doing most of the cooking and cleaning up, but I just knew that I should not speak, certainly not speak about myself." I remembered that the previous spring Allan had used similar words when describing "the mother's voice in my head."

He ended the session with "I wish you had been there to teach me how to talk to people." With those words, I presumed that Allan was feeling some degree of attachment to and support from me. If my supposition was correct, it was time to talk to the introjected voice of his mother. Although I often spot opportunities early in a client's psychotherapy to address an introjected voice or attitude, I prefer to postpone conducting therapy with an introjected parent until the client has a solid bond with me. I am mindful that the client's loyalty to internalized parents may be stronger than the emotional bond with me.

In the next session, we reviewed the gains Allan had made as a result of the previous three years of psychotherapy. He added that he had returned to psychotherapy to "get rid of my mother's criticism of me. Her words paralyze me." This led to my introducing the concept of introjection and how we might proceed (Erskine & Moursund, 1988). I explained that introjection was an unconscious, self-protective identification with the thoughts, feeling, attitudes, and behaviors of a significant other person and how it occurs when a child's physical and/or relational needs are repeatedly left unsatisfied. I explained how a child fills the void of relational neglect by internalizing the features of the person on whom they are dependent (Perls et al., 1951).

By using his own experience and stories of other people, I provided Allan with some illustrations of how the introjected voices, attitudes, and criticisms often returned, years later, as an internal voice, one that repeats the criticisms that the person heard earlier in life and dictates what to feel and how to behave. (See chapters 16 and 17 in Erskine, 2015, for an explanation of the theory and methods of the psychotherapy of introjection.)

Allan and I talked about our psychotherapy contract and how to proceed. We discussed how he could alter or stop the therapy process if it did not fit for him and how the therapy of "the mother in his head" fit into the work we had done about shame, his withdrawing to his internal private place, and his lonely search for someone to love him. Allan and I created some drawings to illustrate the dynamic internal interplay of his relational needs, introjected criticism, shame, and withdrawal from relationships. These provided Allan with visual images of his intrapsychic process and explained what we were doing in our work. Although he was nervous about what he would discover, he said, "Let's do it. It can't feel any worse than how I've already felt." He sighed and withdrew into himself for a few minutes. When he was present again, he said, "Help me get rid of her."

I explained that I would have a therapeutic interview with his mother, just as though she were my actual client. "But," I added, "you are my client. My commitment is to you. At times it may seem that I am empathetic with your mother, but keep in mind that my responsibility and investment is with you." Allan nodded and smiled. I described that in some sessions I would spend between ten and twenty minutes talking to his internalized mother, and then the remainder of the session would be devoted to helping him make sense of what had occurred in my dialogue with her.

In the next session, Allan's internal anxiety was high. He brought several of his photos and used most of the time telling me stories of how he had composed the pictures. In the last fifteen minutes, we were able to talk about his worry that I was going to "interfere somehow, upset things … something will go wrong." I interpreted his comments and accompanying anxiety as an indication that his mother was already internally active and invading our therapy space, just as the memories of her criticisms invaded his internal space. He said that he knew his mother would be "furious with him for talking about her." I responded, "I have no intention of talking about your mother. I will talk directly to her, the mother in your head."

By then it was the second week in October. Allan was nervous and deflected the conversation to the hike he would take the coming weekend. After ten minutes, I interrupted and reminded him about our agreement. I asked Allan to sit in a different chair, and as he was about to do so, I asked him to pause, close his eyes, and then sit like his mother would sit. Allan looked at me and said, "What will I do with her purse? She always has a purse." I said, "Do exactly what your mother does." As Allan slowly sat in the chair, he clutched his arms across his chest as though he were tightly holding a handbag. His left leg began to jitter, and his body was tense. I wondered if Allan was displaying his own emotions or the body reactions of his mother.

I wanted Allan's internalized mother to feel at ease, so I began with a warm welcome, just as though she were a new client. I told her that I needed help in working with her depressed son, that he had been withdrawn and without friends but that he was now changing his life. I told her that she was the person most likely to be able to help. She reluctantly agreed and then said, "He won't change. He was always incorrigible. He's just a loner. No wonder he's depressed. As a kid he sat in his room all the time watching TV." Her voice was cold and condemning. It was my goal to warm her to our cooperative task by having her talk about herself. When I asked her name, she first gave me her married name and then reluctantly gave me permission to call her "Henrietta."

As Allan sat on the chair with his eyes closed, I asked the "Henrietta" ego state where she was from and who was in her original family. She hesitantly told me that she grew up in a wealthy suburb of New York City, was the oldest child, and that she had two younger sisters whom she had always disliked. When Henrietta said "disliked," there was a tone of disgust in her voice. I suspected she was in competition with her sisters. As I inquired, she told me that as an adolescent, she could not wait to be "out of the house and on my own." She bitterly described her parents as "demanding" that she be "proper" but that they spoiled her two younger sisters. She described deciding in early adolescence "to be independent and not need anything from anyone." She quickly added that she was lucky to have a daughter who was not like her own sisters, who was "considerate" and "always an easy child," unlike Allan, who was "a problem to be controlled." As Henrietta spoke, I found myself wanting to recoil from her bitter tone. I could identify with Allan's attempts to hide from her in his room.

After fifteen minutes with "Henrietta," I indicated for Allan to resume his usual place on the sofa and asked him what he was experiencing. He said that he had a sudden clarity that his mother "was always playing a role. She won't tell you the truth. She is just being nice to impress you." He went on to say that his mother had always been "extremely jealous" of her sisters and that she "always criticized people behind their backs." I asked what it was like to live with a mother who had those personality traits. His response was, "I learned to live alone in the same house. The only thing I admired about her was that she was a good cook."

Allan then spontaneously contrasted his mother's attitude toward him with his description of my "accepting and understanding way of being." Immediately he was quiet and turned inward; eventually he spoke about how his life would have been different if he had had a parent like me. Allan's idealizing words touched a tenderness in me as I realized that this type of idealization was an unconscious desire for protection from an introjected mother who treated him as "a problem to be controlled." If I was to be therapeutically responsive to him, I would have to provide a stabilizing protection against his mother's potential lies and caustic tone. I privately renewed my commitment to be with and for Allan. What I provided for him was intangible: my interest, compassion, validation, and presence, in essence, a relationship that was uniquely different from what he had experienced with his mother.

In the next session, Allan wanted to talk about possible changes in his job. But after ten minutes on the job topic, I asked if I could again talk to Henrietta for twenty minutes. I tried asking her about her marriage, but she responded with tangential stories that hid much more than they revealed. In each story, she told me how she was impressed with herself or, conversely, how she was not appreciated, even maligned, by various people. Instead of empathically listening, I changed the focus of our conversation and asked about Allan's infancy. On this topic she was more forthcoming: "When he was a baby he would spit up my milk as I tried to breastfeed him. Even on special formula he was colicky, except if my husband was home. Robert could calm the boy and put him to sleep, but with me he just screamed and threw his arms and legs in the air. He would stiffen up when I tried to put him to sleep. The best thing I did was to let him cry himself to sleep. That took a few weeks, but he finally calmed down."

As she described all this, I again felt a big emptiness in my stomach. Just as in the previous session, I wanted to distance myself from her. I was not scared, but I certainly did not like being with her. I was struck by the intensity of my identifying countertransference; my uncomfortable body sensations and emotional reactions were fundamental in my empathy for Allan. I could only imagine the emotional distress he had endured while living with his mother. I was reminded of Fraiberg's (1982) descriptions of emotionally distressed infants and how they flail their arms and legs or stiffen their body to signal that they are experiencing a relational disruption.

Even though I was resonating with what Allan probably experienced as an infant, I was also curious about Henrietta's story. As I inquired about her feelings when caring for her infant son, she said in a theatrical voice, "He never loved me, never from the start." I responded empathically while she told several examples about being "disappointed" at having "a boy child." While she elaborated on this story, my compassion was centered on Allan. I wanted to protect him. My countertransference, both identifying and responsive, guided me in how to respond empathically to Allan during the concluding twenty minutes of our session.

Allan began the next session with amazement at how "my mother's voice poured out of me so easily," and then he added, "But now I know that the problem is her, not me. I don't remember her saying those things, but I know it's true. I was never wanted or loved by my mother." We spent most of the session with Allan recounting stories of his mother's criticisms and his loneliness in his preadolescent years. He provided a verbal portrait of his mother when he said, "I now realize that she was always self-absorbed. I did not exist. I have always lived in my private wilderness. My only salvation was to be alone."

After thirty minutes, Allan had had enough of our exploration into his past, and it looked like he was going into withdrawal. Preemptively, I asked about what had been happening during the week. He told me about his concern that the company he worked for was merging with another firm. He did not know whether to continue with the new firm or take early retirement. As he was leaving the session, he requested that we have time in some sessions to discuss his future. I wondered if this was a sign that Allan was reorganizing internally or if he was distracting himself from the work we were currently doing.

In several subsequent sessions, I continued talking to Allan's introjected mother. When I asked about Allan's early childhood, school years, and adolescence, her typical, emotionless answer was, "He was quiet. He preferred to be alone." Once, when I asked about Allan's toddler years, Henrietta said, "I had to always tell him 'No.' He liked to get into things." I asked if he ever caused trouble, and she answered: "Well, no, but that's only because I controlled him. I never wanted him to be wild. I didn't want another child. My daughter was all I wanted, she was easy to handle. And I didn't need another male in my life, and certainly not a pigheaded one like my father. Thank God my husband was always away; he worked a lot. When he was home he had no interest in being with me [a one-minute pause]. He died in a car accident when Allan was almost five. I don't like this interview. I never talk about him. He's gone and it's over [another one-minute pause]. The police said he killed himself [pause]. I had my daughter. Until she met her second husband, she was always there for me, not like Allan, who preferred to be alone."

After that conversation with Henrietta, Allan was quiet for several minutes. He propped his elbows on his knees and covered his face with his hands. His posture gave the appearance of defeat. When he finally looked up at me, he said that his stomach hurt. "I'm sad, but I can't cry. It's just the emptiness I always feel, but this time it's in my chest as well. I know that she never loved me." He described how he longed to be loved but felt "great fear that I will be invaded and controlled. I don't like being touched." I reminded Allan of the times he walked the streets of New York City late at night, watching women and lamenting, "Can you love me?" We discussed how Allan's fantasy of being loved provided an illusion of safety; he searched for someone who would be tender, patient, and a companion, and he added, "With no possibility of being criticized or controlled."

In the following two sessions, Allan did not want me to talk to the "Henrietta" part of him. He shuddered as he spoke about hearing the tone of his mother's voice. In the first of those two sessions he said, "What I am remembering now is the sound of her, not so much her words, but the sound of her being disgusted with me. Often I don't hear her exact words, just her sneering tone. When I hear that tone, I know I must hide." We began the next session by talking about how his self-criticism was an effective distractor from remembering the sound of his mother. In both sessions he seemed to require time to withdraw to his private place while I watched over him. After each withdrawal, he told me more memories of his family life.

The next weeks were similar. Sometimes Allan did not want to talk, but he was not withdrawing to his private place. Rather, he kept his eyes on me, watching my face, breathing, and making physical gestures. A couple of times he was surprised that I did not "go away." When I asked what he was sensing in his body during those sessions, he said that he had a lot of muscle tension, stomach pain, and had been biting his lips. Together we hypothesized that these physiological reactions were presymbolic physiological memories stimulated by my conversation with his introjected mother.

I presumed that Allan was quite young, partially regressed, possibly to toddler or preschool age. I was concerned he might have reached an emotional level at which he could not absorb more awareness of the neglect and trauma he had experienced. I watched his pattern of breathing; when it became more rapid and shallow, I assumed that he was close to becoming emotionally overstimulated. When I had that concern, I paused for a while and then changed the focus of our attention to his school-age years when he might have explicit memories. Allan talked about several occasions when his mother castigated him. The details of his story changed depending on what he was remembering, but the themes remained the same.

Allan arrived early one day, distraught by a dream. His face looked flushed as he stumbled over the words to describe his intense body reactions and the dream content. We spent the next several minutes with him focusing on the tight places in his body, breathing into the tension, and finding sounds that reflected what he felt. After several minutes focused on his body, Allan was able to verbally sketch the dream: "I am camping with my hiking group. It gets dark and suddenly no one is there. I was scared and searched for them. Without them, I was terrified of falling off a nearby cliff. I try to run, but all is black. I hear a grizzly bear growling. I know that she will devour me. I cried out, but no one is there to help me. I woke up at the sound of my own weeping. I have never cried like that before in my life."

After a long pause, Allan asked me to help him understand his dream. I began with, "Allan, you HAVE cried like that before." He looked astonished. After a moment's pause, I said, "Several weeks ago your mother told me how she let you cry yourself to sleep when you were just an infant. I imagine that you must have wept intensely many times before you learned to be quiet." His eyes filled with tears. He was quiet for a while, then he asked if I had more to say. I was concerned about having enough time to process the meanings of the dream, so I chose to explain the least problematic part of the dream and save the more malignant part for early in another session. "You have recently made personal connections with some of the people in your hiking group. Perhaps you are more secure when they are with you. In the dream you were scared when you could not find them. I think that part of the dream reflects a desire to be connected to people." Allan nodded his head but said nothing.

In a following session, Allan and I returned to deciphering the dream. I proposed, "In the dream you were without security and all was black. That is how it is for an infant who is left all alone to cry himself to sleep. You must have been terrified." Allan added, "Not only when I was a baby. My mother never comforted me. I have always been alone." We were both silent for several minutes before we discussed the significance of what we had both said. When he was ready to hear more, I added, "Perhaps the grizzly bear represents your mother. You have implied that 'she' is quite ferocious. Your mother must have been terrifying to you when you were a baby and young boy." I paused between each sentence so that Allan had time to evaluate the significance of my words.

We returned to understanding the dream again the next week. I pointed out that when he had originally told me the dream a couple of weeks before, he had described the grizzly bear as a "she." Allan was quick to add, "The essence of me was devoured by my mother's criticisms of me. She was a real grizzly bear." I continued, "You may have been crying for help long before you could understand criticism. At that early age, you could not possibly understand what you know now, but you could feel the absence of affection and protection in the cells of your body. I imagine that you cried until you just gave up on having any human connection." After a pause, Allan offered his understanding: "I spend a lot of time observing and photographing wild animals. With the animals there is no personal connection, we just inhabit the same area. That is how I learned to live, no connections." I interpreted that particular dream, which came at that point in our work, as his mental coalescence and concretization of the implicit and procedural memories that had been emerging in our time together.

We spent a few minutes each week talking at the beginning of each session about Allan's employment situation before we went on to consider what he understood from the work we had done in the previous sessions. Some weeks I reserved ten or fifteen minutes to interview his internalized mother. After each session with Henrietta, Allan and I would talk about his mother's behavior and how he had coped with her coldness and criticism.

As Henrietta's criticisms of Allan continued, I used each derogatory comment she made about Allan to ask her about her childhood. Eventually she talked about her early school years, the secret alcoholism of her parents, contempt for her father, and the emotional neglect she felt as a child. As I listened, I tried to be empathic, but she remained emotionally hidden. The only apparent emotions were disgust and anger.

In one intense session, she remembered being about eleven or twelve years old and coming to the conclusion that "No one loves me," and "I will be independent and not need anyone." In a later session I explored the latter decision, and through a series of phenomenological inquiries she revealed that she wanted her children to be protected by "their independence, not needing anybody." As I questioned her about her criticism of Allan, she confessed that she was teaching him "to manage for himself." I was empathic with her need to be "independent from my alcoholic parents" but challenged how she forced her children to be like her. I talked to her about her emotional neglect of her son and how it resulted in his being depressed and without friends.

I thought it was time to coalesce the work we had been doing, so I began the next session by inviting Henrietta to speak. I empathically reviewed with her the stories she had told about her childhood, marriage, and, importantly, Allan's infancy and school-age years. I was both gentle and confrontational when I described how her behavior had been extremely detrimental to Allan, that he was not a bad child, that he needed her affection, and that her behavior toward him was abusive. I emphasized how lonely and confused Allan was in reaction to all of her criticisms. At first she tried to defend her behavior. I interrupted her justifications by focusing on the effects of her criticisms. I told her how Allan had suffered loneliness and uncertainty all his life, that he was in emotional pain, and that he needed her to take responsibility for how she had affected him.

I then asked Henrietta to imagine Allan sitting on the couch and to talk to him. She began by trying to explain why she had never been emotionally close to him. I confronted her attempt to minimize the significance of her impact on Allan and encouraged her to "be honest with yourself." She began to cry and said, "I never wanted to hurt you, Allan. I only wanted you to be independent." She then told Allan that she had been unhappy in her marriage and wanted out but then discovered that she was pregnant. "I know I blamed you, Allan, but it was not your fault. I was angry at your father."

She told Allan how she longed to be independent from her husband just as she had longed to be free of her family. She disclosed that she did not love her husband but then felt guilty when "he killed himself by smashing the car into a tree." She cried as she said, "You were a lovely boy, energetic, but I stopped you." I then pointed out that she had criticized him from the time he was a small boy until he was a grown man. Henrietta responded, "I should never have done that. I was just so angry at your father, and then guilty. I criticized you, I did it a lot, but inside I was criticizing myself."

Following Henrietta's confession, I asked Allan to sit on the couch and face the empty chair. I encouraged him to respond to Henrietta. At first he had difficulty speaking, and then he blurted out his anger at how she had always criticized him. "You blamed me for your crazy troubles. I had nothing to do with your marriage, and I never deserved your criticisms. You are the one who should be criticized for your cruelty, for making me always be afraid of you and other people. Your words hurt me." Then he wept as his body relaxed into the couch.

In sessions that followed, Allan and I went over each conversation I had had with his introjected mother. He talked about how her coldness and criticism had permeated his life. He went into detail about his mother's voice being "consistent and insistent." We again examined how his self-criticisms had been a way to block out his mother's voice. I talked about "the loyalty of a little boy" and how he had stayed attached to his mother by disavowing his anger and believing her definitions of him. Allan was happy that he seldom heard her critical voice in his head now, but he talked about how he was still inhibited with people at work and in his hiking club. We discussed various strategies about how to connect with people.

Allan was now worried about his current life. Two events were impending: He had an offer to sell his apartment for a large amount of money, and his company was in the process of merging with another firm. He was in a quandary. He could remain employed or he could take early retirement and leave the firm with a payout equivalent to five years of his salary. He had been in the same job for twenty-eight years, and, although he had advanced within the firm, he was not sure what his position would be in the new company. Additionally, Allan was uncertain about selling his apartment because he had lived in the place all his life. He had no idea where to go or what he would do if he retired. The time in our sessions was increasingly absorbed with his concerns about his current life.

I wondered if Allan's concerns were a way of deflecting from the work we had been doing or the result of life's circumstances and the opening of a new chapter in Allan's life. In two sessions we discussed each of these possibilities. In the second session he seemed content when he said, "I've changed inside. My body is more relaxed. Every night I'm busy with my photography work. The voice of my mother is mostly quiet. When I do hear her nasty comments, I tell myself 'That is just the memory of a bitter woman,' and 'She cannot control my life anymore.' If the job and apartment both work out, I want to move out of this city. I've spent fifty-five years in one place. I will have enough money to buy a house and photography studio. I saw a place for sale in Vermont that I might buy. I am going this weekend to see if it will work for me."

We had three more sessions, during which Allan and I reviewed the work that we had done during each year. He shared his vision of a future life as a photographer in a rural, mountain town. In each session he cried as he expressed his gratitude for the quality of our relationship. During those final sessions, I was sad and glad: glad that Allan was creating a new life and sad to be saying good-bye to both the man and the neglected little boy, both of whom I had come to love.

Conclusion

The conclusion of a long case study such as this usually includes a recap of the salient events in the psychotherapy, the discoveries made during the process, and the intricacies of the therapeutic work. However, in this study, I will let the therapeutic narrative speak for itself. My view is that the healing of cumulative neglect (as epitomized in Allan's early life) occurs through the psychotherapist's sustained attunement to the client's affect, unique rhythm, and level of development (Erskine et al., 1999).

As I look back on the four years of Allan's psychotherapy, I am reminded of Modic and Žvelc's (2015) analysis of clients' experiences in integrative psychotherapy. Their research identified which aspects of the therapeutic relationship were most helpful. They found six: (1) the therapist's empathy and attunement, (2) the therapist's acceptance, (3) the match between the client and the therapist, (4) feelings of trust and safety, (5) a feeling of connection, and (6) the experience of a new quality in relationship.

In reflecting on what was central in my relationship with Allan over the four years of his psychotherapy, I was aware of working from a relational (Erskine & Moursund, 2022) and developmental perspective (Erskine, 2019). This perspective is similar to how Bowlby (1969, 1973, 1980) defined the qualities of relationship that facilitate a child developing an internal sense of security. In summarizing Bowlby's three volumes, the French psychoanalyst Didier Anzieu (1993) listed Bowlby's five criteria that are essential in an infant forming a secure bond with the maternal person, the foundation on which all later development rests (Erikson, 1950). These criteria include:

- The exchange of smiles
- The solidity of holding and handling
- The warmth of the embrace
- The softness of touch
- The interaction of sensorial, kinesthetic, and postural signs during breastfeeding and maternal caretaking.

Anzieu added his own sixth criteria: "synchronization of rhythms."

These six criteria, each necessary for an infant to develop both internal stability and relational security, are evident in this case study of Allan's psychotherapy. They are the essential ingredients in the psychotherapy of any client who uses the schizoid process to stabilize and regulate emotions and the distress of unmet relational needs (Erskine, 1998). In reviewing Allan's psychotherapy, I want to emphasize the dimensions that led to a fundamental change in Allan's life:

- Throughout the psychotherapy, I wanted Allan to see a gleam in my eyes that reflected my unswerving interest in his stories, a resolute acceptance of who he was, and my appreciation of his uniqueness.
- I was committed to establishing a relationship with Allan that was authentic, reliable, and consistent.
- I strove to provide a "warm embrace" through my continued presence and to create a relaxed, attentive atmosphere in which Allan was free to be fully himself.
- The softness of my voice, the cadence of my speech, and the respect in the way I talked to Allan provided a therapeutic contrast to his mother's criticizing words and harsh tone.
- My continual attention to Allan's body gestures, muscle tensions, and his tendency to avoid interpersonal contact provided clues as to when I was attuned to his affect and level of development and when I was not.
- When Allan told stories, I listened with curiosity. I waited quietly when he withdrew into his private place and was mindful not to hurry him into interpersonal contact. I remained patiently present. Attunement to Allan's rhythm was essential in healing the relational disruptions that permeated his early life.

References

Anzieu, D. (1993). Autistic phenomena and the skin ego. *Psychoanalytic Inquiry*, 13(1): 42–48. doi.org/10.1080/07351699309533921.

Bowlby, J. (1969). *Attachment and Loss, Vol. 1: Attachment.* New York: Basic Books.

Bowlby, J. (1973). *Attachment and Loss, Vol. 2: Separation—Anxiety and Anger.* New York: Basic Books.
Bowlby, J. (1980). *Attachment and Loss, Vol. 3: Loss—Sadness and Depression.* New York: Basic Books.
Erikson, E. H. (1950). *Childhood and Society.* New York: W. W. Norton.
Erskine, R. G. (1998). Attunement and involvement: Therapeutic responses to relational needs. *International Journal of Psychotherapy, 3*(3): 235–244.
Erskine, R. G. (2015). *Relational Patterns, Therapeutic Presence: Concepts and Practice of Integrative Psychotherapy.* London: Karnac.
Erskine, R. G. (2019). Child development in integrative psychotherapy: Erik Erikson's first three stages. *International Journal of Integrative Psychotherapy, 10*: 11–34.
Erskine, R. G., & Moursund, J. P. (1988). *Integrative Psychotherapy in Action.* London: Karnac, 2011.
Erskine, R. G., & Moursund, J. P. (2022). *The Art and Science of Relationship: The Practice of Integrative Psychotherapy.* Bicester, UK: Phoenix.
Erskine, R. G., Moursund, J. P., & Trautmann, R. L. (1999). *Beyond Empathy: A Therapy of Contact-in-relationship.* New York: Routledge, 2023.
Fraiberg, S. (1982). Pathological defenses in infancy. *Psychoanalytic Quarterly, 51*(4): 612–635. doi.org/10.1080/21674086.1982.11927012.
Modic, K. U., & Žvelc, G. (2015). Helpful aspects of the therapeutic relationship in integrative psychotherapy. *International Journal of Integrative Psychotherapy, 6*: 1–25. https://integrative-journal.com/index.php/ijip/article/view/103.
Perls, F., Hefferline, R., & Goodman, P. (1951). *Gestalt Therapy: Excitement and Growth in the Human Personality.* New York: Julian.

CHAPTER 12

Reflexively exploring the "therapeutic use of self": a response to Richard Erskine's five-chapter case study of Allan

Linda Finlay

I sit down with anticipation to read the five chapters comprising Richard Erskine's latest writings about his work with Allan (Erskine, 2021a, b, c, d, e). His abstract explains how this case study explores depression as a "presenting symptom that reflects an isolated attachment pattern, a core feature in the personality of psychotherapy clients who rely on schizoid process as a form of emotional stabilization." I am aware of my sense of curiosity and excitement. Richard's case studies always inspire; engaging with his text will be a stimulating challenge.

A distant self-critical voice calls out warnings. Richard has invited me to use the work as a "springboard" and share my ideas around psychotherapeutic process. This invitation is a huge honor. But what if I can't make sense of the process? Worse, what if I have nothing to say, nothing to contribute?

Ah. I smile to myself and find my ground once more. This feels a familiar place—a parallel process. That cocktail of assured curiosity and excitement, blended with a touch of (reasonable) professional self-doubt and (less reasonable) personal shame, is exactly my experience every time I sit down with a new client and prepare to go on a journey with them. This time, I'm readying myself to go on a journey with Richard and his client, Allan. I don't know where we're going, or what new vistas will be revealed. But I am eager to step aboard, keen to embrace this opportunity to reflect deeply on psychotherapy process and practice.

I reflect momentarily on my current grounded place which parallels my stance at the beginning of every therapy encounter. The key ingredient here is to grasp and hold a phenomenological attitude. Yes, I think to myself, that is something immediate and specific that I want to talk about. My own approach to relational integrative psychotherapy is similar to Richard's—this is not surprising since he was one of my early teachers. But there are also points where we subtly diverge—mainly concerning his use of psychoanalytic concepts (against my own strong leanings toward existential phenomenological theory and practice).

This lens of focusing on Richard's therapeutic use of self (rather than commenting on Allan's process) with the emphasis on phenomenological insights feels right. I feel an easing in my body, my excitement builds. I have no idea where this journey will take us but, just like the start of therapy, I have opened myself to embracing and exploring whatever should unfold.

* * *

In this chapter, I seek to open up dialogue and debate—both with Richard Erskine and with our psychotherapy community—about the *therapeutic use of self* in integrative psychotherapy. The commentary that follows is a response to Erskine's (2021a, b, c, d, e) five-part account of his therapy with a client called Allan (see Chapters 7 through 11). I've structured my narrative in terms of four phases (the ones typically engaged in long-term therapy). First, there is the initial stage of *assessing and engaging the client* in therapy. Then the focus is on *making contact* (where the client contacts both the therapist and themselves). As therapy proceeds, the process of *making connections* and integration becomes figural; then therapy can proceed toward *endings*.

Assessing and engaging the client

Richard's first impression of Allan is of a shy, pleasant man who is either withholding responses or slow to respond. Through gentle questioning, Richard learns that Allan is a fifty-year-old, "diligent" bookkeeper who has lived in the same apartment since he was a child. His father had died when Allan was in kindergarten. Allan has never married and has lived with his mother until her death (from cancer) four years previously. Although he attends church every Sunday, he remains socially isolated. Mostly flat in his presentation, he comes to life when talking about his hiking and camping vacations in the wilderness (Chapter 7).

Reading Richard's initial evaluation of Allan, I experience a mixture of reactions. There is so much that calls out for attention in just these few, evocatively crafted pages. Not only do we meet Allan, but Richard also models *a phenomenological attitude* (of attunement, openness, and descriptive inquiry). He also engages *clinical reasoning* and demonstrates how to be *reflexively present*. All these processes, which I discuss below, underpin this initial assessing-engaging phase, where both client and therapist commit to the work.

Phenomenological attitude

The phenomenological attitude is open, non-judgmental, and filled with wonder and curiosity about the world. It seeks to hold prior assumptions apart. For therapists seeking to infuse their work with such an attitude, the immediate challenge when entering a therapeutic encounter is to remain open to new understandings: to be present and empathically open to the client, ready to attune to them and simply go exploring. It's important to "bracket" (Husserl,

1936) knowledge and assumptions. Taking its cue from phenomenological philosophy, this bracketing is best understood as non-judgmental focused openness where we are trying to see clients and their lives with "fresh eyes" (Finlay, 2008, p. 29; 2016a, 2022). It's about bracketing in order to be present, while resonating to what is emerging relationally in the here-and-now (Finlay, 2013, 2021).

In his first three assessment sessions with Allan, Richard reveals this ready-to-receive, non-judgmental approach, even if he does not explicitly call it a phenomenological attitude. He is busy opening himself to his client and attuning to Allan's being. "I did not understand his internal processes," Richard says, "but I listened for the covert meaning in his stories. I needed to be patient, attentive, and attune myself (the best I could) to his indistinct and subtle affects" (Erskine, 2021a, p. 30; Chapter 7, p. 103).

Richard favors *phenomenological inquiry* and we see this throughout the therapy and his other writings (Erskine, 2015). For me, phenomenological inquiry is a part of a broader, sustained phenomenological attitude that goes beyond asking questions to being an attempt to describe the "is-ness" of self-states that are emerging (Finlay, 2021).

Novice therapists can all too easily see phenomenological inquiry as simply a technique of asking questions about the client's experiencing in the here-and-now, missing its broader philosophical significance. I suspect Richard has his own philosophical commitments, ones which probably go beyond my preferred humanistic, existential framework. However, based on his previous writings, I believe he privileges phenomenological inquiry over historical inquiry (Erskine, 2015, 2020).

Phenomenological inquiry aims to raise the client's moment-to-moment awareness of their intersubjective experience, meanings, issues, and needs (current and archaic)—all aspects that may have been pushed down or defensively disowned. Through the therapist's respectful questioning and listening, the client can become curious about their own self and gain new insight: the first step toward self-acceptance and growth. For me, the key here is *how* the questions are posed. Especially when working so delicately at the contact boundary with individuals with anxious, avoidant, or isolating attachment patterns, any questioning needs to be done with care and curiosity, ideally with both therapist and client working together on the answers.

Richard notes that with many depressed clients he relies on phenomenological inquiry to focus attention on the client's experience, rather than on their observable behavior. In previous writings, he has explained how to use questions or statements that focus on *bodily* ("What's happening in your body just now?"), *cognitive* ("What sense do you make of that?"), *affective* ("What are you feeling?"), and/or *relational* dimensions ("What's it like to be sitting here telling me that story?") (Erskine, 2021f).

Through his exquisitely patient inquiry, Richard slowly builds a picture of Allan's life. At work, Allan diligently applies himself while being disapproving of his "time-wasting" coworkers. When not at work or attending church on Sundays, Allan takes to the streets of New York City, spending his evenings walking through neighborhoods and observing people from a distance. Saturdays, he sets off alone to hike nature trails. His life is devoid of family, friends, and the warmth of human contact.

Like Richard, I feel sad as Allan's story unfurls. "I felt an emptiness, like a vacuum, in my belly when I imagined that Allan's world was deprived of intimate contact with people," is how Richard describes his feelings. But Richard does not seem to find it easy to tune into Allan's experience. He ruefully acknowledges that in the first three evaluation sessions, his phenomenological inquiry mostly elicited evasion or a non-response. This causes him to wonder if such inquiry might be "more of a hindrance than a help" (Erskine, 2021a, p. 30; Chapter 7, p. 102). I feel some sympathy for him. Those early sessions, marked by Allan's deflections or silent responses, must have been challenging.

Richard keeps reminding himself to be patient. Could there be some irritation and frustration lying beneath the surface: reactions he has not expressed or perhaps does not want to show? He sounds admirably calm. I know from my own work that I can get frustrated and irritated in similar situations and need to redouble my effort to hold on to some compassion and patience. What helps me is supervision or consultation where I can have some space with a valued peer colleague in which to vent and regroup, reminding myself to focus compassionately on the likely terror that lies behind the withdrawal rather than reacting to it.

But there is more here. Is Richard indicating that for some clients (Allan among them) phenomenological inquiry simply does not work? If so, I am not sure I would agree. After all, if Richard had not asked all those vital questions, would he not already be giving up on Allan? I think there is value in showing Allan some of the routes they might take over time, even if the questions look too unappealing or treacherous at that moment. Even if Allan is not responding, the questions are being posed and they can be held in the space, in anticipation of a time when he is ready to take them up. I agree, of course, that care must be taken to not be invasive with the questioning. Part of my version of phenomenological inquiry would be simply to reflect back: "Is it difficult to say what you're feeling just now?" Equally I might engage phenomenological description (what Richard calls "therapeutic description") to begin to raise awareness of the client's process, initially providing some words for the client that they don't yet have, for example, "I sense it is difficult for you to speak about feelings just now" or "I'm sensing there is some scare here. Is that possible?"

I would argue that phenomenological inquiry engaged by a therapist with genuine non-judgmental openness, interest, curiosity, and empathy (i.e., the phenomenological attitude), is an invaluable core stance at all times, even as other therapeutic techniques may be employed. The manner of delivery will emerge and evolve within the specific relationship—over time—as we adapt to the client's needs and the relational context, *and as they adapt to us* (Finlay, 2022). It is hard to tell from Richard's selective narrative, but I would say the bits of inquiry he has already engaged will prove extremely valuable.

Richard's account suggests that he (appropriately) experimented with different kinds of interventions including how he worked toward making more directive suggestions about how Allan might change his behavior or do things differently. Allan's silent responses and/or defensive deflections were in their own way an effective form of communication. Richard evidently heard the message Allan was conveying through his silences, as he changed course and returned (for the time being at least) to gentler, non-invasive phenomenological inquiry:

> I increased my use of phenomenological inquiry, particularly my inquiry about his affect and body sensations. Although he was slow to answer, he usually identified tension in his neck and chest. Somehow that led us to talking about his difficulty in expressing any emotion to people. He said, "I want to remain private. I don't want anyone poking their nose into my business." I asked if that included me. Allan answered, "Yeah, sometimes your questions are too damn invasive." I responded, "What happens inside you when I ask such questions?" Allan shrugged his shoulders and remained silent for the remainder of the session. During the next couple of sessions, he struggled to describe how he became physically tense, expecting me to criticize whatever he said, and how he quickly searched "for the right answer." (Erskine, 2021a, p. 33; Chapter 7, p. 105)

I am struck by this passage—it feels relationally significant. Not only is Allan's difficulty with expressing emotion apparent, but Allan also tells of being primed and alert to the slightest whiff of criticism. Recognizing this watchfulness, Richard grasps the importance of not suggesting any behavioral change that might imply a judgment of sorts. His strategy of simply engaging more inquiry strikes me as helpful since it shows acceptance of Allan's being and choices. As Richard notes, psychotherapy is not happening if the client is simply giving what they perceive to be the "right" or expected answers.

I appreciate Richard's flexibility here. He is responding relationally—titrating his therapeutic use of self to mesh with what Allan is ready to tolerate (Finlay, 2022). Research consistently underlines the importance of tailoring therapy to the individual (Norcross & Wampold, 2018).

In addition to the way Richard is adapting to Allan, I hugely respect his humility and openness to learning. I like the way he allows his client to take on the role of teacher:

> I often overlooked the significance of these subtle signs of the schizoid process. It has taken me a number of years to become sensitive to the unspoken story of such clients, a story replete with fear, shame, disavowed loneliness, self-criticism, and a compulsion to isolate. Allan was one of the clients who taught me to listen for the therapeutically significant story encoded in what such individuals do *not* say. (Erskine, 2021a, p. 37; Chapter 7, p. 108)

Clinical reasoning

Richard notes that Allan fits the picture of a "schizoid" client. I appreciate Richard's rejection of the diagnosis of "depressive disorder." Like other existentially oriented therapists, I resist reductionist, dehumanizing medical model categories, preferring instead more intuitive, phenomenological ways of seeing the client, in the context of their relational world (Finlay, 2016a).

While diagnosis can be informative, it's important to ask what we might miss if we view just through that lens. The lens of "depressive disorder" may lead us simply to peer *within* the person and thereby miss viewing them in the context of their depressing life circumstances. And is there a risk of unduly pathologizing Allan rather than acknowledging it's his way of being and/or our way of seeing him? "When we totalize others, when we reduce them to objects of our knowledge, i.e., to easily labelled categories and stereotypes, we have violated their inherent worth as good in themselves" (Sayre & Kunz, 2005, p. 227).

Atwood and Stolorow (2016, p. 104) also wade into this debate:

> The features of experience and conduct formerly regarded as symptoms of reified psychiatric categorizations or as expressions of decontextualized psycho-analytic character types then become understood as inseparable from the multifaceted relational fields linking the patient to other people, which includes the participating presence of the observing clinician.

Instead of diagnosis, Richard offers a *formulation* of Allan's situation, namely that encoded in Allan's self-descriptions and behaviors are "unconscious relational patterns" that are being lived out in his daily life (flatness, avoidance, and disavowed affect). Apparently devoid of intimacy, these relational patterns are leading him to "despair" and a longing for "peace and quiet." Richard senses that something vital is missing from Allan's life. But he's not yet sure what it is other than appreciating the schizoid process is one of splitting off from the vital and vulnerable child self (Erskine, 2001, 2020).

For my part, I want to hold lightly to this initial formulation (interpretation?). With my reservations about the extent to which anyone can know another, I also want to try to see Allan without reducing and fixing him as a "schizoid patient" who might be treated by preset therapeutic formulae. As Yalom states, taking diagnostic systems and protocols too seriously may "threaten the human, the spontaneous, the creative and uncertain nature of the therapeutic venture" (Yalom, 2001, p. 5).

Being familiar with Richard's work, I know that he too is reluctant to label another and would strive against applying prefabricated protocols. When he uses terms like "schizoid," he is talking about a protective withdrawal process arising as part of a style or pattern of behavior rather than a fixed and pathological "disorder." At the same time, I'm aware of Richard's North American cultural context, where diagnosis is needed for insurance purposes and is often the starting point of framing clinical needs. There is a clear contrast here with my British context and my own experience of private practice. It seems Richard lives more comfortably with psycho-diagnostic labels than I do.

Richard also turns away from taking a fuller phenomenological attitude in his reflections about "schizoid process" and his formulation of what might constitute Allan's "unconscious relational patterns." I suspect I might have done the same—although I would have been working harder to bracket the idea that Allan had a schizoid process. It is here that the difference between theory and the practice reveals itself. It is virtually impossible to completely hold back our assumptions or understandings—a point phenomenological philosophers (e.g., Merleau-Ponty, 1945) stress (Finlay, 2021).

There is a balance to be struck between employing our presence, power, judgment, and expertise as therapists while holding on to unknowing. It takes discipline and courage to sit with uncertainty and not-knowing; it is not easy to let go of power and control toward trusting the process of the therapy encounter (Finlay & Evans, 2009). Richard reveals this in his sincere wish to let Allan's story unfold in the way that it needed to:

> I was curious about Allan, but my inquiries were only partially effective. He answered my questions but often with reticence. I wanted to know him, to know the depth and extent of what he felt, what he had lived as a boy, and how he managed his life. It was necessary to continually remind myself to be patient, to just let his story unfold. (Erskine, 2021a, p. 33; Chapter 7, p. 104)

I agree with Richard that seeking to lift Allan's (so-called) "depression" was unlikely to be a particularly fruitful approach. However, Richard seems to have further concerns about Allan's engagement and their lack of a mutual, affect connection. I, too, wonder about this. It is often the case that some kind of therapeutic alliance is in place by the end of the third session of therapy. Indeed, research indicates that this is necessary for positive outcomes (Norcross & Lambert, 2019). That Richard agreed to carry on with the therapy suggests that he sensed some element of hope, even if it remained vague and intuitive: a sense of the possibility of something positive emerging from the collaboration.

And, importantly, Allan himself seemed more than prepared to commit to weekly therapy for a year. It was essential that he made this commitment. It was an implicit acknowledgment that he was not intending to take his own life (a lurking risk factor Richard rightly checked out). Without mutual commitment on both sides, it would not have been ethical to proceed (Finlay, 2019).

Richard does not say it explicitly, but I have a sense that Allan would not be an easy client to work with. I am reminded that therapy can be hard work—for both client and therapist. Therapy with a client who is flat and lifeless in presentation and who dismissively avoids talking about emotion poses particular challenges where it is hard to keep present and engaged. I am touched by Richard's care and the way he reflects deeply as he makes an "emotional commitment" to meet Allan weekly for a year:

> I wanted our psychotherapy to enhance the quality of his life and provide him with a desire to live. I walked home from the office that night questioning myself: "Was I wanting more for Allan than he wanted or was willing to do?" I knew what was possible in an in-depth psychotherapy, but I had no evidence that Allan knew the commitment, perseverance, and time that would be required to make some fundamental changes in his life. (Erskine, 2021a, p. 32; Chapter 7, p. 104)

The power of this commitment, along with Richard's candor, uncertainty, and doubts, should not be underestimated.

Being reflexively present

Erskine (2015; Erskine & Moursund, 2022) notes there is a duality to the therapist's presence: a simultaneous attending to client and to self (in terms of being emotionally available and self-aware). The therapist de-centers from their own needs, making the client's process the primary focus. Here the therapist is mindful of the client's experience, watching every little gesture, listening to each word, and being with the client's silence. At the same time, the therapist's history, relational needs and sensitivities, theoretical stance and professional experience all enter into building therapeutic presence (Erskine, 2011; Erskine et al., 1999).

More than a duality, however, I would argue that the best relational work in psychotherapy is characterised by a *triality* (or, to apply my preferred metaphor, seeing with three eyes). As Richard has indicated, one eye is focused firmly on the observing-sensing the client; the second eye is engaged with reflexively observing-sensing oneself. The new third eye element is an explicit monitoring by the psychotherapist of the emerging relationship between the client and the therapist. Here, I follow Hycner's (2017) dialogic Gestalt approach, which underscores the need to be present to all these three points of focus. Sometimes we are deeply immersed in holding a client's story; then we switch our attention to our own embodied experience and also toward reflexively monitoring what is happening in the relationship. We focus on ourselves and the relationship, not out of narcissistic motives, but reflexively as a way of furthering our appreciation of the client's process.

I believe that Richard engages this three-way focus when he makes his regular, explicit *sensorial searches* of his own internal process while monitoring the moment-to-moment dynamics of the relationship with Allan. At these times he recognizes the importance of maintaining his own vitality and curiosity (particularly in the face of any deadening deflections from Allan).

Being *present* in this way involves being grounded in one's own embodied self in order to receive the client's experience (Geller & Greenberg, 2002). Opening ourselves to whatever is emerging moment-to-moment in the therapeutic encounter in open, alive, curious ways is central to our work as therapists (McWilliams, 2017; Schneider, 2008). It is about being present to new possibilities, ready to be awed and surprised as we touch—*and are touched by*—the other. Placing our trust in the therapeutic process, we strive to be energetically present, inviting, alive to creative possibilities, and ready to share ourselves as we join with our client and go exploring (Finlay, 2016b).

Richard's "relational needs" work (and I include here his writing colleagues) (see Erskine, 2021f; Erskine & Trautmann, 1996; Erskine et al., 1999) attests to the importance of being focused on the therapeutic relationship while being solidly grounded, attuned, aware, responsive in order for the client to feel adequately held and attended to. It can also be powerful for the client to see they have impacted the therapist. The less the therapist is present, the more anxiety-provoking the situation is likely to be for the client, who may feel shame and/or abandonment in the face of therapist withdrawal or perceived lack of interest. In turn, the client is likely to want to withdraw and/or dissociate. In other words, "the presence of the therapist invites the client to be present" (Finlay, 2022, p. 39).

Richard has written elsewhere (2001, 2020) about being the security-in-the-relationship and engendering a sense of security in the client so that they do not need their self-created withdrawal defense. The point I would stress here is that this is a cocreated relational process. The therapist does not just create a "safe space." Instead, somehow the therapist needs to involve and negotiate with the client, trying to work out together what would be a safe space.

With Allan initially struggling to be fully present to himself and his therapist, Richard's presence becomes more important. He needs to be present as a safe presence in order to invite Allan to be present. He does this by holding a welcoming therapeutic space where Allan can feel accepted, respected, and empathized with. In a way, Richard is like a welcoming, gracious host who offers a special kind of spacious hospitality (Finlay, 2022):

> The guest ... client comes seeking sanctuary, a safe place of protection where wounds can be carefully cleansed and healed. But where is the sanctuary, if not fundamentally in the heart of the host or therapist who is willing to face this living encounter and courageously open to it? (Kapitan, 2003, p. 74)

Making contact

> The challenge to the therapist is to meet the client at that point of contact in a manner that encompasses that resistance, rather than threatens it. It is to genuinely see the resistance as a point of contact between rather than as merely an oppositional force. (Hycner, 1991, pp. 151–152)

Over the course of the first year or so, the therapeutic alliance between Richard and Allan builds. As the two men explore Allan's world together, their contact deepens. They are engaged in something of a dance at the contact boundary as they explore the space between intimacy and distance, insight, and resistance. At first, their dance is stiff, the steps uncertain. But then their ease with the movement builds. Richard glides through a series of improvised steps with Allan, movements whose sharp shifts of focus and rhythm are more reminiscent of a tango than a graceful waltz. At times they move together; at other times Allan pulls away and then is gently brought back.

A question lies between them: *Just how close is it safe to be*? Would their tenuous interpersonal connection prove sufficient to prevent Allan reverting to his old isolated-isolating patterns? Richard recognizes that Allan's avoidant withdrawing pattern is part of his survival strategy in the face of an unresponsive, critical mother. With this compassionate empathy to the fore, Richard takes care to be patient and respectful; he strives to lessen the likelihood of

Allan closing down. I applaud this approach: honoring Allan's defenses is, paradoxically, likely to result in him relinquishing them.

In this critical dance-of-contact phase, four dimensions of the therapeutic use of self stand out for me: *dwelling*, *resisting contact*, *transference*, and *titration*.

Dwelling

The art of engaging a proper phenomenological attitude and inquiry involves a special attentiveness that dwells with the situations the client describes and attends to (even magnifies) details (Finlay, 2021; Wertz, 2005). The aim is to focus on the implicit meaning of the situation as it presents to the client. At the same time, the therapist takes a slowed, savoring approach which involves intuitively sensing, moving with, empathizing, responding, and resonating with their whole body-self. George Atwood and Robert Stolorow (2016, p. 103), both phenomenologically oriented psychoanalysts, characterize dwelling as an "active, relationally engaged form of therapeutic comportment" geared toward healing emotional wounds. In dwelling, they say, we don't just seek to understand the other's world. Instead, "one leans into the other's experience and participates in it, with the aid of one's own analogous experiences" (p. 103).

Time and again through the case study, I see Richard sensitively embodying this dwelling approach (though he may not use that word or see it, as I do, as being linked to the phenomenological attitude). For instance, I really appreciate the way that Richard engages Allan's dreams (over the years). He does this in a layered way, excavating meanings when it seems Allan is ready to face them. These dream analysis sequences are powerful, and I suspect pivotal, as Allan learns about the richness of his internal world.

Early on in therapy, whenever Allan mentions a dream Richard invites him to find his own meanings. Allan appreciates this; as he notes later on in therapy, "You allowed it to be my dream, my meaning" (Erskine, 2021b, p. 44; Chapter 8, p. 113).

In his account, Richard suggests that he might have offered interpretations about Allan's intrapsychic life had he had more information. My view is that interpretation would be an unnecessary embellishment and that working phenomenologically is sufficient at any stage. Interpretations, I feel, take away from the very dwelling inquiry which was now beginning to bear fruit. As Richard acknowledges, what is important is the client's meaning and growing awareness.

Allan's tortured inner world is further revealed in his disclosure that when he leaves the therapy session, the volume of his self-criticism rises. Richard makes a point of working with such insights, showing that he is resonating with Allan's affect or unarticulated relational needs:

> I encouraged him to let me hear what was happening inside him, even to shout the criticisms out loud. When he finally spoke, the forcefulness of his words was lethal: "I'm useless," "I'm a weakling," "No one's interested in me." (Erskine, 2021b, p. 48; Chapter 8, p. 117)

This Gestalt technique of amplifying inner dialogue, Richard notes, is effective precisely because intrapsychic conflict is diminished when it is externalized (Baumgardner & Perls, 1975; Perls, 1973).

In time, the source of those shamed–shaming judgments is traced to Allan's disdainful, fault-finding mother. This insight emerges as Allan acknowledges that his trust in Richard is precarious; it seems that Allan has *expected* Richard to criticize him. Richard explains how Allan is transferring emotional memories of his mother's responses onto his therapist and is perhaps compensating for the damaging effects of his mother's criticisms by imagining Richard's criticism. However, we do not learn how exactly this is communicated to Allan. I find such interpretations are best delivered cautiously rather than authoritatively and best posed as an open question for exploration.

Resisting contact?

Allan's reluctance to talk about his relationship with his mother speaks loudly to Richard. But given the intensity of Allan's pain and anger, it is crucial that Richard continues to be patient while persistently trying to access Allan's feelings.

In the initial stages of therapy, Allan remains reticent, unwilling to modify his behavior, or talk about his feelings and his early life experiences. Weekly therapy sessions seem to follow the same pattern, one in which Allan simply shares his stories about his irritations at work, night treks in the neighborhood, or his nature hiking. It seems that what was important to him was to stay with the familiar and safe—his routines helped to stabilize and protect him. It is not clear from the narrative if Richard made attempts to bring the functions of Allan's repetitions to his awareness.

Unlike many therapists, Richard notably avoids the term "resistance" when he talks about Allan and his response to therapy. The fact that he does not critically label Allan as resistant is significant. The concept of resistance in psychotherapy has been hotly contested, with different schools having different understandings of what it is and how to work with it. Since its introduction to the psychoanalytic field there is general agreement that resistance can be understood as a defensive, protective response to threat.

However, if we take a humanistic-relational perspective, we understand that interpersonal contact is always a cocreation (Erskine, 2015). This being the case, resistance cannot be understood just as a refusal by one person to engage. I would challenge this pathologizing characterization of the client as the "problem." Rather than seeing resistance as unidirectional, negative, and an oppositional move by a recalcitrant client, I prefer the Gestalt approach to seeing resistance as a potentially wonderful *creative adjustment* that needs to be respected, honored, and even celebrated. Then, it can be gently managed (McFerran & Finlay, 2018). The relational therapist will want to create a safe-enough space where client self-protection is met with non-judgmental compassion. By naming, not judging, the battle between avoidance and self-insight, therapists can establish themselves as able to contain expressions of the subjective life of the client, which then allows these expressions to emerge more freely (Atwood & Stolorow, 2014; McFerran & Finlay, 2018).

I am interested in Richard's observation that initially he did not attend to the sarcastic swipes Allan aimed in his direction. I see this as evidence of Richard's experience (and robustness) coming into play. While we all have a need to feel helpful (we may even yearn to be needed or appreciated), usually experience helps us to avoid taking criticisms too personally. It's likely that any negativity or rupture has arisen out of a relational process to which both client *and* therapist are contributing. Reflexively exploring underlying dynamics more deeply will help enrich the work and strengthen the awareness or choices of both therapist and client.

Richard rightly starts to probe the function of Allan's habitual criticism of both himself and others. Do Allan's projections offer momentary relief from his own raucous self-criticisms? Are his criticisms the active outward expression of all that he has introjected from his mother and sister? Exploring these questions explicitly in therapy results in Allan having a profound insight: that his self-criticism is a way of drowning out his mother's voice:

> We talked about how his self-criticism became more prevalent and vociferous than his mother's and a distraction from the emotional pain of a mother's words. His posture changed, and the tension in his face and shoulders relaxed as he cried (Erskine, 2021b, p. 52; Chapter 8, p. 120)

Transferential responses

From his previous writings, I recognize that Richard's therapy model of *contact-in-relationship* (Erskine et al., 1999) is in play. It is a model that draws on transactional analysis, behaviorism, Gestalt therapy, systemic, relational psychoanalysis, and developmental-attachment theory.

Perhaps the biggest challenge for any integrative psychotherapist is how to blend competing—even contradictory—perspectives (Finlay, 2016a). One potential contradiction in Richard's model is the place of psychoanalytic understandings of unconscious processes and transference. Humanistically inclined therapists reject the idea that the unconscious, irrational, instinctive forces determine human behavior. Some even deny the existence of an unconscious as such, preferring instead to talk about material that is not yet in conscious awareness. I wonder where Richard sits in this debate as he attempts to straddle psychoanalytic and humanistic assumptions. Perhaps he manages to avoid the problem of contradiction by his use of transactional analysis, since that theory is implicitly integrative and smoothly blends interventions that work with both archaic and here-and-now needs. From his other writings (Erskine, 1991), I understand that he follows Berne's (1961) early TA formulation seeing transferential transactions as "externalized expressions of internal ego conflicts between exteropsychic and archeopsychic ego states" (p. 66). More specifically, transferential transactions may be both a projection of child needs and intrapsychic conflict, and an overt transaction from either exteropsychic or archeopsychic ego states.

I do not disagree with Richard here as my model of working draws heavily on his model and the use of transactional analytic concepts and processes. However, it can be problematic when practitioners inadvertently misuse the model by naively claiming to be simultaneously psychoanalytic, behavioral, *and* humanistic in their approach. More critical discussion is needed about precisely *how* competing theories, with their contradictory underpinning philosophies and assumptions, can or should be integrated (Finlay, 2016a).

I like Lynne Jacobs's dialogic Gestalt approach where she finesses apparent contradictions in her concept of "enduring relational themes" (Jacobs, 2017). Here she highlights how clients' patterns of relating derived from historical experience can become embodied-emotional perspectives on the world. Here, she embraces a thoroughgoing humanistic focus on the intersubjective here-and-now, without assuming that past relationships somehow get unconsciously displaced onto the present. Transference and countertransference are reframed as a cocreated relationship of mutual responding where the histories of both therapist and client shape our hopes, longings, or dreaded expectations. This position, focusing more on the relationship as opposed to an individual's intrapsychic world, would probably find acceptance with many contemporary relational psychoanalysts and relational integrative psychotherapists more generally.

I suspect Richard would feel comfortable enough with Jacobs' position. At the same time, he is explicit about his work with transference and his psychodynamic interests. In this case study, I'm interested in the way Richard usefully and clearly categorizes his countertransferential responses as *reactive, responsive,* and *identifying* (Erskine, 2012, 2013a, 2013b). That he deeply and reflexively challenged himself to explore his internal experience is significant, and I appreciate his honesty in recognizing his own unrequited relational needs and identifications, as well as his desire to offer relational healing.

Allan's developmental attachment history is palpably present, both in his own responses and in those of Richard. Richard treads carefully, given the way inquiries about Allan's childhood have been largely rebuffed ("I don't remember my childhood"). He is forced to fall back on his own observations and "intuitive sensings" of possible unconscious relational patterns from childhood. In session after session, as he listens to Allan's detailed stories of his nature hikes or nightly "low-down" treks, it seems that Richard gets the message that he needs to show a "fatherly" interest: "I began to form a developmental image of Allan as a six- to eight-year-old boy, a child without a father to take an interest in his adventures" (Erskine, 2021a, p. 34; Chapter 7, p. 106).

This developmental image, Richard says, evoked feelings of compassion within him and increased his interest in Allan's stories. He took care to ask factual questions about Allan's hiking and to use his face and body gestures to indicate that he was present and attentively engaged. I feel touched when I hear that Richard wants to go hiking with Allan, to smell the forest, to see the woodland trail, to be a companion. I appreciate his care in listening so intently. I feel happy for Allan that he has finally found someone who can mirror, witness, and validate him—and be the companion he has never had.

I am aware of my own powerful developmental image of a caring father and (no longer lonely) little boy walking hand-in-hand through the woods. I recognize that my own enduring relational themes have become figural, and that in a parallel process this could be understood as my own reactive and identifying countertransference.

Titration

The somatic therapist Peter Levine (2011) has developed a systematic approach to working bodily with trauma which involves helping clients progressively access bodily energies and sensations a little bit at a time to build up their tolerance. Borrowing from the field of chemistry, he calls this process "titration."

We can observe titration in action in the way psychotherapists constantly adapt their therapeutic use of self, making subtle adjustments (Finlay, 2022). Research consistently emphasizes the importance of adapting therapy to the individual. "The clinical reality is that no single psychotherapy is effective for all patients and situations no matter how good it is for some" (Norcross & Wampold, 2018, p. 1893).

"As therapists, we make deliberate choices about how and when to intervene. We continuously adapt and pace the levels of tenderness, formality, spontaneity, emotionality, challenge, support, self-disclosure, intimacy, and directiveness we offer" (Finlay, 2022, p. 3). Early in the therapeutic relationship, we might choose to engage more phenomenological inquiry and/or description, and simply listen in a reserved, slow, quiet, empathic way. A client's withdrawal (to self-stabilize) might be supported and even encouraged. As therapy unfolds, we may become more present, animated and/or inject more challenge or self-disclosure (Finlay, 2022).

Throughout the case study, we see Richard making subtle adjustments in his approach, adapting to what Allan can tolerate. When even phenomenological inquiry proves too much, Richard eases back to be simply an appreciative listening-witnessing ear for all of Allan's stories. When Allan experiences Richard as too invasive or critical, Richard again backs off and is respectful of Allan's silent withdrawal.

Of course, it is not always that easy to attune to the precise level of tenderness, silence, empathy, challenge, directiveness, and so on, the client can handle. Some clients can find too much attentiveness overwhelming and invasive; feeling unworthy themselves they become uncomfortable with too much warm appreciation (Finlay, 2022). Allan, it seems, found any inquiry about his affect uncomfortable (or confusing?), which resulted in him deflecting by changing the topic.

It seems that Richard got the balance about right. He helps Allan begin to express himself by accepting the deflections or silences in a non-judgmental way. Any other approach (e.g., being more directive or challenging) would have resulted in Allan disengaging, I suspect (although perhaps a cognitive behavioral therapist would disagree with me).

As the months and years of therapy go by, I again appreciate Richard's artful titrating of his therapeutic use of self where he invites relational connection and makes contact with Allan's vulnerable parts. Sometimes he leans in and offers challenge, at other times he pulls back to give more space to Allan. He continuously adjusts his responses—relationally.

We can see Richard regularly and reflexively monitoring his use of self. This is particularly evident at times when he realizes his intervention may be a mistake. Importantly he does not beat himself up:

> I was disappointed in myself because I had missed the significance of his various criticizing comments. But, unlike Allan, I did not chastise myself. Instead, I wondered what was happening within Allan, what was unexpressed, and the functions of his criticisms of others. (Erskine, 2021b, p. 51; Chapter 8, p. 119)

I am struck by this passage where Richard states he does not chastise himself (unlike Allan). I suspect this more self-accepting stance grows with experience. We all make mistakes. It is part of the process—possibly even a necessary part. It is best to view our so-called mistakes with curiosity and compassion and see them as potential opportunities. Many arise out of therapists' genuine concern; if at times we try too hard it is because we care. Ideally, we catch any errors, repair any ruptures, and manage arising wounds over time. Both therapist and client have the opportunity to learn and grow (Finlay, 2022).

Making connections

> The client is becoming whole. Contact with the self, with all its complexities and capacities, so long split and fragmented, is being re-established. Feelings and thoughts and perceptions rush in, often with surprising intensity. And each of those long-repressed, long-hidden parts of self has a kind of fragility, like a flower bud freshly opened or a butterfly newly escaped from its hard cocoon. (Erskine et al., 1999, p. 172)

Integrative psychotherapy aims to facilitate a sense of wholeness in a person's being and functioning, at intrapsychic, mind–body, relational, societal, and transpersonal levels (Finlay, 2016b). We strive to enable our clients to gain insight into their experience and to have a sense of feeling at home with self, at ease with others (i.e., both internal and relational integration). There are, of course, limits to the extent to which any of us can be deemed "whole," but integration remains the driving spirit of our project—particularly so in the case of longer-term work.

Relationally oriented therapists believe that healing integration occurs through relationships (with the therapist and with others). The therapeutic relationship acts as a particular catalyst, enabling a client's growth. It is the unfamiliar experience of being deeply connected in a relationship that allows previous ways of being to be understood and laid to rest, enabling new ways of being to be brought to life. In later stages of therapy, the focus goes toward helping the client own previously disowned parts, find ways to emotionally self-stabilize, and become aware of new possibilities and life choices.

The case study demonstrates this theory beautifully. Over the years that follow, trust, intimacy, and connection between Richard and Allan deepen, just as Allan's connection with himself solidifies. For me this distinguishes the most artful level of relational integrative work where the client's connections *both* externally and internally are enabled (Finlay, 2016a).

As Richard and Allan begin to more closely examine and work through the effects of Allan's mother's disapproval at each developmental age and his efforts to hide from her Allan experiments with using a relationship with Richard as a microcosm of his world Allan is able to allow the surfacing of issues around trust, shame, and feeling criticized. As Allan connects with his archaic experience, his self-criticism becomes louder. At last, he can acknowledge his shame and the harsh intense grip of self-criticism is loosened.

The work Richard and Allan engage in is so profound that there is much to comment on and explore further. I would like to open up two aspects: *working creatively* and with *multiple parts of self*.

Working creatively

> The flow of therapy should be spontaneous, forever following unanticipated riverbeds; it is grotesquely distorted by being packaged into a formula that enables inexperienced, inadequately trained therapists (or computers) to deliver a uniform course of therapy. (Yalom, 2001, p. 34)

Curiosity, warmth, passion, permissiveness, courage, and heart-and-soul commitment are among the qualities that often animate the best relational work. It is important to remain creative rather than follow therapy recipes. We need to engage our own vitality if we are to help enable another's to come forth. Being mechanical or formulaic in our work stultifies the dynamic, growth-enhancing potential of therapy (Finlay, 2022). As Yalom (2001) advises, we should create a *new therapy* for each patient, one tailored to their needs.

Richard shows this creativity again and again. I would like to highlight three instances shown in the way he: i) challenges Allan to talk about his relationship with his mother; ii) works with another dream; and iii) encourages Allan to withdraw to a safe internal space.

Being challenging

First, I appreciate the way Richard makes a few deliberate inquiries about Allan's relationship with his mother in each session. That deliberately provocative challenge of his brought a smile to my face. Although Richard does not openly liken their relationship to a battle, there is certainly a battle of sorts (a battle for Allan's soul?) at work.

Richard's persistence eventually pays off—Allan shares more about his early life; his awareness of the impact of his mother's abusiveness grows.

> I continued to inquire about his body sensations, and it became evident that each time he held his breath for a moment and then sighed that he had heard an internal criticism such as "You can't do that," or "People don't want you bothering them." With several phenomenological inquiries, Allan was able to tell me that it sounded just like his mother's disapproving voice. We talked about how discouraging it was to constantly relive his mother's criticism. I asked him to make those comments again, and loudly, like he was talking to little Allan. He repeatedly yelled his mother's words, then he lowered his head and was silent for several minutes. When he again looked at me he had tears in his eyes. (Erskine, 2021b, p. 52; Chapter 8, p. 120)

In this quotation, the embodied creativity of Richard's interventions is revealed where he makes direct contact with Allan's vital, vulnerable child self (Erskine, 2001, 2020). He has shown some courage in bringing that somewhat scary mother into the room. But the intervention has poignant results. At last, little Allan has a witness for his mother's abuse.

Allan now feels safe enough with Richard and sufficiently protected to let his mother appear. In Richard's place I might have considered engaging psychotherapy with his introjected mother, perhaps as a future possibility when the solidity of the therapeutic relationship was more firmly established. Otherwise referred to in the literature as a "parent interview" (Erskine, 2015; Erskine & Moursund, 2022; Erskine & Trautmann, 2003), this technique offers a way of giving in-depth therapy to the introjected other (e.g., internalized parent ego state) with the aim being for the client to experience a resolution of the intrapsychic conflict. I wonder if this also was Richard's thinking. Such carefully chosen and calibrated timing of interventions is characteristic of the work of "master" practitioners.

Dream work

Second, Richard's creative approach is demonstrated when he works with another of Allan's dreams. When Allan explicitly asks Richard for his interpretation of one particular dream, it seems important for Richard to try to respond to this request. Richard hears a young boy ask his father, "What does it mean?" Somewhat challenged, Richard tries to find a heart-to-heart way to offer a "duplex transaction" (Berne, 1961), where the therapist talks simultaneously to the client's child and adult ego states. This is not easy to do, and I'm reminded once more of Richard's considerable sensitivity and skills.

I am touched by his intuitive spontaneous empathetic approach where he reflected back the story of the young boy (taking the form of a locomotive train) who carried a heavy load and was stopped in its tracks by a threateningly "large faceless woman" (possibly representing his "mother").

That Richard and Allan dwell with this dream over several sessions is important. I appreciate Richard's decision to properly record the dream as Allan was telling it so that details can be pulled out in subsequent sessions.

Eventually, Allan is ready to hear the message of the dream more directly:

> I said, "It must have been impossible for you as a young boy to have a real face-to-face contact with your mother, particularly if she was criticizing and misdefining you. It seems that your mother could not face your uniqueness and vitality. Nor was she sensitive to your vulnerability … but she was able to stop your locomotion. Just like in the dream where the faceless woman stopped the steam locomotive." (Erskine, 2021c, p. 64: Chapter 9, p. 129)

As Allan's trust in Richard and connection to himself slowly grow (i.e., external and internal relational connections made), he is able to face his shame and demons and begin to find his uniqueness and vitality. Allan disclosed that he had held back a shameful secret: that on his nighttime neighborhood treks he follows women.

The story that eventually unfolds over several sessions is thoroughly heartrending. It turns out that spotting a woman, and following her, allows Allan a few moments of fantasy: the make-belief that she might be kind to him. The question he has repeatedly asked into the silence is, "Can you love me?" Over time, Richard and Allan come to interpret the mantra of "Can you love me?" as a lament. Through this question, Allan has been facing the reality and grief of being an unloved, neglected yet controlled child who yearned to be loved.

Initially hearing about Allan's stalking behavior, I could feel my alarm stirring. Richard was clearly also concerned and confronted a huge ethical dilemma. Weighing up the risks, he made a choice to stay with patient empathic listening rather than being more directive, critical or challenging (Finlay, 2019). While I feel uncomfortable about this decision (like it seemed Richard did), I agree with Richard's therapeutic response given the women were not—it would appear—being actively damaged. And I wonder if in Richard's place, I would have been able to contain my judgments and aversion to Allan's potentially threatening obsessive behavior with women. I would be interested to hear more about Richard's process of navigating this delicate and tricky ethical dilemma.

Encouraging withdrawal to a safe internal space

Third, I value the way Richard employs a special creative strategy of actively encouraging Allan to withdraw to a safe internal space *during* sessions. Then, he shows a touching attunement to Allan's silence. This is perhaps the most significant and powerful technique Richard uses when working with schizoid processes (see also Erskine, 2001, 2020).

Richard becomes aware that in highly charged emotional moments during therapy, Allan seemed to withdraw, automatically returning to a private internal place. By inviting a deliberate withdrawal, he raises Allan's awareness of this approach to emotional self-stabilization and regulation. Recognizing the safety of this space, Richard encourages Allan to withdraw at will during the therapy sessions. It seems that Richard saw this process as a way for Allan to internally hide and keep himself safe lest someone damage his soul once again—a vital ingredient when working with schizoid process. Together, they make the discovery that, watched over by a caring, attentive (but non-invasive) presence, Allan could safely get in touch with many painful and suppressed memories. They also discover that, after being replenished by his private space, he is more relationally contactful and spontaneously vital.

I appreciate the way a therapeutic space has been opened up through Richard's attunement to silence, allowing Allan's memories to surface *in their own time*. Allan has also been given a new resource: a space where, rather than engaging in defensive withdrawal, he can explore his past in more positive and helpful ways.

Multiple parts of self

During the fourth year of therapy, Allan is beginning to feel less depressed and self-critical. Is it now time to wrap up the narrative and celebrate the progress? Or is there more work to be done? What is in Allan's best interests?

Such are the questions Richard now confronts. But at this point he discovers that Allan is hearing his mother's critically harsh voice ever more loudly. For this reason, Richard suggests one further year of work. It could be beneficial, he thinks, to begin working explicitly with that introjected parent.

Many of us routinely refer to different metaphorical selves within us (such as our "inner critic" or "rebellious adolescent"). Sometimes it can feel like different parts within us are at war with each other (such as the conflict between the "industrious student" part of self and the "playboy" who just wants to have fun). For some people, the internal splits are more extreme and disturbing, for instance, when a suicidal part acts out in self-destructive ways. Sometimes an individual might embody different personas in dissociative ways without conscious memory of their actions (as in dissociative identity disorder) (Finlay, 2022).

In the field of trauma work, different theories that embrace a multiplicity of "selves" tend to subscribe to the idea that people who have a history of trauma show evidence of internal fragmentation (e.g., splitting or dissociation), even if they have perfectly crafted, adaptive social selves which they show the world, or do not have an actual dissociative identity disorder. Here, we might include theories such as: transactional analysis and ego state theory (Berne, 1961; Watkins & Watkins, 1997); internal family systems (Schwartz, 2001); self-pluralistic perspectives of person-centered and experiential psychotherapies (Cooper et al., 2004); and parts work in Gestalt therapy. The metaphorical representation of selves or parts-of-self in these therapies can be a useful way of containing the fragmentation and exploring problematic aspects (which may or may not be owned) toward integration (Finlay, 2022).

In the case study, Richard doesn't talk explicitly about using the metaphor of parts of self, other than mentioning "little Allan," and then latterly in the in-depth way he engages Allan's internalized "mother" therapeutically. His version of working with parts here is thus to think in terms of transactional analytic ego states. (See Erskine, 1991, for an in-depth elaboration which applies Berne's (1961) original definitions to integrative psychotherapy.)

While it is difficult to spot clear differences between what I can see of Richard's practice and my own, I suspect that, with Allan, I would have done more to engage parts work early on and done so more explicitly, beyond thinking in terms of ego states. Parts work figures regularly in my own relational integrative practice (Finlay, 2016a, 2022) when I work somatically and existentially with longer-term clients, particularly when shame and trauma are involved. The question for me is which parts of the client (and myself!) are coming forward. Who is talking to whom? Our relational connections are usually multiple with different attachment and relating styles between us being revealed.

"The theory makes sense to me as it mirrors my internal landscape and my own therapeutic journey" (Finlay, 2022, p. 135). I see parts in myself and perhaps that sensitizes me to see them (or look for them?) in others. "I appreciate the way that parts work calls forth an integrating, self-compassionate, creative energy. When a new part comes forward (and is recognized by my client or myself), the moment of insight can resemble an inspirational epiphany" (Finlay, 2022, p. 135). With this integrating awareness the client becomes aware of the possibility of choice, change, and escape from habitual ways of responding. The ability to turn down the volume on cacophonous choruses of strident voices becomes a realizable goal (Finlay, 2022).

DeYoung (2015) has highlighted the role of relationally validating connections based in "right-brain-to-right-brain communication" when working with clients who experience chronic shame. Highlighting the role of respect and compassion when working with chronic shame, DeYoung recommends engaging multiple parts of self:

> Bringing shame to light often illuminates a needy part of self who is despised by a tough, independent part of self. Listening respectfully to both parts and helping each to find compassion for what drives the other brings better balance and harmony to the whole self system. ... Parts of self can find space to speak the unspeakable about need, longing, and humiliation, and in their speaking and being heard, integration happens. (2015, pp. 132–133)

Work with the parts which represent internalized others is potentially the most powerful, transformative, imaginal technique we have at our disposal. I know from his previous work that Richard is a master when it comes to this way of working (Erskine, 2015; Erskine & Moursund, 1988, 2022).

While hugely aware of the healing promise of therapy with internalized others, I'm also mindful of its potential to be intense, stirring, disorientating, and unsettling. This is not an intervention to be used superficially as a technique or gimmick. It needs to be handled carefully so that plentiful time and space are given to processing the material. I know from my own experience how terrifying it can be to have the problematic internalized other come into the therapy space. The therapist needs to ensure the client feels safe and supported while the internalized other is being worked with. At the same time, the "parent"/other needs to be acknowledged and respected for their own struggles while being challenged to take responsibility for the impact of their behavior.

Richard did all these things—of course. But I am struck afresh at the care he took *initially* to explain the process; then again, *during* the work he took care with his sensitive, tactful handling of both Allan and his "mother"; and *after*, he gave plenty of time to explore the revelations. In particular, Richard worked with Allan's child's response to work with this "mother" enabling him to express what had not been previously expressed, helping to free his child confusion and the old attachment bonds. That the work was layered, and carried on over several sessions, is particularly interesting to me. Most of my previous experience with this sort of work has been as a one-off "parent interview" and I am now intrigued about the possibilities of engaging in-depth psychotherapy with the introjected other and discovering how this way of working may unfold when engaged long-term on an ongoing basis.

I also appreciate Richard's evident skills in helping Allan work through some of his relational trauma, his sense of betrayal and anger at the neglect and disparagement he received. I particularly like the empty-chair work where, first, Allan's "mother" was invited to explain her treatment of Allan and challenged to take responsibility for it. Then Allan was invited to take the cathartic step of sitting in the chair and replying to his mother.

Richard's summary shows something of the extraordinary, completed Gestalt that was achieved:

> In sessions that followed, Allan and I went over each conversation I had with his introjected mother. He talked about how her coldness and criticism had permeated his life. He went into detail about his mother's voice being "consistent and insistent." We again examined how his self-criticisms had been a way to block out his mother's voice. I talked to Allan about "the loyalty of a little boy" and how he stayed attached to his mother by disavowing his anger and believing her definitions of him. Allan was happy that he seldom heard her critical voice in his head now. (Erskine, 2021e, p. 84; Chapter 11, p. 146)

Endings

The decision about when to end long-term therapy is never easy. Then a further layer of difficulty must be worked through to ensure the end is handled in a constructive, healing way. Clients and therapists alike face the challenge of separation and the grief that results from severing a special bond. Ending therapy can also trigger a reexperiencing of past loss, rejections, and unresolved grief (Finlay, 2016a, 2019). It is not surprising there are sometimes missteps along the way. Either therapist or client may begin to think it is time to end. Then suddenly it isn't. They may disagree, tussle, or find a way to compromise. Richard and Allan also had to face this negotiation.

The key process in this ending phase involves enabling a client to work through any arising pain. In strategic terms, it is about allowing the client to deal with unfinished business. Therapy should not add to the list of a client's experiences of problematic endings (Finlay, 2016a).

I am intrigued to learn that Richard builds in a summer break vacation when doing long-term work—something I have never done (choosing instead to take a week or so off periodically). I now see that having a formal, built-in break offers interesting grist for the mill. For one thing, there is an opportunity to practice the eventual ending process, which could otherwise be avoided or resisted. This happens, for example, when clients ask, "Can we keep in touch?" or—worse—when a therapist says, "Come back if it doesn't work out." Any ending, says Romanyshyn (2006, p. 31) is "always a petit mort." Even if we don't go as far as thinking in terms of death and grief, at the very least, having a summer break can offer time for reflection and therapy can be reset accordingly.

Perhaps helped by their formal breaks, both Allan and Richard seem well prepared when the end of therapy eventually occurs. That Allan was leaving therapy because he was moving away to fulfill a dream helped with the positive forward-looking momentum.

I am not sure I can say the same about being prepared for the ending myself; I am aware that I want to find out more about Allan. Is he enjoying his new life? Has his photography taken off? Has he found some nice nature trails nearby? Has he made some new friends or supportive acquaintances? Ruefully, I acknowledge to myself that I am not quite ready to let them go. (And, yes, this is another parallel process—I often feel something similar at the end of therapy.)

Richard does not expand on what the loss of Allan means to him personally. He does not mention if part of him was reluctant to let Allan go, or whether he was tempted to invite a continued correspondence. Maybe I project my own difficulties with endings here. After all, Richard had many months in which to work through the ending.

Yet at the end of his writing Richard strikes me as retreating a little abruptly into theory. I wonder if that intellectualization helped him move away from the loss and grief he might have been experiencing. Perhaps, too, the act of writing up his case study was another way to "let go" while also celebrating Allan's growthful journey.

I respect Richard for ensuring what sounds like a good (relationally connected) ending with Allan. As he says of the last few sessions:

> In each session he cried as he expressed his gratitude for the quality of our relationship. During those final sessions I was sad and glad: glad that Allan was creating a new life and sad to be saying good-bye to both the man and the neglected little boy, both of whom I had come to love. (Erskine, 2021e, p. 85; Chapter 11, p. 147)

I find it almost unbearably poignant to hear Richard say he had come to "love" Allan. I appreciate his authentic honesty and the way he both owns and gives voice to the special kind of love we can feel in the therapy room—one that we do not often talk about publicly. That love stands as a testament to their profound relational work. I wonder if Allan was eventually able to feel he was truly loved by Richard—both the man and the little boy.

As therapists, we carry the privilege and the responsibility associated with endings. Our role is to help clients face the pain of the good-bye as part of embracing life. We celebrate the client's growth with them as they take their new discoveries into the rest of their lives. And then we need to let to let go with *grace* (Finlay, 2016b, 2019).

I am honored by this opportunity to work with this story of Allan's therapy. Like others, perhaps, I feel privileged and humbled being given such an intimate glimpse into Allan's trauma; witnessing the healing process through which the accumulated impact of his neglect is healed through the therapeutic relationship with Richard. Dwelling with their story has helped me identify both with Richard and with Allan. I had a strange sense of being a part of their relationship where tendrils of vicarious healing unfolded for me as well.

I started this project of dialoguing with Richard's writing with excitement and curiosity, and yes, some uncertainty. I believe I have managed to unfurl some interesting aspects of their journey and learned more about the therapy process (a lifelong quest!).

There is much more, had space allowed, that I might have said but I hope I have conveyed the deep respect I feel for Richard's work. It's not just that he engaged some wonderfully attuned and care-full therapeutic interventions with the right balance (for Allan) between inquiry and challenge; it's the artfulness of his exquisitely sensitive choice and timing of those interventions and the way he uses himself therapeutically, in service of Allan's growth.

Their work has touched me deeply and, although I leave it now with some sadness, I remain grateful for and enriched by Richard's gift.

References

Atwood, G. E., & Stolorow, R. D. (2014). Undergoing the situation: Emotional dwelling is more than empathic understanding. *International Journal of Psychoanalytic Self Psychology*, 9(1): 80–83. doi.org/10.1080/15551024.2014.857750.

Atwood, G. E., & Stolorow, R. D. (2016). Walking the tightrope of emotional dwelling. *Psychoanalytic Dialogues*, 26(1): 103–108. doi.org/10.1080/10481885.2016.1123525.

Baumgardner, P., & Perls, F. (1975). *Gifts from Lake Cowichan: Legacy from Fritz*. Palo Alto, CA: Science and Behavior Books.

Berne, E. (1961). *Transactional Analysis in Psychotherapy: A Systematic Individual and Social Psychiatry*. New York: Grove.

Cooper, M., Mearns, D., Stiles, W. B., Warner, M., & Elliott, R. (2004). Developing self-pluralistic perspectives within the person-centered and experiential approaches: A round-table dialogue. *Person-Centered and Experiential Psychotherapies*, 3(3): 176–191.

DeYoung, P. A. (2015). *Understanding and Treating Chronic Shame: A Relational and Neurobiological Approach*. New York: Routledge.

Erskine, R. G. (1991). Transference and transactions: Critique from an intrapsychic and integrative perspective. *Transactional Analysis Journal*, 21(2): 63–76. doi.org/10.1177/036215379102100202.

Erskine, R. G. (2001). The schizoid process. *International Journal of Integrative Psychotherapy*, 31(1): 1–6. doi: 10.1177/036215370103100102

Erskine, R. G. (2011). Attachment, relational-needs, and psychotherapeutic presence. PhD keynote address, International Integrative Psychotherapy Association Conference in Vichy, France, April 21. https://integrativetherapy.com/en/articles.php?id=73.

Erskine, R. G. (2012). Early affect-confusion: The "borderline" between despair and rage. (Part 1 of a case study trilogy.) *International Journal of Integrative Psychotherapy*, 3(2): 3–14.

Erskine, R. G. (2013a). Balancing on the "borderline" of early affect-confusion. (Part 2 of a case study trilogy.) *International Journal of Integrative Psychotherapy*, 4(1): 3–9.

Erskine, R. G. (2013b). Relational healing of early affect-confusion. (Part 3 of a case study trilogy.) *International Journal of Integrative Psychotherapy*, 4(1): 31–40.

Erskine, R. G. (2015). *Relational Patterns, Therapeutic Presence: Concepts and Practice of Integrative Psychotherapy.* London: Karnac.

Erskine, R. G. (2020). Relational withdrawal, attunement to silence: Psychotherapy of the schizoid process. *International Journal of Integrative Psychotherapy*, 11: 14–29.

Erskine, R. G. (2021a). Depression or isolated attachment? Part 1 of a 5-part case study on the schizoid process. *International Journal of Integrative Psychotherapy*, 12: 28–40. https://integrative-journal.com/index.php/ijip/article/view/207/113.

Erskine, R. G. (2021b). Internal criticism and shame, physical sensations, and affect. Part 2 of a 5-part case study on the schizoid process. *International Journal of Integrative Psychotherapy*, 12: 41–55. https://integrative-journal.com/index.php/ijip/article/view/208/114.

Erskine, R. G. (2021c). Isolation, loneliness, and a need to be loved. Part 3 of a 5-part case study on the schizoid process. *International Journal of Integrative Psychotherapy*, 12: 56–65. https://integrative-journal.com/index.php/ijip/article/view/209/115.

Erskine, R. G. (2021d). Therapeutic withdrawal and painful memories. Part 4 of a 5-part case study on the schizoid process. *International Journal of Integrative Psychotherapy*, 12: 66–74. https://integrative-journal.com/index.php/ijip/article/view/210/116.

Erskine, R. G. (2021e). My mother's voice. Part 5 of a 5-part case study on the schizoid process. *International Journal of Integrative Psychotherapy*, 12: 75–88. https://integrative-journal.com/index.php/ijip/article/view/211/117.

Erskine, R. G. (2021f). *A Healing Relationship: Commentary on Therapeutic Dialogues.* Bicester, UK: Phoenix.

Erskine, R. G., & Moursund, J. P. (1988). *Integrative Psychotherapy in Action.* London: Karnac, 2011.

Erskine, R. G., & Moursund, J. P. (2022). *The Art and Science of Relationship: The Practice of Integrative Psychotherapy.* Bicester, UK: Phoenix.

Erskine, R. G., Moursund, J. P., & Trautmann, R. L. (1999). *Beyond Empathy: A Therapy of Contact-in-relationship.* London: Routledge, 2023.

Erskine, R. G., & Trautmann, R. L. (1996). Methods of an integrative psychotherapy. *Transactional Analysis Journal*, 26(4): 316–328. doi.org/10.1177/036215379602600410.

Erskine, R. G., & Trautmann, R. L. (2003). Resolving intrapsychic conflict: Psychotherapy of parent ego states. In: C. Sills & H. Hargaden (Eds.), *Ego States: Key Concepts in Transactional Analysis, Contemporary Views* (pp. 109–134). London: Worth.

Finlay, L. (2008). A dance between the reduction and reflexivity: Explicating the "phenomenological psychological attitude." *Journal of Phenomenological Psychology, 39*(1): 1–32. doi.org/10.1163/156916208X311601.

Finlay, L. (2013). Unfolding the phenomenological research process: Iterative stages of "seeing afresh." *Journal of Humanistic Psychology, 53*(2): 172–201. doi.org/10.1177/0022167812453877.

Finlay, L. (2016a). *Relational Integrative Psychotherapy: Engaging Process and Theory in Practice*. Hoboken, NJ: Wiley-Blackwell.

Finlay, L. (2016b). "Therapeutic presence" as embodied, relational "being." *International Journal of Psychotherapy, 20*(2): 17–30.

Finlay, L. (2019). *Practical Ethics in Counselling and Psychotherapy: A Relational Approach*. London: Sage.

Finlay, L. (2021). Phenomenological "use of self" in integrative psychotherapy: Applying philosophy to practice. *International Journal of Integrative Psychotherapy, 12*: 114–141. https://integrative-journal.com/index.php/ijip/article/view/167/123.

Finlay, L. (2022). *The Therapeutic Use of Self in Counselling and Psychotherapy*. London: Sage.

Finlay, L., & Evans, K. (2009). *Relational-centred Research for Psychotherapists: Exploring Meanings and Experience*. Hoboken, NJ: Wiley-Blackwell.

Geller, S. M., & Greenberg, L. S. (2002). Therapeutic presence: Therapists' experience of presence in the psychotherapy encounter. *Person-Centered and Experiential Psychotherapies, 1*(1–2): 71–86. doi.org/10.1080/14779757.2002.9688279.

Husserl, E. (1936). *The Crisis of European Sciences and Transcendental Phenomenology*. Evanston, IL: Northwestern University Press, 1970.

Hycner, R. (1991). *Between Person and Person: Toward a Dialogical Psychotherapy*. New York: Gestalt Journal Press, 1993.

Hycner, R. (2017). What does it mean to be a relational psychotherapist? [Lecture]. Scarborough Counselling and Psychotherapy Institute, Scarborough, UK, September 8.

Jacobs, L. (2017). Hopes, fears and enduring relational themes. *British Gestalt Journal, 26*(1): 7–16.

Kapitan, L. (2003). *Re-enchanting Art Therapy: Transformational Practices for Restoring Creative Vitality*. Springfield, IL: Charles C. Thomas.

Levine, P. A. (2011). *Waking the Tiger: Healing Trauma—the Innate Capacity to Transform Overwhelming Experiences*. Berkeley, CA: North Atlantic.

McFerran, K. S., & Finlay, L. (2018). Resistance as a "dance" between client and therapist. *Body, Movement and Dance in Psychotherapy, 13*(2): 114–127.

McWilliams, N. (2017). Core competency two: Therapeutic stance/attitude. In: R. E. Barsness (Ed.), *Core Competencies in Relational Psychoanalysis: A Guide to Practice, Study, and Research* (pp. 87–104). Abingdon, UK: Routledge.

Merleau-Ponty, M. (1945). *Phenomenology of Perception*. C. Smith (Trans.). London: Routledge & Kegan Paul, 1962.

Norcross, J. C., & Lambert, M. J. (Eds.) (2019). *Psychotherapy Relationships that Work, Vol. 1: Evidence-based Therapist Contributions* (3rd edn.). New York: Oxford University Press.

Norcross, J. C., & Wampold, B. E. (2018). A new therapy for each patient: Evidence-based relationships and responsiveness. *Journal of Clinical Psychology*, 74(11): 1889–1906. doi.org/10.1002/jclp.22678.

Perls, F. (1973). *The Gestalt Approach and Eye Witness to Therapy*. Palo Alto, CA: Science & Behavior Books.

Romanyshyn, R. D. (2006). Therapy and the theater of soul: The drama of performance. Keynote address: New Zealand Association of Psychotherapy, February 23–26. http://robertromanyshyn.com/Therapy%20and%20the%20Theater.pdf.

Sayre, G., & Kunz, G. (2005). Enduring intimate relationships as ethical and more than ethical: Inspired by Emmanuel Levinas and Martin Buber. *Journal of Theoretical and Philosophical Psychology*, 25(2): 224–237. doi.org/10.1037/h0091260.

Schneider, K. J. (2008). *Existential-integrative Psychotherapy: Guideposts to the Core of Practice*. New York: Routledge.

Schwartz, R. C. (2001). *Introduction to the Internal Family Systems Model*. Oak Park, IL: Trailheads.

Watkins, J. G., & Watkins, H. H. (1997). *Ego States: Theory and Therapy*. New York: W. W. Norton.

Wertz, F. (2005). Phenomenological research methods for counseling psychology. *Journal of Counseling Psychology*, 52(2): 167–177. doi.org/10.1037/0022-0167.52.2.167.

Yalom, I. D. (2001). *The Gift of Therapy: An Open Letter to a New Generation of Therapists and Their Patients* (revised and updated edn.). London: Piatkus.

CHAPTER 13

The role of shame in the development of the schizoid process

Lynn Martin

Some years ago, I received a call from a woman who was desperate for me to work with her adult daughter Carmen who had just been discharged from a psychiatric unit. Normally I would expect an adult client to make their own contact and request for therapy but the desperation in her mother's voice convinced me to make an exception. It was also clear that her daughter did not have the capacity to make the request for herself due to her deeply depressed state and inability to connect with the world in any meaningful way.

Carmen had made several attempts to take her own life and had a history of chronic abdominal pain dating back to her adolescence, the cause of which could not be established despite seven exploratory laparoscopies. A small amount of endometriosis had been found but not nearly enough to justify the level of pain that Carmen was experiencing.

Carmen had first engaged in counseling for two years at school when she was between fourteen and sixteen years old. She had more counseling during her university years followed by three blocks of cognitive behavioral therapy, through her doctor's surgery, in her twenties. None of the therapy she had been offered so far had been useful.

She was in her early thirties, and on long-term sick leave from her work in the pharmaceutical industry when we began our work together. Her therapy is ongoing as I write this chapter and we have talked about the potential impact of my writing, including the possibility that her agreement to my using her material came from a compliant, transferential place. We have considered that we might use this text in her ongoing therapy, slowly exploring and dealing with the inevitable shame that is stimulated through our exploration of her therapeutic journey so far.

At the beginning of the work Carmen was taking a total of eleven different types of prescribed medication including two antidepressants and an antipsychotic, high doses of opiate medication and other analgesia, hormone treatment and a nerve block every few months, none of which appeared to have any impact on her level of physical pain or her depressed mood. Whether the physical pain was a manifestation of her psychological pain or vice versa was an important consideration for me. The word pain comes from the Latin *poena* meaning punishment or penalty so I wondered if Carmen's physical pain was a form of unconscious self punishment or a kind of self destructive behavior, although Carmen described it to me during one of our sessions as "a big hug."

> We discover that in the course of the child's development, pain and relief of pain enter into the formation of interpersonal (object) relations and into the concepts of good and bad, reward and punishment, success and failure. Pain becomes par excellence a means of assuaging guilt and thereby influences object relationships. (Engel, 1959)

While the link between somatic and psychogenic pain has been well discussed in the psychiatric literature for many years (Bass, 1990; Blumer & Heilbronn, 1982; Engel, 1959; Tyrer, 2006), Carmen's physical pain and depressive symptoms had been treated individually and separately since their onset in her adolescence, without success. Her pain and her suicidal intent would always increase when the status quo was threatened and especially if anyone suggested that she was getting better. When I suggested to her that taking responsibility for the management of her medication represented a step forward, she described my comment as a "slap in the face." This was an example of my misattunement to her relational needs (Erskine et al., 1999) in that moment. I believe that she really needed to continue to define herself, and for me to be accepting of her without judgment, instead of validating her change in behavior which meant that I was defining her.

My first impression of Carmen was that she was overweight, unkempt, and older than her years. Much of the excess weight was a side effect of her medication. Through her heavy sedation she found coherent thought difficult and her ability to verbalize was initially exceedingly difficult, at times impossible. For an intelligent woman, this inability to articulate her thoughts and feelings stimulated shame and reinforced her script beliefs of being "useless, worthless and unable to do anything right." During this first phase of therapy my task was simply to be a stable, dependable other who had no agenda and no expectations of Carmen. I imposed no time scale where she was expected to be well and returning to work. My focus was on careful rhythmic attunement, not too fast so that she felt overwhelmed and not too slow so that she felt abandoned. It took many sessions of my sitting and waiting for her to feel safe enough in our relationship for her to begin to emerge.

All the psychological assessments and offers of therapy from the psychiatric services that Carmen had not found helpful simply increased her shame and belief that everything is her fault. She told me that her husband had constantly shamed her for not being able to do anything right. If she vacuumed the carpet, he would find pet hairs that she had missed. If she chopped vegetables, he would claim that they were the wrong size. He told her that it was her fault that their marriage had failed. At work, if she was summoned to her manager's office, she always assumed that she had done something wrong.

Her final attempt to hang herself came after a failed attempt by hospital staff to carry out a nerve block. She naturally believed that this was her fault and the failed nerve block, coinciding with my absence at a conference, overwhelmed Carmen and suicide seemed to be the only way she could withdraw far enough. Yontef (2001) suggests,

> Suspended in the death-level conflict between total isolation and being swallowed up, these individuals often feel tired of life and the urge for temporary death. This is not active suicide, just exhaustion from living a life with insufficient nourishment. (p. 11)

However, for Carmen, after so many years of a battle to which she could see no end, it was another active attempt at ending her life.

Fairbairn (1952) suggests that people who develop a schizoid process are bought up by parents who were unable to demonstrate tender, loving emotions, causing the child to experience rejection and to withdraw into an inner world, which is safer, but lonely.

Carmen was the only child of professional parents who Carmen experienced as having no time for her. She had a clear script message that she was always "in the way."

Both Masterson (1988) and Yontef (2001) describe the cold, disconnected childhood experience of someone who develops a schizoid process. On several occasions Carmen told me that her father's view of children was that they were a "sexually transmitted disease." When she first told me this, there was no feeling in her voice, as if she had just told me that it was raining. Over time, with each new telling the distress and shame that this view of herself caused her became more and more apparent. She was eventually able to connect with an appropriate angry response to being defined in this way by her father. Each new appropriate expression of affect, especially anger, coincided with an improvement in her mood and a decrease in her physical pain.

Through careful attunement to Carmen's capacity to connect with her own outrage, my role during this time was to assess what would be an appropriate response from me. If I had expressed my own indignation too soon, I would have been at odds with Carmen's response, and offering my judgment on the parents who she still relied on so heavily would have been counterproductive.

I attempted to get a picture of Carmen's childhood and early adult life through historical inquiry, which was difficult due to the heavy doses of medication which made her barely able to stay awake in our first year or so of therapy. I felt as though I was just "holding" a space where there were no demands, no criticisms, no definitions. The first real breakthrough came after nearly two years when she said, "I'm not worth anything." Then immediately, without being prompted by me, she changed the statement to, "I don't *believe* I'm worth anything." This shows that her self definition was changing and she was becoming more aware of the script decisions that she had made early in her life.

Often during the first few years of therapy with Carmen I would think to myself that we were just chatting. We "chatted" about birds, gardening, wildlife, anything as long as it was a safe subject that didn't require any deep self exploration or expression of affect. I took this to supervision regularly and always felt criticized by my supervisor's response which was to question my lack of working at depth and challenging Carmen. This of course stimulated my own shame within the therapy room, paralleling Carmen's shame for getting it wrong.

I always returned from my supervision sessions resolved to challenge Carmen to go deeper and to express more of what she was experiencing phenomenologically. I was aware that sometimes I felt irritated by Carmen's inability to work at greater depth and I was at risk of projecting my shame onto my client and blaming her for her lack of progress in the therapeutic work—a blame that was, of course, familiar throughout Carmen's life and which would have confirmed her script that it was all her fault.

From what I now know about working with someone who has such a profound schizoid process my intuitive way of working was exactly what Carmen needed, providing an attuned, holding environment (Bowlby, 1969) which she had never experienced as an infant, so that she never developed an emotional attachment to her mother or father. My aim was to encourage a healthy attachment to me that would act as a template for developing other healthy emotional attachments.

I believe that what appeared to be somewhat superficial conversation also had a protective function. It kept us away from any deep connection that might allow an exploration of affect that was deeply buried, for fear of the impact it may have on her ability to manage relationships within which she experienced a considerable amount of ambivalence. These relationships included her parents, her husband, and possibly me as well. It also reflects Guntrip's (1962) "schizoid compromise" where we could be in relationship providing the level of intimacy was superficial.

Another profoundly harmful script belief was that she was "in the way." Both her parents were successful career people and toward the end of her primary schooling they both were appointed to new posts in a different town. Carmen was left at the family home during the week, cared for by a neighbor, while her parents worked away. They returned each weekend, but Carmen's memory was of no attempt to engage with her needs, rather expecting her to fit into the activities in which they engaged.

Later in her therapy she connected with some intense rage toward both her parents and her husband. As a child she relied entirely on her parents. She rarely mentioned extended family and as an only child they were all she had. At the beginning of her therapy she continued to rely on them as they held her medication, delivering one day's supply at a time, so she was unconsciously replaying her childhood dependence.

As she began to get in touch with her anger toward her husband, she realized that he had never made her a priority. For example, he refused to take a day off work when Carmen needed to go into hospital for a surgical procedure. She would not be able to drive herself home again and the anesthetic meant that she was advised not to be alone for twenty-four hours after the operation. He arranged for someone to pick Carmen up from the hospital and drop her at the door to their house.

Sometimes as I reflected on our work, I would notice the changes that she was making and found it hard to understand how "chatting" could possibly help to make those changes. Now I understand that the importance of our chatting was that it enabled the secure bond to form with no threat to Carmen's integrity. It was a place where there was no risk of her being shamed and provided a relationship where she felt accepted and respected and where there was nothing demanded of her. Just to sit in silence with Carmen would have been shaming as she would have believed that she was bad for not being able to fill the silence.

Nathanson (1992) describes a number of defenses against shame including withdrawal and attacks on the self, and I had to learn the importance of both rhythmic and affective attunement in avoiding a schizoid withdrawal when making any phenomenological inquiry. Her inability to express her phenomenological experience would lead to shame. The defense against shame is the denial of the need for relationship and consequent withdrawal (Erskine, 1995).

Erskine (1995) suggests that shame is a complex process involving:

1. A diminished self-concept, a lowering of one's self worth in confluence with the external humiliation and/or previously introjected criticism
2. A defensive transposition of sadness and fear, and
3. A disavowal and retroflection of anger.

Her disavowal of anger was absolute, and I considered that part of my role was to help Carmen to reconnect with her retroflected anger at a pace that was tolerable and acceptable within her script beliefs. In the first few years of her therapy, any mention of anger would send Carmen into a defensive withdrawal as she experienced anger as shameful and leading to conflict. If I mentioned anger she would always respond with, "I don't like conflict." In the relationship with her parents she would go to any length to avoid expressing her anger toward them, sometimes cutting her legs with scissors as a way of retroflecting her anger, particularly toward her mother.

Any attempt at phenomenological inquiry in the early years of her therapy would result in Carmen looking frightened. Being unable to answer my questions about what she was experiencing internally led to her feeling shamed because she thought that she "ought" to know. So, when I noticed the tension in Carmen's body and the darkness of her frown I would tentatively say, "As you say that, you sound angry." Her response in the early part of therapy would be to twist her fingers, her feet would point inwards and be raised up to give the impression that she was so small that her feet couldn't reach the ground, and she would respond with, "But I don't feel angry" in the very high-pitched voice of a young child. The obvious defensive position that she adopted at these times was a clear message to me that I had overstepped the mark in noticing the anger that terrified her and had been disavowed. It was a clear misattunement on my part that would result in a schizoid withdrawal for Carmen. However, without those gentle invitations to notice her anger, no progress could have been made. Gradually, through my noticing when either her tone of voice or her body language suggested that she was experiencing an angry response to something or someone, she slowly began to recognize her affect and she gradually learned to express her feelings more authentically.

As I was working in conjunction with local psychiatric services, I attended Carmen's case reviews at her request. I met with her psychiatrist and community psychiatric nurse; her GP and parents were initially also present. At these meetings I received a lot of criticism for not working in a more solution-focused and time-limited way. The reports that were written following these meetings continually reiterated that open-ended therapy was not effective and that "a planned and managed ending that is a focus from the onset is of most therapeutic value." Throughout our work, any suggestion that her therapy needed to be time-limited would stimulate a schizoid withdrawal and an increase in physical pain for Carmen. As Guntrip (1962) states, "There is certainly no quick and easy way of making a stable and mature adult personality out of the legacy of an undermined childhood" (p. 273).

Her psychiatric diagnosis was of avoidant and dependent personality disorder with recurrent depression and I'm reminded of Johnson's view of the continuum from schizoid personality disorder at one end and the avoidant style at the other (Johnson, 1994). In his description of the early development of the schizoid process, Johnson suggests that,

> The hatred of the caretaking parent will be introjected and will begin to suppress the life force of the organism, such that movement and breathing are inhibited and there develops an involuntary tightening of the musculature to restrain the life force. (1994, p. 75)

Whenever Carmen felt any challenge from me, no matter how small or gentle, I would notice that she had stopped breathing. Also, when she first began to feel the tears pricking behind her eyes, she became so overwhelmed that she would completely stop breathing and tense her whole body as if she were trying to disappear. For a long time I had to gently remind her to breathe whenever she began to cry. Initially her crying was silent and clearly painful as it resulted in a tensing of every muscle in her body in an attempt to prevent the tears flowing. Reminding her to breathe resulted in a huge intake of breath followed by a loud, body wracking sob.

Throughout the first few years of therapy Carmen would panic at any suggestion that she was getting better. Any suggestion that she was improving would send her into a spiral of increased physical pain and suicidal thoughts. Her pain and incapacity had become part of her identity without which she said that she didn't know who she was. She saw herself not as someone who was experiencing pain, but that she was the pain. She also said that she was afraid that if she got better, no one would like her.

During this first phase of therapy, when she was still taking large doses of medication, she made collections of her tablets as an insurance that if life became too unbearable, she could end it with certainty. Initially I talked with her about how she could give up the medication collection to me to dispose of. The second collection she agreed to take to her doctor's surgery. Relinquishing this "insurance" increased her anxiety and after the second collection had been surrendered, I was greatly concerned about her physical safety. As I reflected on our work I realized that I was not attuning to Carmen's needs. In telling me about her collection of medication she was attempting to paint a picture for me of the existential dilemma of someone who has developed a schizoid process. My focus had been much more about what I considered to be my ethical duty to keep my client safe and prevent her from completing suicide. In fact, I realized that my over-simplistic method of keeping Carmen safe, by removing the lethal collection of medication, was similar to how her parents would respond, rather than an empathetic consideration of what was really best for my client by attuning and inquiring.

I then realized that Carmen would probably be safer if she was allowed to keep her "insurance" because she would be in control. Without the collection of medication she would look for other ways that she could kill herself and as she had already attempted strangulation a number of times, this was a real danger. Having written to her psychiatrist, explaining the situation and my thinking, he responded by agreeing with me and Carmen was allowed to hold her collection until she was ready to give it up. This had the effect of immediately reducing her level of anxiety, which gave us an opportunity to focus our efforts on strengthening her sense of self as potent in the world.

Carmen has gradually learned to identify her angry response, almost as though she was learning a foreign language, and through my assurances that her anger is justifiable she has learned how to express herself, in an appropriate way, which enables her to maintain relationship with the person who is the object of her anger.

Laing (1960), in describing the schizoid person says,

> Such a person is not able to experience himself "together with" others or "at home in" the world, but, on the contrary, he experiences himself in despairing aloneness and isolation; moreover, he does not experience himself as a complete person but rather as "split" in various ways, perhaps as a mind more or less tenuously linked to a body, as two or more selves, and so on. (p. 1)

Carmen had spent her whole life isolated from other people. She just had no idea how to be in an intimate relationship. Her husband fit her life script as he clearly had similar interpersonal difficulties and although we didn't explore their relationship at any depth, I believe they probably had interlocking scripts. This made their divorce inevitable as Carmen became more able to enjoy being in relationship and developed a healthy autonomy. She had very few friends at school and when she began to work, she also found it difficult to relate to others. When she came into therapy the only people she described as friends were the friends of her parents. She has been on sick leave from her job in the pharmaceutical industry for a number of years and was eventually made redundant. This gave her the freedom to begin to volunteer in a variety of roles in her local community. This gradually led to part-time paid work in a local primary school working with some of the more challenging children, and latterly a more substantial role in another primary school, again, supporting children who display challenging behavior. She still has a rather small friendship group but one of the most exciting developments for me was when she began dating and found a new partner with whom she has a sound, loving, mature relationship.

In summary

> The greatest need of a child is to obtain conclusive assurance (a) that he is genuinely loved as a person by his parents, and (b) that his parents genuinely accept his love. It is only in so far as such assurance is forthcoming in a form sufficiently convincing to enable him to depend safely upon his real objects (parents) that he is able to gradually renounce infantile dependence without misgiving. In the absence of such assurance his relationships to his objects is fraught with too much anxiety over separation to enable him to renounce the attitude of infantile dependence: for such a renunciation would be equivalent in his eyes to forfeiting all hope of ever obtaining the satisfaction of his unsatisfied emotional needs. Frustration of his desire to be loved as a person, and frustration of his desire to have his love accepted, is the greatest trauma that a child can experience. (Fairbairn, 1952, pp. 39–40)

Carmen never received such assurance from her busy, professional parents. She felt "in the way," "not important," and everything was her fault. She is now living fully independent of her parents with whom she now has a more robust adult–adult relationship within which she is able to express her needs as well as her feelings toward them. She has no problem expressing healthy anger toward them and other people in a respectful, relational way.

As our work has progressed, she has gradually ceased taking all medication and is now mostly as pain-free as the general population. She has now learned to associate an increase in physiological pain to unexpressed emotions, especially anger and disappointment.

Two years ago, she joined a group where she is using artistic expression. She has shared some of the creative work that she had been completing in this group. This art work has really helped her to connect with some deep anger and sadness. As she spoke about the images, I thought I detected an unspoken question in her voice as she was describing the meanings behind the images. "Why did we not use these techniques earlier in my therapy?" I looked at her and asked if my thinking was correct. She nodded, looked thoughtful for a while, then without me saying a word, she just said, "I would have been completely overwhelmed!" I felt an element of relief here as I had heard my supervisor's voice for a moment criticizing me over the years for not challenging Carmen much more robustly.

I am deeply grateful for the opportunity that working with Carmen has given me to learn about the role that shame plays in the development of a schizoid process and I feel privileged that she trusted me enough to stay with the process through my learning how to be with her that enabled the healing of the split within herself. Her courage to stay alive when she believed that there was no hope of anything ever changing has been inspirational for me to experience. I have also learned to consider that for some people, suicide might just be the ultimate schizoid withdrawal.

References

Bass, C. (1990). *Somatization: Physical Symptoms and Psychological Illness*. Oxford: Blackwell Scientific.

Blumer, D., & Heilbronn, M. (1982). Chronic pain as a variant of depressive disease: The pain-prone disorder. *Journal of Nervous and Mental Disease, 170*: 381–406.

Bowlby, J. (1969). *Attachment and Loss, Vol. 1: Attachment*. New York: Basic Books.

Engel, G. (1959). "Psychogenic" pain and the pain-prone patient. *American Journal of Medicine, 26*: 899–918.

Erskine, R. G. (1995). A Gestalt therapy approach to shame and self righteousness: Theory and methods. *British Gestalt Journal, 4*(2): 107–117.

Erskine, R. G., Moursund, J. P., & Trautmann, R. L. (1999). *Beyond Empathy: A Therapy of Contact-in-relationship*. London: Routledge, 2023.

Fairbairn, W. R. D. (1952). *Psychoanalytic Studies of the Personality*. London: Routledge & Kegan Paul.

Guntrip, H. (1962). The schizoid compromise and therapeutic stalemate. *British Journal of Medical Psychology, 35*(4): 273–288.

Johnson, S. M. (1994). *Character Styles*. New York: W. W. Norton.

Laing, R. D. (1960). *The Divided Self*. London: Penguin.

Masterson, J. F. (1988). *The Search for the Real Self: Unmasking the Personality Disorders of Our Age*. New York: Free Press.

Nathanson, D. J. (1992). *Shame and Pride: Affect, Sex, and the Birth of the Self*. New York: W. W. Norton.

Tyrer, S. (2006). Psychosomatic pain. *British Journal of Psychiatry, 188*(1): 91–93.

Yontef, G. (2001). Psychotherapy of schizoid process. *Transactional Analysis Journal, 31*(1): 7–23.

Part III

Clients' perspectives on the psychotherapy

CHAPTER 14

"Come closer … but keep your distance": a client's perspective on the psychotherapy of schizoid process

Leigh Bettles

> *"Well, come back and have tea with us," said Moon-Face. "Silky's got some Pop Biscuits— and I've made some Google Buns. I don't often make them—and I tell you they're a treat!"*
> —Enid Blyton

I entered the profession of psychotherapy with an intense desire to help people heal from the relational disruptions and traumas that they had endured in their lives. Little did I realize that I also had a troubled child inside of me, who required a healing relationship in order to feel alive and authentic. In doing my psychotherapy training I was able to understand the relational conflicts that shaped the adult I had become. Importantly, with a couple of attuned psychotherapists I was able to give that troubled inner child a voice, understanding, and a sense of inner peace.

This chapter is a sharing of the positive outcomes of some of the psychotherapy work I have done over the years. I particularly want to share with colleagues what I have learned from one specific hour of intensive therapy—that had a profound impact on my life to the extent that I no longer need to withdraw in social relationships; I no longer feel alone, as I am at peace within myself. This chapter contains an unedited transcript of an hour-long therapy session, which I did during a five-day professional training program with Richard Erskine. I was initially attracted to Richard's training programs because I was impressed with his writings on the theory and methods of a developmentally based, relationally focused psychotherapy. He was offering a series of workshops in the UK on the psychotherapy of shame and self-righteousness, narcissism, the early affect confusion of the borderline client, and the psychotherapy of the schizoid process. I wanted to know so much more about the practice of a relational oriented psychotherapy, so I signed up for the extensive training program.

As Richard described the *schizoid process,* it was as though he was talking about me. His illustrations of the "schizoid compromise" put words to my emotional distress, my self-criticism, my loneliness, my emotional withdrawal in many social situations, and, importantly, when I needed to connect with a sense of inner peace (Erskine, 2001). The psychotherapy session that I describe below helped me to know, not just cognitively, but in the depths of my body, that I am not alone.

I lived my childhood in an environment of secrecy. I was unable to freely talk about what was happening in my family and certainly not what was happening within me. I was brought up in a society that did not recognize or talk about what went on within the family and certainly not the domestic violence between my parents. I had grown to believe that I must not talk about my experience and if I did, bad things would happen. I was fearful about talking because in my fantasy I would lose the people around me who I depended on for my survival. The combination of the brutal conflict between my parents and my fantasy led me to feel isolated and alone.

I felt a sense of deep shame, as I had internalized the belief that I was bad and that there was something wrong with me. In my school class I cowered in my chair, terrified of being seen and unable to raise my hand or use my voice to speak out. I can remember answering the teacher's questions in my mind, but by the time I could find the words to answer, the class had moved on to the next question. I was so scared of getting it wrong. One day I was asked to stand up in class and talk. I accidently said a word wrong and the whole class laughed at me. I felt ashamed and stood there blushing and wishing I could disappear. Each time I went over this event in my mind it reinforced my script belief that "I should not speak out."

I remember my mother attending parents' evening. An evening that I dreaded because I struggled academically. But I thought that at least I would get a good review from my geography teacher. I loved to hear about different countries and how landscapes formed with meandering rivers. But on this evening my mum came back and said that my teacher told her that I showed a lack of interest in the lessons and was always looking out of the window or not paying attention. I was upset by this. He had misinterpreted the times that I was struggling to do the work and be part of the class. This led me to feel like I did not belong, I was the odd one out. When I struggled with the work, I would look out of the window and wish I was somewhere else and not there, or I would go to my "sanctuary," my special place of internal quiet, for a break from the anxiety and pressure of feeling that I had to get things right.

My parents did not have high expectations of me. I knew that my brother was the "brainy one" and in response I developed a strong internal critic telling me "I can't learn," "I'm stupid." I also told myself "I'm fat and ugly." As I grew older and got a job, my internal critic intensified. I told myself again and again, "I'm stupid and boring," "Nobody wants me as a friend."

As a result of these script beliefs, I could not trust anyone. Consequently, these script beliefs led me to adapt my behavior. I separated myself from people around me. I stopped myself from getting close with anyone; and I concluded that I desperately needed to protect myself from people. I told myself, "I can't trust anyone"; "People will hurt me"; "If people really know me, they will shame and reject me." Although I desperately wanted to be liked, I avoided anything that would make a conflict and possibly lead to a break in the relationship. All through this time, I knew that I had the ability to go inside myself to my "private sanctuary." At a party I could look as though I was enjoying the music and dancing, but I had the ability to "space out"; I would go to my special place of peace and quiet.

I wanted a family and children, but marriage brought the realization that I needed help to deal with my past and to be able to form lasting relationships. My partner was not a talkative person, which was OK in the beginning because I too was silent much of the time. But as I did my therapy and training, I started to be able to use my voice and express myself. I realized that I needed to be with someone to whom I could talk openly. Over time I got more frustrated and angrier. I struggled with the question, "Why would he not listen or talk to me." I hated seeing him sit in his chair with a massive newspaper up over his face. The paper reminded me of an iron wall, leaving me on the outside. There was no face or connection. I felt alone again!

An intense therapy session

It was the afternoon of the third day of a five-day professional training workshop that Richard Erskine was conducting in Manchester, UK. I had previously attended five, five-day training workshops with Richard. In these professional development workshops Richard would lecture on specific topics, engage the training group in discussions about personality theory and how it applied to their clients, invite us to present cases for peer discussion and supervision, and demonstrate various psychotherapy methods with members of the group who volunteered to have an hour of psychotherapy with Richard. As usual in the training group, the colleagues were sitting on several comfortable chairs in a large oval. I was looking for a place to sit where I could watch and learn. The group had asked Richard to demonstrate how he would work with a client who uses relational withdrawal as a way to manage their emotions. Richard asked for a volunteer, specifically for someone who may have identified with what he had been teaching the previous three mornings.

While Richard had been teaching about the qualities of a psychotherapy that are essential for healing the various splits in a client's sense of self, I was thinking "I know what he is talking about." Earlier that day I had several memories of the times when I hid myself from people, searching for a secure place in my mind. I timidly said to Richard, "I kinda want to work," and at the same time I was prepared for someone else to volunteer. In my mind anyone else would be more worthy of the opportunity to work with Richard than me. My old self-criticism was coming into play. My wish was to conform to what the other person wanted of me: to avoid conflict and competition; to maintain the appearance of relationship by always being quiet and pleasant. I was frozen in place. It took me almost half a minute to move toward Richard. I instinctively knew that the confidentiality and intimacy, so central to this unique training group, provided the necessary security for me to be vulnerable, to expose what had been my personal secret for many years. I needed the gentle, patient strength that I saw Richard provide to others in the group and I also needed to reveal myself in front of a group of colleagues whom I respected. As a reader, you may wonder if I was in transference with Richard and the group. Yes, indeed, I was in an emotional transference with both the group and Richard. I desperately needed a healing relationship, someone on whom I could rely—someone who would understand my nonverbal story, who would validate my inner experiences. I also needed the group members' acknowledgment and acceptance of who I am; I needed a new group experience in order to counteract my intense sense of shame.

The following is an uncut, word-for-word, transcript of our therapeutic transactions.

Richard: Come sit over here, so that I'm not twisting my neck around and we're facing each other.

As I approached, I was aware of my apprehension. I was feeling unsure and somehow younger. What would happen? What should I say? Could I do this? The sensations in my arms, legs, and neck indicated to me that my body was stiffening.

Leigh: I'm still a bit curious about our eye contact, as I still find it hard and you're really staring at me now.

My voice was a little shaky and I gave a nervous laugh. I was feeling so uncomfortable about the way Richard was looking at me. His face seemed intense. He looked interested as though he wanted to know what I had to say. There was a sense of confusion as he gave me his full attention and the look of someone who "cares." I just was not used to being looked at like this. It crossed my mind that I may not be able to stay looking face to face with Richard.

Richard: I want to see you.
Leigh: Yeh.

My tone of voice suggested that I was half agreeing but half surprised that he had said this. I didn't know how to react to Richard's comment. I wanted to move on, away from me being the focus of his attention, but I did volunteer. I thought "It will be OK." An important reaction that was my way of calming myself.

Richard: I never realized how blue your eyes were before.
Leigh: I think it depends on what I wear as well. Sometimes they stand out a bit more.

I was making polite conversation. I had been brought up to do this social skill and thought it was the right thing to do. At the same time, I was able to calm myself, as I knew what I had said was appropriate.

Richard: But you said that you were identifying with …
Leigh: I was identifying with um (nine second pause) … I suppose withdrawing with people and um (six second pause) … and because of the eye contact with you, like going into my own place and not connecting with people. Coz I was saying about … how in the previous five-day workshop I was … I was kind of … um … very aware of how, I didn't make contact with you … um …

I had been aware of deliberately not making contact with people on the previous five-day workshop. At that time, I had needed to keep myself separated. My internal critic was causing me to hesitate. My cheeks turned red hot; I was full of shame as I admitted to myself that I had done this. But I needed to take a few seconds to think about what had made me volunteer. Why was I sitting there?

Richard: Do you think I demand it?
Leigh: Um. Do you think you demand it?

I started to have difficulty focusing on what Richard was saying and I felt confused. I was returning to my adult self and was trying to concentrate on the questions, so that I could get the answers right. "Demand" seemed like a harsh word and I was feeling uncomfortable in my stomach. As I tried to repeat his question his words didn't make sense to me or seem to connect with what we were talking about.

Richard: No. Do you think I demand that you be in contact?
Leigh: No. I'm not aware of it anyway … um.

I didn't think Richard was being demanding in any way. I was now aware of the people sitting around me. I was listening to the questions and desperately struggling to give Richard the right answers.

Richard: Did you feel pressure to do so?
Leigh: No. When I think of the previous five-day workshop, I think we worked well. I went away and I didn't feel overwhelmed, as maybe I have been in the past, so it was good.
Richard: You had been concerned about that before and I wanted to take your concern into consideration.
Leigh: (eight second pause) Mm … Yeh.

Richard had read the email I had sent to him about my intense feelings after a previous workshop. He remembered that I did not want to go away from the workshop overwhelmed. It felt reassuring that he had taken my request seriously. I felt more comfortable and secure sitting with Richard. In the past I had been the quiet one, not giving an opinion, going along with what others wanted to do. Because of this I never made a direct impact on anyone. My friends were organizers and sorted out what we were doing, and I just complied with their decisions. I was amazed that my request had been heard and responded to by Richard. I realized that I had made an impact on Richard. His response was so different from what I had experienced in other relationships.

Richard: I wonder what would happen right now, if you took some time to go to a safer internal place … with my support and encouragement?
Leigh: What's coming into my mind is … um … going away will mean getting in touch with the loneliness. Which is really hard.
Richard: So you don't go all the way away … go halfway away?
Leigh: Are you saying that I just go halfway away? Or do I go all the way?

I was returning to a younger age. Again, I felt confused and anxious, my senses were not working. My hearing deteriorated and I could not understand what Richard was saying. The words become fuzzy. Like when I was young, what was being said didn't make sense. When I got confused my anxiety increased. It was a vicious circle because when I was a child it was necessary to get it right, but if I was anxious, I could not understand and therefore I could not get it right. I was frightened, lonely, and sought refuge in silence.

Richard: Yes … You said if you go all the way away you'll get in touch with the loneliness.
Leigh: I guess it depends on the situation.
Richard: Well, see what would happen if you just close your eyes.
Leigh: OK.
Richard: And see if you can go away, even while I'm here watching over you. … (six second pause) And I'm not going to do anything abruptly or fast. … I'm not gonna surprise you … (five second pause) I'm going to stay right here, watching over you.

Richard's facial expressions seemed really important to me at that moment. It stimulated a memory of waiting for my father to come home. If he had a normal, stress-free happy face it was OK to go and greet him, but if he had that angry menacing look it was a sign that I needed to quickly retreat to my bedroom for safety, as it was likely that he would cause an argument with my mum. The arguments never were about important matters; in his mind she did things against him on purpose.

I was aware of Richard's calm, slow, caring voice. My breathing had become deeper, slower and I relaxed my shoulders. I felt safer with the knowledge that Richard was taking care of me. I felt reassured that he would not let anything bad or shocking happen. His voice gave me the sense of being held safely. I was aware he was not too close and not too far away. Richard created a safe environment that was a great contrast to the chaos around me during my childhood.

As a child there was no one to help regulate my emotions and to help me to understand what was happening. I needed the adults to stop the overwhelming shouting between them; I was caught in their violence. I did not have any control at those times of what was going on, neither outside nor inside my body.

> Leigh: (fifteen second pause) It feels like I want to open my eyes to just check that you're still there.

As soon as I shut my eyes I was in a different place, dark and alone. I could not see Richard's face to gather any information or reassurance that all would be OK. Everything was black and I was alone. No longer was I in the familiar room with my colleagues. And I could not find my peaceful "sanctuary" place. It was cold and dark. My body became alert, and I began to panic. I needed to see Richard's face for reassurance, to hear his calm reassuring voice in order to feel safe.

> Richard: I'm right here and I'm going to stay here. … (eighteen second pause) I'm paying attention to how fast your heart is beating. So, I suspect you're scared.
> Leigh: I'm just anxious really.
> Richard: Anxious.
> Leigh: Because it feels like I'm on my own, with my eyes closed.

Over the years I have developed the ability to diminish the significance of my anxiety by saying to myself that I am "just" anxious. I often convinced myself that "the current situation is not so bad." These little phrases help me to stop myself from becoming overwhelmed. These self-regulating techniques had helped me in many situations, but they had not solved the underlying issue of being both terrified and lonely. I longed for resolution of my terror and loneliness and that was why I was taking the risk of revealing my true self to Richard.

> Richard: … (seventeen second pause) Alone. … (twenty-five second pause) And I'm going to be right here with you, while you're on your own.
> Leigh: … (six second pause) It kinda doesn't matter if you're there or not because I know I can … I can just be in my head and be OK.

What I did not say out loud was: "It's OK because I can go to my 'sanctuary' where I can feel calm and safe, and no one need know that I have gone." Most of the time it seemed like going to my sanctuary just happened. But with the help of my ongoing therapy, I uncovered the three ways in which I would retreat to my sanctuary: I became still and said nothing; I stared into space without any focus; or I would focus on the sensations in my body. With each of these three ways I could slip into my sanctuary where I would be temporarily safe from the potential of invading chaos. After this psychotherapy with Richard, I realized that repeating words over and over again, like a mantra, was another way to ease into my private place of peace and quiet.

Some of my clients who used dissociation to handle overwhelming emotions have described their out of body experiences where they are observing the abuse inflicted on them but without physical sensations or emotions. To these clients it is as though the trauma did not happen to them, an "it's not me" experience.

My experience of withdrawing into my sanctuary was different from dissociation. I would go to my internal "no place," a place without people. But I was not dissociated; I was always me, still in the room and watching, but I was not in emotional contact with anyone. Friends did not notice; they could not see my internal struggle. I was "spacing out" which was how I described what I was doing to myself. In some threatening situation my withdrawal seemed to happen almost automatically, like flicking a light switch. On other occasions going to the "no place" was much slower, like turning the dimmer switch for a light.

My sanctuary provided me with calmness, peace, and a place to be me. Although a disadvantage of retreating to my sanctuary was that I lost my sense of time. Often, I did not notice that I had withdrawn into my private place. I worried about my "spacing out" and how it may be affecting my life. I knew that it was often necessary to record training workshops and supervision sessions because I was afraid I would space out and miss important information and not understand what was being presented. I remember that in my early therapy sessions I frequently had an intense pull to withdraw into my sanctuary.

Richard: … (eleven second pause) So *it* doesn't matter. … (eleven second pause) Such an important phrase. … (seven second pause) "Doesn't matter if you're there."

When I heard Richard emphasize the words "doesn't matter" I felt intensely sad. I couldn't tell him how desperately I want and need someone, him, to be there. There was a high risk of being controlled, criticized, or invaded again. It felt like a real threat and I needed to hide from any threat. I was in constant conflict between wanting to be closer to Richard and desperately wanting to pull away.

Richard: (seventeen second pause) And I'm going to stay here watching over you. Even if you say, "doesn't matter."

I was relieved that Richard was not leaving me alone. A longing and hope for relationship kept me from completely withdrawing. There was a constant push, a desperate need to stay in relationship and experience the care I never had at those fearful times. At the same time there was a constant urge to pull away from the painful criticism, control, and invasion that I feared would happen if we were in a close relationship.

I have seen the way other people have formed relationships and supported each other in the five-day training workshops. The sight of other people supporting and hugging each other reminded me of how painfully alone I was. At that time, I couldn't imagine having that relationship with others even though I periodically had some hope for satisfying connections with people. I was stuck. If I pushed Richard away, I thought that I would lose my chance for any relationship with him. If I let myself be close with Richard, he might take over and control me. That immediately brought up memories of being hurt in previous relationships. Withdrawal to my sanctuary was the best solution.

Richard: ... (forty second pause) The feeling must be intense. ... (forty-nine second pause) But it must be wonderful to have a place to hide. ... (six second pause) To have a hiding place that provides some security. ... (eleven second pause) A safe place to go where there's no conflicts with anybody. ... (four second pause) Must be wonderful.

I was listening to Richard's soothing voice and agreeing. Internally I was acknowledging the truth of what he was saying: he was describing my internal experience, how it was for me. It seemed like he understood because he was talking to the child I once was.

It was important that he didn't ask factual questions or inquire about my feelings because I was too young to answer. I didn't have the language to explain what was happening. Richard was giving me a vocabulary to help me understand and explain my experience. He was confirming why I had been protecting myself. Nobody had done this before or had been interested in where I went to feel secure. Not having to think and answer questions helped me to be calm. I was not aware of the other people in the room, except for the occasional turning of a page or someone taking a drink. I felt calm, I was back in my sanctuary, but this time Richard was nearby, relaxed, and at my pace.

Leigh: ... (seven second pause) It's just peaceful (I clear my throat to be able to speak) It's peaceful.
Richard: Oh! So necessary to find peace. ... (fourteen second pause) The noise that you'll hear in a moment is just me straightening my leg. I'm not going to invade your peace; I'm just moving my leg. ... (ten second pause) It must have been so necessary, to find a peaceful place. ... (fourteen second pause) So much feeling when I say that. ... (twenty-one second pause) Must be sad to have to search for a private peaceful place.

It felt reassuring when Richard told me that he would move his leg. He was doing what he said he would do by going slowly and taking care not to surprise or shock me with loud noises or sudden movements. Richard seemed to understand the importance for my need for security. He let me know that he wouldn't invade me in any way. His words were comforting; they gave me a sense of security which increased my trust in him.

Leigh: ... (eight second pause) It's because things are so overwhelming outside, that I have to go inside.

I recalled my parents fighting. Mum would scream for help. My father was bigger and stronger than she was, so instead of fighting back she would scream back at him, things she knew would hurt him emotionally. It was her only way of getting back at him, even though it meant she got hurt more.

Richard: Of course. That's why I used the word wonderful before. … Wonderful that you found at least some place, to have a little bit of peace. … (ten second pause) Overwhelming outside.

I was crying as I recalled past overwhelming experiences. Richard passed me a tissue. His gesture was soothing.

> … (nine second pause) Overwhelming and anxious making, perhaps frightening, perhaps confusing.

As Richard spoke I could I feel my jaw tightening and my lips pushing together. Memories of needing to escape the domestic violence in my home were coming in and out of consciousness but surprisingly I was not feeling overwhelmed. In the past I always felt emotionally overwhelmed when I had these memories, but now I felt calmed by Richard's slow understanding voice.

> … (twenty-eight second pause) Overwhelming. … (fourteen second pause) So necessary to create a peaceful place. … (twenty-one second pause) To have some quiet. The preciousness of quietness.

It sounded like Richard understood how bad it was and why I needed to hide. At the same time, he validated my need for peace and quiet. I sat very still, the same way I did when I was a child, not moving, not wanting to be seen, not sure if I could speak.

> … (twenty-four second pause) There's no rush. We are not going to do this work in a hurry. So, there's no need to think about being quick here to satisfy me. I'll adjust to your rhythm.

As I listened, I slowed my breathing and found the pace I needed. I was aware that I was not under pressure to do or say anything. It helped that I was not compelled to think of answers because I always perceived questions as either invasive or controlling. Richard's reflective comments where reassuring and validating.

> … (twenty-five second pause) To have some time to really appreciate the peacefulness is so important. … (sixteen second pause) So necessary to escape the confusion

     and chaos. … (eleven second pause) To go to a place where there is no criticism. … (twenty second pause) I'm going to listen even if you don't talk, I'm listening to your breathing, listening to your body vibes and yet I know you must have a lot to say. Even though it seems impossible to talk.

  Leigh: … (seven second pause) It feels like I lose my voice sometimes. I can't talk.

I recalled seeing the violence in my family and wanting to shout and scream "Stop!" But I had no sound. Sometimes I thought that I had screamed but then later I was aware that I had not made a sound. I was invisible and soundless as the family violence played out in front of me.

Richard: … (five second pause) Em … em … Can't talk. … It must be very hard to be hiding in your peaceful place and talk at the same time … because if you talk people might invade your peaceful place. … (four second pause) They might invade. … It seems better to never speak.

While Richard was talking, I was having quick flashes of watching my father, not knowing if he would kill my mum. I could not physically shout out "Stop." I was too terrified of drawing any attention to myself. I was six to twelve years old and had a realization that I was regressed to a much younger age. I was terrified that my father would turn his rage on me because I was sure that I would not survive his temper. The only way I could cope was to find my own sanctuary.

Richard: (eighteen second pause) I'll listen to your silence. Because I think there is a big story in the silence. A sad story and a fearful story.

Richard acknowledged the importance of my silence. It felt like *he knew* my inner world. It was so important to me that someone could know that my fears were real; he validated the importance of my sanctuary.

  Leigh: (twenty-two second silence) I'm just aware that sometimes I don't want to be on my own. I want somebody to be there.

Prior to my psychotherapy I lived in a state of anxiety, not knowing what would happen next. I would force myself out of the house to be with friends as much as I could manage and then I dreaded going back to the house. I spent hours in my bedroom reading and enjoying my life in a world of fantasy. When I was younger books such as Enid Blyton's *The Magic Faraway Tree* (1942) provided an opportunity to escape to distant lands with Moon-Face and Silky, through the clouds at the top of the magic tree. The fantasy took my loneliness away for a time, but I could not escape what was happening around me. Fantasy was not enough to take away the fear of what I witnessed; for that I needed to withdraw to my sanctuary.

Richard: (four second pause) But not to be invasive.
Leigh: That would be too scary.

I knew that I had to sit still; it was as if moving would shatter my peace and bring the chaos back. Being physically still was a way of not being seen; I was physically tight and rigid as a result of my fear. I was remembering some of the arguments and how once the shouting had stopped, my mum would come into my bedroom and sleep on the floor by my bed. Although it was good to know she was OK, it was terrifying because "what if he came in the room?" I was scared stiff while watching the crack at the bottom of the door. I was waiting to see if his shadow was outside the door, waiting to see when the light went off, an indication that he had gone to bed. Yet, even if he had gone to bed, I was always expecting that he would come into my room.

Richard: To be present ... if you had an absolute guarantee that there'd be no invasion, no controlling, ... then it might be nice to have somebody there. ... (six second pause) But not the invasive, not the critical, not the controlling.

I was silent, remembering the invasiveness, being controlled, and used. I had been used as a form of communication between my parents: my father would say, "Tell your mother ..." If I was slow, he would shout, "Tell her," even when she was in the same room. He was so controlling, and I was so confused, perhaps even angry. But I could not dare to express any anger because that was dangerous. I was suddenly filled with the same scary feelings that I had known from the past.

Leigh: ... (six second pause) It's too scary ... I have to keep everybody out.
Richard: Well, that's what I'm going to do today. ... I gonna keep everybody out. ... And make sure that nobody here does anything that's invasive or critical. ... Because I know how sad you are.
Leigh: It's because I'm on my own, it's only because I'm on my own.

I desperately needed someone there. The loneliness was intense, like a deep hole in my body, and at the same time I was full of fear. I longed to hear the kindness, caring, and reassurance that Richard was giving me. But it was so important that he was respecting my boundaries and was not controlling or telling me what to do. If he had done those things, it would have been hard not to see him as my father.

Richard: No, I don't think so ... I see how scared you are ... but I hear the criticism. ... Right now, I heard the criticism, of blaming yourself ... but I think you were a frightened little girl, frightened and sad and probably very lonely. ... (twelve second pause) Lonely! ... (eight second pause) But it must seem easier to blame yourself than to feel that loneliness. ... (forty-seven second pause) I'm right here watching over you and there's no need to be in a hurry about this. ... (nineteen second pause) There's so much feeling inside. Feeling that never gets put into words.

I was crying as I became increasingly aware of just how frightened I was as a child. My eyes were closed but as I listened to Richard's voice, I sensed in my body that I was safe. The calmness of Richard's voice, his attunement to my pace, and his understanding and consideration of my boundaries gave me a reassurance that I could trust him. This was a great contrast to how my father had treated me.

Leigh: (nine second pause) I'm just thinking that I have blamed myself for things that have happened in the past.
Richard: Of course.
Leigh: Because maybe, it is easier.

Blaming myself made sense to me; how could I blame my dad?
   He was my dad. And my mum, she was doing what she could to protect us. It was always so much easier if all the conflicts were my fault. I told myself: "I did things to make my dad angry"; "I didn't do anything to stop him hurting my mum"; "I should have done better at school." These chastising comments occupied my mind; they kept me distracted from realizing the reasons for my terror and loneliness.

Richard: Of course, so much easier to blame yourself. Than to feel that loneliness. ... (eighteen second pause) There's so much feeling inside. Feeling that never gets put into words. ... (seventeen second pause) Lots of criticism, lots of self-blame, but lots of sadness. Lots of loneliness too.

At this point I was crying because it felt safe to let the tears come. I had criticized myself for years, blaming me for all the troubles in the family. With this cry my body was relaxing, things made sense, my mind went quiet.

Leigh: (one minute, three second pause) I'm not really thinking of anything.

It was strange to just sit there with nothing to say and Richard was still there. Then I started to worry, "Can he really be interested in me?"; "When will he get angry?"; "Who is going to laugh at me for being ridiculous?" Yet Richard stayed there, listening to me. He did not move. This was not what I would have expected to happen.

Richard: It's OK, I'm still listening. ... Listening to your heartbeat, to your breathing, to your vibes. And your words when you're thinking. ... I'm also listening to your silence ... The silence that tells a thousand stories.

I couldn't understand what Richard was doing. Why was he staying with me, still listening, spending so much time with me, and not disappearing? I was unsettled by this unfamiliar experience, and yet, I didn't want Richard to stop.

Richard: (twenty-three second pause) What I'm feeling is, the sadness … and I'm feeling the loneliness.
Leigh: And how hard it is to reach out.
Richard: Yeh. Almost impossible to reach out, coz the fear is so great … It's so wonderful to be in a hiding place that's peaceful. That in the beginning feeling so good, until the loneliness builds up then it gets lonelier and lonelier, if you reach out it's so frightening, because there's all the chaos again. … (fourteen second pause) It's so wonderful to have a hiding place that's peaceful and so terrible to feel that loneliness … Peaceful, lonely.

Naming my dilemma was so important to me. Up until that moment I had lived my dilemma, but I hadn't acknowledged the internal struggle between having a peaceful hiding place and the painful loneliness. Richard put my internal conflict into words when he said the phrases "so wonderful to have a hiding place" and "so terrible to feel that loneliness." The words were new but somehow, they were familiar and comforting because they described me, the struggle of my life. I felt trust.

Richard: (forty-four second pause) I'm right here.
Leigh: (twenty-eight second pause) I want to reach out but I'm too scared.

At that moment, my body froze. I wanted to reach out and touch Richard, but a rush of intense fear made it impossible to take that risk. I was certain that no one could possibly know how terrifying it was to want to touch and yet to freeze with fear. I was trapped in a body that was trying to protect me.

Richard: Of course … Too scared to reach out and so lonely … but it must seem dangerous to reach out … so maybe it's better to accept the loneliness. At least then it's peaceful.
Leigh: (five second pause) It's not better.
Richard: Not better … But you know that loneliness. You've known that for years and years and years. … It's better than invasion.
Leigh: I don't need to be scared anymore.
Richard: Say that louder.
Leigh: I DON'T NEED TO BE SCARED ANYMORE!
Richard: Are you sure?
Leigh: (five second pause) No.

Richard: (eight second pause) People do mean things. People become critical, controlling.
Leigh: (five second pause) I feel I need to reach out and touch you, but then that's enough. Because I need to know you're there.

The urge to know that Richard was fully present was really strong. I needed reassurance that I would be OK. I was feeling braver. Testing out that Richard is not going to harm me. He reached out and briefly touched my hand.

Richard: Just a little pat like that? Or is that too much?

At that time a pat was not enough but my body was frozen. I could not reach out. I needed Richard to initiate. I wanted him to take my scare away. I needed his calm voice and slow movements. Any fast movements would have scared me away. I could not separate the past and the present. Although I knew it was different. Richard was gaining my trust and was doing everything that he promised.

Leigh: I want to reach out my hand, but I can't, because I can't move my arm.
Richard: Shall I come to you?
Leigh: (eight second pause) I'm scared.
Richard: I'm going to come closer. If you don't like it you can push me away … It will be OK with me if you push me away … So lonely and so scared … So scared of invasion … then so lonely, … how terrible it is inside to have both. … (one minute, fourteen second pause) … right here with our finger-to-finger contact.

As Richard touched my hand, I quickly started to feel overwhelmed. I was unable to regulate my body sensations. When I was a child there was never anyone there to teach me how to calm myself. The only soothing thing I knew was to withdraw into my sanctuary. I pulled my hand away.

Leigh: That's enough now. That's all I need.

I felt an embarrassment that we had touched hands, that I needed the contact, and some guilt that I could only stay for such a short period.

Richard: That's important for you to say, that's all I need. To say no, that's enough. If it's true.
Leigh: (ten second pause) (I laugh nervously. I feel alone again.)

Instantly I was back in a lonely place. As I type this transcript, I feel so sad. I recall wanting to hold Richard's hand, but the desire was gone in a flash because I was overwhelmed with fear. I immediately pulled away.

Richard: I'll stay with you while you're all alone. Go back to that quiet place, you know that so well. ... (one minute, ten second pause) I'm right here. Paying attention to your loneliness, ... and your sadness and your fear. ... (thirty-five second pause) I'm right here. ... Paying attention to your loneliness, ... and your sadness and your fear. ... (thirty-six second pause) It must be very difficult and brave to say those words, "Hold my hand."

I took a deep breath to ease the tension in my body.
 I was sad and confused. But it was different with Richard there. I was able to tell him what I was thinking, and he did not doubt or question me.

Leigh: (seven second pause) I don't want to be hurt again.
Richard: Of course not ... Never again. Why, that was the purpose of hiding, the purpose of going to that peaceful place.
Leigh: Like running away.
Richard: Running away to never be hurt again. ... (twenty-two second pause) So deeply hurt. ... (twenty-one second pause) So scared.

Again, Richard validated my experience. I felt the tensions leaving my body. Until this moment no one had understood my deep hurt and responded in such an authentic way.

Leigh: (nine second pause) It's scary when there's no one there.
Richard: Yes, almost as scary as when someone is going to be controlling, or hurtful, or invasive. ... Two kinds of scared. ... (twelve second pause) Impossible to protest. ... Impossible to say Stop it or No! or I don't like it. ... Because then it gets worse.
Leigh: (nine second pause) I can't say it. I couldn't say anything.

Again, it was difficult to talk because my body started to freeze, and my voice was barely audible. I suddenly lost my ability to speak just as I did when watching my father hit my mum. The fear took over once again, my lips tightened, and my jaw tensed.

Richard: Dangerous to say "Stop it." Dangerous to say "No," frightening to say, "I don't like it."
Leigh: (fifteen second pause) It's OK, it's OK, it's OK, it's OK, it's OK.

I repeated "it's OK" over and over. I was surprised as I started to say the same mantra that I used repeatedly as a child. I suddenly made the connection that I used the words "it's OK" all through my life to stabilize myself.

Richard: I hear the words, "it's OK, it's OK, it's OK, it's OK" ... I hear that mantra when I know it's not OK. ... It's not OK inside. ... I hear the words "it's OK, it's OK, it's OK." I know you're scared, very scared.

Leigh: Just block everything out, block everything out.
Richard: Yeh, "block everything out." "Block everything out" and go to your peaceful place. Just go to your peaceful place.
Leigh: It's OK, it's OK ...

I continued to say my "it's OK" mantra very quietly. I was desperately trying to reassure myself, to regain control. I was giving myself what I needed to survive, the sound of a reassuring voice. It may have been my own voice, but it felt reassuring; it was distracting me from being overwhelmed. Once I was reassured, I could again focus on what Richard was saying.

Richard: That peaceful place where you can say "it's OK, it's OK." Don't talk, don't say anything, don't protest, don't say no.

My mantra also served the purpose of keeping me quiet, calming, stopping me from protesting.

Leigh: It's peaceful again.
Richard: Never say those words, ... never shout back, ... just keep quiet and good, ... quiet and good. There's safety in being quiet and good ... So important to find safety ... So necessary to have a safe place to hide ....

I could not respond to Richard. It was hard for me to hear him saying those words—words that I only said to myself. I was full of emotions and body reactions as Richard spoke: he was saying the same things that I repeatedly said to myself; he was voicing my internal criticism—"keep quiet and good." These were some of the critical words that compelled me to remain silent.

Leigh: (fifteen second pause) I couldn't have survived without it.
Richard: Survival inside. ... But then it gets so lonely. ... You started itching for something.

I was scratching my skin. I needed to feel something on the outside of me because I was feeling so intensely inside. Even now, as I write this there are no words to describe what I was feeling. I was just struggling to survive. The same survival struggle that was with me every day in my childhood.

Leigh: (fifteen second pause) I need to feel.
Richard: Mmm?
Leigh: I need to feel something.
Richard: Yeh!
Leigh: (five second pause) I can feel your hand. ... (seven second pause) I can feel your hand.
Richard: (twenty-nine second pause) Very important to stay quiet and not to define yourself. Not to protest, keep those lips sealed. It's the only safety. ... (one minute, sixteen

Leigh: second pause) I'm right here … watching over you. Even though it's necessary to be in your peaceful place.
Leigh: Why am I here?
Richard: "Why?" What a wonderful question. For safety. … So necessary to be in a peaceful place for safety. … So necessary to be in a peaceful place, for safety. … You know that answer more profoundly than my words express. … You know it in all those tight muscles, … in your back, in your arms, and in your pelvis, … and in your jaw, … those muscles know that answer. So important to be seen. To find peace from all the chaos, all the noise. … (forty-six second pause) I'm listening.
Leigh: (thirteen second pause) I'm amazed that you're still there.
Richard: I want to be here. … But I want to make sure I'm not invasive.
Leigh: (six second pause) Why are you there when nobody else was there?
Richard: Some questions I cannot answer. But I heard what you said. "Nobody else was there." That's quite a story, you're just giving me the headlines. The headlines are "Nobody else was there."
Leigh: I don't understand.
Richard: Yes you do. "Nobody else was there."
Leigh: When I was alone and scared, I needed someone, and nobody was there.
Richard: Oh! When you most needed someone when you were alone and scared. And nobody else was there. Alone when you most needed it.
Leigh: So why are you there?
Richard: I want to be.
Leigh: It doesn't make sense. It's confusing. I don't understand, I don't understand anything.
Richard: You're so familiar with nobody being there, so familiar.
Leigh: I needed someone to be there.
Richard: (seven second pause) Of course … someone to be there. … To *really* be there. … Without being controlling.
Leigh: (seventy second pause) Thank you.

I felt a sense of gratitude to Richard for staying with me, for not invading my space, for sticking to his words, and for understanding me. His way of being with me provided me with a new sense of trust—trust in another person, and trust in myself. Richard's way of being was so different to how my father behaved. My internal reactions were a mixture of disorientation and relief; my body was relaxing. I felt fully present.

Richard: My commitment.
Leigh: (one minute, thirty-six second pause) It's peaceful again.
Richard: Yes, I feel at peace too.
Leigh: It's strange but when we started it felt like you were on the outside, and it feels like I briefly allowed you to come into my quiet place.
Richard: Thank you for the privilege.

It was a daunting experience to have an intense psychotherapy session like this in the middle of my training group. I was suddenly worried that the group members would now see me as crazy. My internal critic said, "They could not see me as a capable therapist after witnessing what I had said. Then I looked around. I didn't see what I expected. I saw the faces of people who cared about me, they were on my side. Although it was difficult to look in their faces, it was necessary because their smiles and kind words provided evidence that they accepted me. Their presence and interest in me silenced my internal critic.

Near the end of my psychotherapy session, while I was in my peaceful sanctuary, there were a few moments when I sensed that the therapist was there with me. The knowledge that he was keeping me safe from harm, his patience and presence, made it possible for me to trust him. Even to this day, deep in my body, I retain this feeling of safety, a sense of confidence that I am OK, and the knowledge that I am not alone anymore. I remember the feeling of having someone watching over me, keeping me safe.

I learned so much, professionally, from this intensive psychotherapy session. My practice of an in-depth, relationally focused psychotherapy has been enhanced in several ways. Now I:

- Understand the necessity of resonating (Erskine, 2015) with the client's body and maintaining a consistent attunement to their rhythm.
- Realize how important it is to watch for subtle clues indicating that the client may be on the verge of becoming emotionally overwhelmed. And the importance of adjusting the therapeutic transactions so that the client can integrate their affect and cognition.
- Provide the necessary physical distance between client and myself so that the client can have access to their private space, and yet also sense that they are in the presence of someone who is safely watching over them.
- Identify when a client can benefit from the use of respectful touch, and I carefully secure their permission to focus on their body sensations (Erskine, 2015).
- Appreciate the use of therapeutic description and how it is effective when working with a client who relies on relational withdrawal as a form of self-stabilization (Erskine, 2020).
- Maintain a genuine interest in the client's internal experience and appreciate how it may be both similar and different than mine.

In my practice of psychotherapy, my aim is to develop an attuned therapeutic relationship so that my clients feel safe with me. Together we discover their unique experiences and identify which relational needs (Erskine, 2021) are not being met in their current lives. We explore how they can get today's relational needs satisfied in their day-to-day relationships with family and friends.

This intensive psychotherapy session where Richard sensitively attended to my schizoid process has been extremely important to me. As a result of this session, I have changed in several ways. I have gained a deeper understanding and appreciation of my schizoid process. I have increased confidence and trust in myself, and that other people can be there for me. Ultimately, I am able to feel an inner sense of peace and that I am not alone.

References

Blyton, E. (1942). *The Enchanted Wood.* https://quotes.thefamouspeople.com/enid-blyton-5350.php (retrieved from the internet February 25, 2021).

Erskine, R. G. (2001). The schizoid process. *Transactional Analysis Journal, 31*(1): 4–6. doi.org/10.1177/036215370103100102.

Erskine, R. G. (2015). *Relational Patterns, Therapeutic Presence: Concepts and Practice of Integrative Psychotherapy.* London: Karnac.

Erskine, R. G. (2020). Relational withdrawal, attunement to silence: Psychotherapy of the schizoid process. *International Journal of Integrative Psychotherapy, 11*: 14–28.

Erskine, R. G. (2021). *A Healing Relationship: Commentary on Therapeutic Dialogues.* Bicester, UK: Phoenix.

CHAPTER 15

From inner safety to contact-in-relationship: analyzing the psychotherapy of the schizoid process

Silvia Allari and Eugenio Peiró Orozco

In this chapter we will explore the schizoid process by analyzing a psychotherapy session conducted by Richard Erskine for a client named Pablo. Pablo is a professional colleague who attended the same training workshop held in Barcelona that both of us, Silvia and Eugenio, attended. The name, Pablo, is a pseudonym because our colleague asked to remain anonymous even though he was active in our analysis of his psychotherapy session.

It was Sunday, the third day of a five-day professional training workshop. After teaching about relationally focused integrative psychotherapy, Richard invited participants who were interested to engage in a psychotherapy session as a demonstration of the concepts and methods. As Richard started therapy work with our colleague, Pablo, I intuitively knew that it would be an important session so I decided to write down every word that both Richard and Pablo said. I wanted to have some exact examples for our group discussion that followed the therapy session.

When the workshop concluded I asked both Pablo and Eugenio to help me write about the concepts and methods that Richard used in his work with Pablo. We thought that Pablo's psychotherapy session was a valuable example of relational psychotherapy of a client's schizoid process. We want to share our analysis of the psychotherapy session with our professional community because we realize that this is a valuable form of research.

Our analysis has shown that the therapeutic interventions are like a dance between the therapist's understanding, intuition, and attunement and his ability to translate into words the client's affect and implicit memories. From the patient's point of view, it is the journey within oneself in the presence of the other; it is an unprecedented path which opens new options of contact within oneself and in interpersonal contact with the other.

Central in this psychotherapy session, as in the therapy work with all clients who engage in a schizoid process, is the psychotherapist's respect for silence. Silence within the therapy dialogue provides an opportunity and relational space for something meaningful to gestate. This relational space is demonstrated in Richard's not asking many questions. Instead of using phenomenological and historical inquiry he uses *therapeutic description*—statements that reflect the client's not-verbalized inner experiences.

Through therapeutic description Richard clarifies Pablo's script beliefs, the definitions that he has previously formed of himself. Each time Richard reflects Pablo's story and definition of himself, Pablo needs silence—the time and space to contemplate his own sensations and reactions. During these moments of silence we observe that Richard, although quiet, is consistently present with Pablo, constantly watching his body and creating a therapeutic environment for something to happen but not making something happen. Richard's watchfulness is like a parent sitting up at night watching a sick child with a fever, watchful of every breath and movement but not prematurely waking the child.

Organization of our research

We have organized the written transcript and our observations on five levels:

- The first level of our analysis is in the presentation of the verbatim transcript that provides the reader with both the therapeutic dialogue and context of the psychotherapy session.
- The second level of our analysis includes the findings that emerged during the interview that we did with Pablo two weeks after his psychotherapy session and immediately after he read the verbatim transcript. To make it easy for the reader, we have included an abbreviated version of Pablo's reflective comments in italics and bracketed with quotations marks. These are the exact words he used to describe his internal responses to Richard's therapeutic interventions. They are marked as Comment 1 through 20.
- We continue with Pablo's own words in a fifth level where we provide some additional comments that Pablo made in the follow-up interview. These final remarks are an extension to what we include within the transcript. In the interview we inquired about what the therapeutic work had stimulated within Pablo, such as his awareness of a sense of self, his experience of change, and his openness to relationships with others. We have categorized his answers into seven specific points at the end of this chapter.
- A third level of our analysis is in our descriptions and interpretations of the therapist's interventions. These are indicated with an arrow adjacent to various sections in the verbatim transcript.
- Importantly, as a fourth level in our analysis, we have included an indication of the length of time for most of the silent moments during the psychotherapy. These silent moments are essential in the psychotherapy for clients who rely on a schizoid process to manage relationships and stabilize their affect.

The psychotherapy session

In the transcript of an hour-long psychotherapy session that follows, P stands for the client Pablo while T stands for the psychotherapist, Richard Erskine. Please note that Pablo had previously attended several psychotherapy training workshops with Richard. Richard had some understanding of Pablo's way of being in relationship after watching his interactions within the group discussions. As the work begins, the workshop participants are seated in a circle. Pablo responds to Richard's invitation to the group, "Who wants to do some personal therapy?" Pablo silently gets up and sits in front of Richard.

P: I didn't think about anything.

> Comment 1: *"It was a pivotal point, I hadn't prepared, I hadn't thought of a theme as is often the case when you propose yourself as a client in a workshop. It was the condition that allowed me to be there, to be in the present, to get inside myself, in touch with me without giving myself a task. Simply being."*

(approx. one minute silence)

T: Close your eyes and look inside. I am listening to you, even if you are silent, I am listening. You will have my full attention, you don't have to produce anything. I will listen to you. I think you have a lot inside, things that are difficult to say because you have the feeling that they will be criticized.

> → Pablo had been looking intently at Richard as though he was searching for some clue as to how to proceed. Richard responds to Pablo's long silence by inviting him to make internal contact. Richard declares his presence and attention without a demand that Pablo produce something.

P. My head feels like it's shaking.

> Comment 2: *"It's like an electricity, like the brain is shaking, I feel like that when I'm especially well, it's a reaction to Richard's introduction, because he proposes the possibility of really being myself and immediately the body responds."*

T. It is shaking. You must be feeling something important.

> → In the previous comment Richard reaffirms his presence and communicates a message of, "I see you, I'm here for you." "Your internal process is significant."

(approx. fifteen second silence)

P. I used to feel a pain here (Pablo points to chest).

> Comment 3: *"My feelings were twofold: my head was shaking with the possibility of being listened to and in contact without performance—listening, presence; my chest was aching because being in contact can be risky."*

(approx. one minute silence)

T. Take your time. You don't have to be alone. You have spent a lot of time alone in your life. (pause) Your body is telling a story. (pause) Your facial expression is expressing it, too. (pause) Alone, in your private place. It's so private that it's hard to talk about. (pause) It's always hard to put words to it, especially if you think they won't understand you.

> Comment 4: *"Wow. He's putting into words what I'm thinking, what I'm feeling and what I'm not able to say. I don't have the words to say it. I feel perfectly understood, I can get into my internal place … but then I'm alone. Richard reads my need to experience my functioning."*

> → We observe that through therapeutic description Richard provides a verbal avenue for internal experiences and implicit memory to become explicit. Pablo's awareness begins to take shape, it forms into concepts that identify and reflect his private history and experiences.

P. The feeling is that if I ask … I won't get it. Then I give up and remain sorry. … What I ask for I won't get.

> → Since the beginning of the psychotherapy Richard's affect attunement and understanding of a child's attempts at self-stabilization allow the therapy to reach a new, intimate depth wherein Pablo begins to trust and follow Richard. He keeps his gaze on Pablo the entire time while matching his breathing to that of Pablo's. Richard's physiological resonance and attunement to Pablo's rhythm has a stabilizing effect.

T. And will I be criticized?

> → Richard vocalizes Pablo's anticipation of criticism. In doing so, Richard's nonverbal communication is, "You are not alone. I Understand." This is a form of cognitive attunement, a putting into words what he senses Pablo's unspoken experience to be.

P. Yes, of course, not understood … misunderstood … It's best not to say.

> Comment 5: *"In that moment I felt strange, in touch with myself, in relationship with Richard, with the group listening to me … a whole new experience!"*

T. That is an important conclusion: it's better not to talk … not to share, so as not to be criticized and not understood.

> Comment 6: *"That's exactly what it's about: more than talking, my problem is sharing, talking about me. Throughout the session I feel torn between the desire to share and the fear of being misunderstood, criticized."*

(approx. forty-five second silence)

> → Richard puts Pablo's implicit script conclusion into concrete words, "If I am not understood and criticized it is better to not share." In our observation it appears that Richard understands and is reflecting Pablo's unspoken experiences.

P. It is familiar to be in here.

> Comment 7: *"I am having a unique experience for me: I can be inside myself and, at the same time, be accompanied, be in relationship and share. It's a reassuring condition. I express myself but I'm not in the performance, the pace is slow. Richard accompanies me."*

T. That's why they call it the safe place.

> → We observe that Richard tunes into Pablo's slow rhythm. He puts words to Pablo's unspoken experiences and confirms the significance of having a safe place. By calling it a "safe place" Richard is normalizing Pablo's urge to withdraw.

(approx. fifteen second silence)

P. There's a lot going on in here. There are more things in here than in life … fantasy … my space … imagination.

> Comment 8: *"I may not be able to have what I want on the outside, but I am allowed to have what I want inside of me … with imagination … with fantasy."*

T. They are especially protected if they are not expressed. Perhaps you still hope that they will appreciate what you have inside.

> Comment 9: *"Richard still helps me by defining, giving words to my experience that was for me only something perceptible in sensations, but without words."*

P. I still have hope. … It's scary, I also have fear.

T. It is important that the other person listens to you with interest.

> Comment 10: *"He's perfectly describing what I'm feeling inside!"*

(approx. fifteen second silence)

> → Throughout this part of the psychotherapy Richard continues to mirror Pablo, to use therapeutic description, and provide cognitive understanding. Richard is helping Pablo integrate his physiological sensations, affect, and cognition while fostering an intimate relationship.

P. I learned not to get it.

> Comment 11: *"At this point I feel that I deeply understand. Richard knows my coping path. I finally understand myself!"*

> → Pablo has come to an understanding of his childhood coping decision. This is an important step in being able to redecide how to manage relationships.

T. You learned not to have the need.

> Comment 12: *"Actually I have ignored my needs. I had never realized it was about my needs."*

(approx. thirty second silence)

> → Richard describes how Pablo coped with his situation by disavowing his various needs, particularly his need to be listened to and respected. In doing so, Richard helps Pablo define himself.

P. (Pablo turns his head to the right; there is no eye contact.)

(approx. thirty second silence)

T. Maybe the solution is better than not being understood, it's better to feel alone. Between not being understood and feeling alone you chose to feel alone.

> Comment 13: *"I feel the stress, the fear. Richard gently walks me through it."*

(approx. one minute silence)

> → Richard describes Pablo's childhood conclusion, to feel alone is better than not being understood. Then Richard remains silent but his gaze is on Pablo even though Pablo has turned his head away and is not speaking. The act of being present together in silence is an important aspect of this psychotherapy. This is a "pregnant pause" that allows Pablo's affect and realizations to emerge.

P. I had to hope for a long time.

T. Lost desire. Sometimes when people lose their desire they experience a sense of being desperate.

P. Me also.

T. I want to understand the loss of desire. I guess it covers many, many years.

> → Richard is interested and inquires; he is demonstrating his involvement, something that was missing in Pablo's early life. The silence that follows is an essential part of Richard's involvement; it is a form of respectful connection—a being with the other in their silence.

(approx. thirty second silence)

P. I feel shame.

T. Shame keeps us quiet. Shame doesn't allow us to speak.

P. I think I was trying to avoid criticism.

T. More than just being criticized … I think of humiliation.

> Comment 14: *"Yes, the word humiliation matches me; it's a deeper level than criticism."*

(approx. one minute silence)

T. And sometimes there's no protest. Hiding is a good thing when you think you're going to be humiliated. It's important to hide to avoid the criticism … to hide where everything is quiet. The memory of criticism. The memory of humiliation.

(approx. thirty second silence)

> → Richard is validating the internal effects of criticism and humiliation. He articulates the path that led Pablo to withdraw from relationships and to create instead a safe place within himself.

P. This has been my life, to be in here, in my safe place.

T. I know, you spent five years showing it to me. I still don't know you, but I want to.

P. Now I want to change. I want to come out from the inside but I feel a lot of shame.

T. Yes, of course.

P. I paralyze myself.

T. Can you describe what you feel? … (pause)
The world is outside of you. Can you touch it with your hand?

(approx. thirty second silence)

P. I'm changing, I'm doing a lot of things, but I also think there are a lot of things I can't do.

> Comment 15: *"Richard changes the plan, gets in the here-and-now and that has a big impact for me."*

T. That you can't or that you don't know?

P. I don't know why I can't.

> Comment 16: *"It was a fundamental clarification, that's right, I can't do because I don't know how to do it."*

T. It would take someone with more experience to teach you how to ride a bike. The best thing is to have a teacher.

Comment 17: *"Richard shows me the way to redecide; starting from my experience he defines what I can use to satisfy my need to do: having a guide."*

P. I have always wanted guidance. My feeling is that I'm always late to things.

→ Richard is responding to Pablo's relational need to have someone who is reliable, consistent, and dependable to serve as a guide.

T. When I guide you in this dialogue between us your eyes light up.

P. Yes, they do.

T. I, for example, like to travel, but not alone. I think it's a natural need to have a guide.

P. For me coming to the workshop is part of that, the guidance is important to me.

→ Richard affirms and normalizes the need to depend on someone for guidance. Pablo states that this is why he has attended the workshops for the past five years. Richard is responding to Pablo's unsatisfied childhood need to have someone on whom he could depend for support, information, and guidance while at the same time satisfying Pablo's current need to rely on someone whose advice and direction is reliable.

T. How would you describe the way you study?

Comment 18: *"Richard concretely becomes my teacher, my guide."*

(approx. twenty second silence)

P. I need to see and try in order to repeat.

T. So your learning is hands-on, putting your hands in.

→ Richard puts the client's way of learning into words, another form of normalization.

P. With this training I get guidance. Same for practicing sports.
For me the most important thing is to make mistakes. For me it is important that you tell me, "This is a mistake, find the different form." I need guidance.

T. And who didn't understand that you need guidance?

(approx. twenty second silence)

P. My father, my teachers, my friends, my brothers. I learned everything on my own.

T. Take a few moments and go back inside your silent place.

> Comment 19: *"Another very significant moment. I was actually tired, felt the need to rest."*

(approx. one minute silence)

→ Pablo has been on a journey of self-discovery. Richard invites him to return to his safe place. Richard validates the positive function of Pablo's safe place—a place of peace and re-stabilization.

T. I'm here. … Maybe we are going too fast. … I want to find the right rhythm for you. … You have my full attention.

(approx. one minute silence)

P. I'm OK now, Richard.

T. Feeling?

P. I don't feel the need to talk.

T. But, I think you need me to understand you. … To appreciate you for your uniqueness. … And you need me not to criticize you, not to falsely define you. … And you need to define yourself, to express yourself. … And that's a need for all of us.

> Comment 20: *"Richard is saying what I need to hear."*

(approx. forty second silence)

→ Richard is again acknowledging, normalizing, and validating Pablo's relational needs.

P. Lately I've been thinking … I often ask to be accepted, but first I have to accept myself. I have to define myself first … ask myself what I want from myself.

T. It is important to express your personality and be accepted.

P. It seems impossible to me. I can see it now, though.

T. Can you name the need?

P. Yes, when I was thirteen I was with my friends and I didn't know which people I liked, it was impossible. Now I do.

T. That's a big step.

> → Richard invites Pablo to name his need. Instead of directly answering Richard's question Pablo tells a story about how he was unable to identify who he liked when he was an adolescent. Rather than returning to the question Richard acknowledges that Pablo has made a big step. Early in the training workshop the group had been talking about the type of music they like. In the next transaction Richard makes use of that previous conversation to address the difficulty Pablo has had in identifying and expressing his relational needs.

P. For me it is.

T. I saw that you were struggling when I asked you what music you liked.

P. Yes, these are personal questions. For me music is not a song but the whole story that led me to choose that song.

T. Can you tell me which song you like? Then I'll tell you which one I like.

P. "Selve amiche," composer is Alessandro Parisotti. The musician is Antonio Caldara.

T. Is that an aria?

P. Yes. I was preparing a concerto by Cajkovsky with the boys.

T. Music is often a metaphor for internal sensations.

(Richard then asks the group to put on music and dance. The group members jump to their feet and begin to dance with Pablo.)

> → Richard makes use of music and dance at the end of this psychotherapy session. It has several purposes: the use of music and dance serve as physical metaphors of Pablo's internal change; the dance helps Pablo move his body that has been tense throughout this session; and, the dance unites the group in an activity that is important for Pablo.

The dance allows his whole nervous system to readjust and relax. At the same time the dance subtly conveys several important messages: "It is important to express yourself"; "It is good that you seek out people with whom you can share your experiences"; and, "It is necessary to have someone on whom you can rely for support, encouragement, and guidance."

Pablo's reflections

We conducted a two-hour interview with Pablo two weeks after his psychotherapy session with Richard. We wanted to evaluate the progress of his psychotherapy and to understand his phenomenological experiences, what it was like to be the recipient of the psychotherapy. We discovered that this psychotherapy session allowed Pablo to have several important experiences. Rather than report the interview in its entirety we condensed Pablo's reflective comments and organized them into the following seven categories.

- **Internal contact with a vital and vulnerable self:** Pablo described the contact with Richard as facilitating an *"acceptance of what happens in each moment, improvising, experimenting, in therapy and in life."*
- **Psychotherapist as a witness:** Pablo says that the therapeutic relationship allowed him to *"retreat to my safe place and a chance to be comfortable there. A chance to accept, with curiosity, whatever happens within me without any criticism. I got scared at first; that's what my physical sensations were telling me. Then I knew I could calm down. Now I do the same internal calming just as it happened to me in the session with Richard."*
- **The experience of acceptance of a self with parts:** Pablo describes it as *"My way of being, of being inside and outside, is fine, I don't have to exclude a part. They each have an important purpose."*
- **A desire for change:** Pablo adds, *"The awareness and acceptance of my internal functioning allows me to choose and affirm what I want to change. I don't have to be my old self all the time."*
- **Having a guide to accompany the change:** Pablo articulates, *"I realize that I want to change but I didn't know how to do it. I needed a teacher to help me find ways to do things the way I want to do them and not the way I used to do them. I was always trying to imitate what others did in order to be part of the group."*
- **Sharing with others:** Pablo declares, *"When I realize that there is nothing wrong with me, that I have a normal process, I am no longer ashamed and I can share it with the group without the shame of feeling inadequate."*
- **Manifesting a wholeness of the self:** Pablo concludes, *"When I realize that I'm OK, I can go out into the world and take what I need in a different way, I know that I can be myself, I don't have to hide."*

Pablo ended our interview by saying, *"The psychotherapy session was tiring but so important. I felt an intense tension but I also felt safe. I needed the slow pace of Richard's comments in order to open up. It is like I have permission to relate to myself and other people in a new way. I have more of a connection with both my internal and external worlds."*

Pablo's final comment was, *"This psychotherapy session has made it possible for me to make a meaningful redecision. … I want to change and I can do it with the help of a guide who will accompany me."*

Conclusion

Writing this chapter has been an intense, complex, and exciting journey for each of us, the two authors, and Pablo. Our research was compounded by working in three languages, yet the doing of it was exciting and informative. As a result of the psychotherapy training workshops, we were professionally stimulated and encouraged to investigate the healing factors of a relationally focused, integrative psychotherapy for clients who stabilize their affect by engaging in a schizoid process.

In this chapter we have presented and analyzed a psychotherapy session in which the psychotherapist attended to the client's schizoid process. Our objective was to gain insight into the client's phenomenological experience of the psychotherapy and to track the relational qualities of how the therapist interacted with the client. In this hour-long psychotherapy session we observed that the psychotherapist made his relationship with the client central. He was present, patient, and attuned to the client's affect and relational needs. The therapist built a healing relationship by following and respecting the client's rhythm and helping him to define, think about, and accept his previous ways of functioning—a necessary step prior to focusing on change (Erskine, 2021).

The pace of this psychotherapy was slow; it provided the client with the necessary time to feel his inner sensations and affect, to experience the presence of the psychotherapist, and to make some important decisions about how to be in relationship with people. The result was a deep encounter between the client and the psychotherapist in which they coconstructed a fulfilling outcome. We have observed that the psychotherapist's empathetic presence, timing, and therapeutic comments—all without pressure or demand—provided the client with an opportunity to accept and appreciate both a vulnerable self that is withdrawn into a "safe place" and a social self that is able to reveal his needs and share himself with others.

In this psychotherapy session we witnessed Pablo emerging from his safe hiding place. In our opinion Pablo emerged because he experienced being understood, accepted as he was, and that his needs were normal. He made an important redecision. No longer was his belief *"I have to do it alone. There is no one for me,"* but he now had the relational support to make a redecision, *"I want to change and I want to be accompanied in the change. I need a guide."*

Endnote

We would like to thank Marta Schicchitani and Barbara Revello, two colleagues, for their invaluable contribution in correcting and clarifying some parts of this chapter.

Reference

Erskine, R. G. (2021). *A Healing Relationship: Commentary on Therapeutic Dialogues.* Bicester, UK: Phoenix.

Part IV

Theory into therapeutic practice

CHAPTER 16

Louise: social facade, depression, relational withdrawal

Richard G. Erskine

*P*erplexed, challenged, tender, patient, gratified, sorrowful*—these words portray the variety of countertransference feelings that dominated my therapeutic involvement with Louise. As I tell you the story of Louise's psychotherapy journey, I want to share my jumble of internal sensations so that you can have a richer sense of the affectively based, nonverbal, intersubjective dynamics between the client and me. So much of what was crucial in Louise's psychotherapy defies language because the essential healing aspects of our interpersonal contact were in the facial expressions, body gestures, and timing of our therapeutic dialogue. These nonverbal interactions, along with our therapeutic dialogue, profoundly influenced and impacted each of us.

Louise came for psychotherapy in order "to try it for a while" because she was "fed up with constantly being depressed." She said, "No one at work, or even my friends, would think I'm depressed. Sometimes I am not completely depressed because I continually push myself to be active." In these first few sessions Louise frequently described her social life as "active." She said, "I go to many theatre performances and I have a subscription for two people to the entire season of the symphony orchestra. I always invite someone to join me."

Over the next couple of months, I noted that Louise arrived precisely on time, impeccably dressed in stylish business attire. She carried herself with an elegant posture. I imagined that her appearance induced both women and men to turn their heads for a second look. In each of our sessions Louise talked in great detail about how she had mastered the intricacies of trading on the stock market, the lucrative transactions that she made, and how her clients profited because of her skill. She seemed to enjoy the prestige of working in the financial market. "I'm not depressed at work. There I have a good businesswoman's way of thinking."

Throughout the first few months Louise talked extensively about her wealthy clients and her love for symphonic music. Her conversation was usually about her accomplishments. She said, "The job requires me to be very personable … but it is all an act." I was left to wonder if Louise was authentic with me or if her stories and genteel behavior were also an "act."

I felt perplexed; we were not talking about her "depression," which is what she initially said was her reason for engaging in psychotherapy. As I made inquiries about her depression her responses were evasive. She was intent on telling me about the day-to-day activities in her life.

In the early months of our weekly psychotherapy sessions Louise was resistant to my inquiry about her feelings; she was offended when I inquired about her physiological sensations. She arrogantly rebuffed my inquiry about her childhood with "The past is the past. I don't believe in dredging it up." She approached psychotherapy as though talking about her social life, shopping for fashionable clothing, and believing her business successes would somehow relieve the "depression" she felt at home. I had an inkling that her self-aggrandizing stories provided a momentary antidepressant. It was ten months before Louise was willing to tell me anything about either her family history or what she experienced internally. From time to time, she would allude to her "depression" but then would be elusive in response to my inquiry.

Narcissistic style

Throughout the first year of our psychotherapy, I considered the possibility that Louise's behaviors constituted a *narcissistic style* (Johnson, 1994) and that her relational withdrawal was her way of coping with an absence of emotional validation throughout her early life. Similar to how I approach psychotherapy with narcissistically inclined clients, I began to respond to her with consistent empathy rather than comment on the content of what she was telling me (Kohut, 1971). I chose to not focus on her behavior or offer any conceptualizations; I refrained from making any interpretation or confrontation. I felt challenged by this daunting task ahead of me. Several case reports describing effective therapeutic involvement indicate that it is necessary to provide the narcissistically inclined client with consistent empathic responses to their needs for validation and self-definition prior to exploring their early life experiences and comprehending how they compensate for early childhood relational disruptions (Bach, 1985; Basch, 1988; Kohut, 1977; Stolorow et al., 1987; Wolf, 1988).

My primary way of trying to connect with Louise was by being fully present, carefully listening to each word she said, and responding empathically to her stifled affect. But I had no evidence that she felt my presence. Although Louise continued to come for psychotherapy there was very little emotional contact between us. I was left to ponder the question raised by Marye O'Reilly-Knapp in her 2001 article, "What is required in a therapeutic relationship so that the uncommunicable, walled-off parts can be spoken, heard, and understood?" (p. 44). It became clear to me that my task was to open the door for interpersonal contact and then to wait patiently until she peeked through that relational door.

My quiet, empathic responses to Louise's self-aggrandizing stories seemed to have an effect. After the first six months Louise's bragging about her accomplishments diminished. She began to tell me vignettes about her "secret depression." "I don't want anyone to know what I feel." Although she professed to know many people, the central feature of her stories was that she was alone. She did not speak directly about being lonely—she hid her vulnerability—but I could sense that something was amiss; her life was devoid of intimate relationships.

Each time Louise talked about being alone I responded to her with facial expressions and body movements that mirrored her unspoken affect. Although it was not initially her word, I introduced the term "lonely" as a way to refer to and clarify the "depression" she described—a depression that enveloped her when she was in her apartment. During these sessions in which we talked about her "depression" and "loneliness," the rapid speed in which Louise usually talked decreased. She was increasingly vulnerable and far less social in her dialogue with me. In response I could feel a growing sense of tenderness within me. My rhythm of interactions slowed; I became more protective. I wanted to connect with the vulnerable and vital facets of Louise.

I reflected on the possibility that my sensitivity to Louise's need for validation, my attunement to her loneliness, and my adjustment to her pace were changing the nature of our communication. To paraphrase the previous quotation by Marye O'Reilly-Knapp, I had the hope that the previously uncommunicable, walled-off parts of Louise were beginning to speak because she was being heard by me and that we were forming a communication between us in which she felt understood.

Early in our psychotherapy sessions Louise had said that she had an "active social life," but as I repeatedly inquired, it became clear that she had no close friends, no one with whom she could talk heart to heart. Although she frequently invited a guest to accompany her to a symphony concert or theatre, she and the other person never talked about the play or music after the performance. She would just go home with the excuse that she had much to do the next day and, once in her apartment, she would become "depressed." Eventually I discovered that Louise often spent the entire weekend "alone, sleeping most of the time and then playing on the internet." She recounted, "There are times when I can be charming and active with people but then it all gets to be too much. I need to retreat and replenish."

In other sessions I explored the quality of Louise's friendships and her personal interactions with clients and colleagues. As I listened to her stories it seemed to me that all of her interpersonal contacts were superficial. Louise made a noteworthy comment: "I am friendly to everyone but I don't say anything about myself." In response to my questions about her possible romantic life she reluctantly said, "Several years ago I had a boyfriend who lived in Minneapolis. We talked on the phone each week and we would vacation together twice a year. But for some unknown reason we both lost interest." When I asked if she missed him, Louise wasn't sure: "I miss the boating we always did. We were always very active. But I don't know if it is him I miss or if I miss all the activities he arranged." Another day she said, "Frequently men ask me out but I'm not really interested. I don't want to get into a relationship. Life is easier alone."

I repeatedly inquired about Louise's sense of "depression." She told me how she sometimes dreaded going home after work and that she would regularly go to the same restaurant "because the waiter likes serving me. I reserve the same table every time. After dinner I just go home to my stupid internet." Then Louise lowered her head, stared at the rings on her fingers, and remained silent for several minutes. When she again looked in my direction Louise said that she wanted to end this session early. I encouraged her to stay and focus on what she was feeling. Her shoulders slumped, her breathing became shallow, the contours of her face changed: she suddenly looked many years older. After several minutes of silence she said, "This is what it is like in my apartment. No matter how beautiful I decorate it, I still feel depressed." After a long pause she added, "I don't want you to see me like this." The door to her vulnerability was open for a few minutes, then it was abruptly closed.

I thought about Louise's "depression" and wondered if it was similar to Marye O'Reilly-Knapp's description of her schizoid client's "isolated attachment." For clients who rely on a schizoid process to emotionally stabilize themselves, relationships with other people are difficult to sustain. Therefore, they are often overwhelmed by a profound sense of depression, "cut off from people and the world, cut off from his or her needs and wants, the person withdraws so far into 'nothingness' that no one is there, and even the sense of one's being is nullified" (2001, p. 49).

An isolated attachment pattern is revealed through the quality of interpersonal contact made by individuals who use withdrawal to manage relationships. In my psychotherapy practice I have found that clients who use emotional withdrawal to manage relationships report that significant caretakers were consistently misattuned to their physiological rhythms, misinterpreted their emotional expressions, and were controlling or invasive of the client's sense of identity. To be vulnerable is sensed as dangerous. The child may then develop patterns of relationship marked by a social facade, psychological withdrawal, intense internal criticism, and the absence of emotional expression (Erskine, 2015). Clients like Louise, with an isolated attachment pattern, have an implicit fear of invasion.

Schizoid pattern

Could Louise be diagnosed as having a *schizoid disorder*? Probably not.

However, Louise does fit the profile of someone with a *schizoid pattern*—a pattern of behavior and emotional reactions that shape most of her life and all of her potential relationships. When in dialogue with me, Louise curtailed her affect; with other people there was an absence of emotional involvement, and she spent a considerable amount of time in her internal world. Any affect that she may have felt was hidden by a well-polished social facade. Louise was the only one who knew her misery. The frequency, intensity, and duration of both her relational withdrawal and social "act" are certainly more acute than in someone with a *schizoid style*.

On many weekends Louise isolated herself in her apartment, "usually depressed." She said, "Even when I'm on the internet it often seems meaningless in the end." Louise reported how she had to be "charming and engaging at work" and then added, "Being with people exhausts me. Yet, when I am alone, I am not happy. But it is better to be unhappy alone than to be swallowed up by people." Ronald Fairbairn (1952) and Harry Guntrip (1968) aptly termed this internal conflict the *schizoid's dilemma*. Ray Little vividly describes this dilemma when he writes, "Retreating from contact leaves the individual isolated, lonely, and in pain. In some cases the longing for contact will reemerge and the person may move toward others; however, such movement also brings with it the anxiety of being close" (2001, p. 39).

Gary Yontef clearly illustrates Louise's schizoid pattern when he says,

> It is dangerous to move into intimate connection if you cannot separate when needed. If you think you are going to be caught up, devoured, or captured in the connection, it is terrifying to move into intimate contact. On the other hand, if you do not feel connected with other people, especially if you do not believe you can intimately connect again, the separation or isolation is both painful and terrifying. (2001, p. 9)

Louise certainly had a narcissistic social presentation in that she sought continuous affirmation of her value. While her narcissistic characteristics were obvious, her schizoid pattern of emotional withdrawal constituted the undisclosed, yet dominant, features of her personality. Louise is a good example of how schizoid withdrawal and narcissistic self-aggrandizement may be contemporaneous and congruent—together they form a narcissistic/schizoid matrix. Ronald Fairbairn (1952), in writing about his schizoid clients, identified three salient characteristics: an attitude of omnipotence; preoccupation with an internal life; and, detachment from relationships. These three attributes are also used to describe narcissistic clients (American Psychiatric Association, 2013; Masterson, 1981).

It is interesting that the British object relations literature tends to emphasize schizoid phenomena (Fairbairn, 1952; Guntrip, 1968; Khan, 1974; Laing, 1960) while the American psychoanalytic literature emphasizes narcissistic dynamics (Bach, 1985; Johnson, 1987; Kernberg, 1975; Kohut, 1971, 1977; Masterson, 1981). These two bodies of psychoanalytic literature, the British and the American, apparently exist in isolation from each other even though they seemingly refer to two coinciding personality constellations (Melniker, 1988).

Louise's narcissistic traits were a manifestation of her lifelong struggle to self-regulate and maintain some semblance of relationship while her relational withdrawal was a manifestation of desperate attempts to self-stabilize (Erskine, 2021a, 2021b). Her narcissistic-like persona was an effective disguise of her schizoid traits. If we theorize these two constellations of behaviors with the metaphor of "splitting," as illustrated in Ray Little's 2001 article, we can concretize each of these as constituting a *split in the sense of self*, and therefore manifestations of both a social self and a vulnerable/sequestered self.

Phenomenological inquiry and therapeutic description

On several occasions I noticed that Louise seemed annoyed whenever I engaged in any phenomenological inquiry or asked any questions about her life when she was a child. Each time I inquired about her annoyance with me she was even more irritated. She eventually said, "I don't like your controlling questions." I was surprised by her depicting my inquiry as "controlling"; that was far from my experience. I asked myself if she was giving me useful feedback about my therapeutic methods. I had to make a quick assessment of both my intentions and the effects that my inquiry had on Louise. It was clear to me that the impact of my inquiry was more significant than my intentions; therefore, I needed to change how I interacted with Louise.

At the same time, I surmised that Louise was transferring old relational conflicts into our therapeutic relationship. By reacting so strongly to my phenomenological inquiry she may have been revealing a relational pattern formed with other people in another time. Through the transference Louise was demonstrating the relational needs that had been thwarted, how she has compensated, and what was needed in our therapeutic relationship (Erskine, 1991; Little, 2011; Stern, 1994).

After a thoughtful pause, I made a statement, "Perhaps you have a strong reaction to being controlled." She responded immediately with, "You're just like my mother. She was always poking her nose into my life. She asked me question after question; she is so controlling." Louise continued to talk about how her mother "tried to know everything I felt, thought, or did." I replied with words that I hoped would describe her inner experience, "I imagine that you must have felt invaded." After a long pause she softly said, "My teenage years were awful. I had no personal space. My mother wanted to know everything about me." Then she looked down at her lap and was silent for a few minutes. Louise's expressions of annoyance with me, and her telling me about her mother's controlling behavior, was the most open she had been up to this point in her psychotherapy. This transferential encounter was the beginning of our exploring the effects of her mother's "controlling behavior" at various developmental ages.

In response to Louise's annoyance with my inquiry I changed the nature of how I constructed my questions; rather than phrasing my inquiries in an interrogative form, I rephrased them in the form of an indefinite declarative. Instead of phenomenological inquiries such as, "What are you feeling when you want to be alone?" I changed the structure of the sentence to, "You must have various feelings when you are alone." As an alternative to phenomenological inquiry (Erskine et al., 1999) I used *therapeutic description*, a non-authoritative, tentative voice that hopefully allowed her to dismiss or disagree with my statement. Like other clients who struggle with internal criticism and use relational withdrawal to self-stabilize, Louise responded to my inquiries about her feelings, physical sensations, or thoughts as though they were a criticism. When I rephrased my inquiry as a description of how I imagined Louise felt, she was more revealing.

Criticism and shame

Throughout the second half of this first year, it became apparent that Louise was distressed by self-criticism. At first, her self-criticisms were subtle, in the form of little disparaging remarks or self-putdowns, usually veiled in the midst of a story. In response to my inquiry about her internal criticism Louise would change the topic or lapse into silence. On a December day in the second year of her psychotherapy, Louise was caught in a cold rainstorm without an umbrella or protective clothing. She came into my office with her clothes and hair completely wet, her makeup running down her face. She immediately fled to the washroom. I could hear her cursing herself with, "Stupid me," "I'm a mess," "I can't do anything right."

When she finally emerged from the washroom Louise did not speak, she evaded eye contact, she hung her head. I was intrigued by the contrast between the self-chastising comments she made in the washroom and the silence in our therapy room. I realized that she was probably feeling shame. After a few minutes of silence I said, "When a person is defined as 'stupid' or 'a mess' they often feel a sense of being unworthy, ashamed of who they are." She looked up at me and nodded her head in agreement.

I added, "I picture a little girl who is being criticized and doesn't know what to do because she is full of shame." She remained silent but again nodded her head in agreement. I said nothing more about shame in that session. She had allowed herself to be vulnerable in my presence. I too remained silent; I didn't want to encourage her to reveal more of herself before she was secure in our relationship. I would follow her lead.

On that rainy day when Louise was shivering from the cold, I offered her a blanket and invited her to curl up on the couch. She pulled the blanket up to her knees and cuddled under the warmth of it. Although I initially spoke to her about the self-criticism, the remainder of our session was in silence. With the blanket pulled up around her neck, she watched me intently. During the last fifteen minutes of the session she periodically closed her eyes for several moments. Louise removed a facade; I could now see a different facet of her.

When Louise returned the following week I had the blanket folded, on the couch. As she sat down, she pushed it aside with a scornful expression on her face. After a long pause I said, "You must have a lot of feelings today." She eyed me suspiciously and then eventually said, "I don't want to talk about it." We both sat in silence for several minutes and then I said, "Talking about feelings is difficult, particularly if we expect to be ridiculed." After another long pause she continued, "I was a mess last time. I hate it. I have been upset all week." I asked her to tell me more about being "upset." Louise added, "I could not sleep a couple of nights knowing that you would think I was acting like a helpless little child."

Rather than address this transferential comment directly I continued with, "Perhaps you are feeling shame … shame because I saw how distraught you were." As I said these words, she began to stroke the fabric of the blanket. Her gesture reminded me of a very young child seeking soothing by clinging to something soft. After a short pause I added a validating comment, "You seemed so natural cuddled up with the blanket." With that comment, Louise picked up the blanket and clutched it to her chest. After a pause she said, "I'm torn. I just want to curl into the blanket but that's just being a stupid kid." I added, "I think your need to be comforted is so important. I wonder if you were humiliated for having natural needs." We spent the rest of the session in silence while Louise pulled the blanket around her.

As we sat in silence, I was reminded of Gary Yontef's comment:

> shame is a fundamental process for schizoids. They are easily shamed, although that is not always obvious because they deny that they are attached or that they need anything. When they feel safe enough to start exploring their shame, they manifest a great deal of loathing for their needy self. (2001, p. 12)

This led me to reflect on the many things I had learned about shame from other clients, such as, when a child grows up in a relationship tainted by criticism, ridicule, or other humiliating behaviors, the result is an increased vulnerability in all relationships. They tend to withdraw—to hide their vulnerability. They also disavow their anger and focus instead on two other aspects of shame: the sadness of not being accepted as they are; and the fear of abandonment in the relationship because of who they are. They either comply with how they have been defined, or they engage in self-criticism, and/or they become self-righteous, arrogant. As a self-protective strategy a person will use either shame-filled relational withdrawal or self-righteous arrogance as a protective dynamic to avoid the vulnerability of being humiliated again. (For an elaboration on the psychotherapy of shame and self-righteousness see Erskine, 1994, 1995.)

As I look over my notes it is clear that on the day Louise got drenched in the rainstorm, she and I entered a new phase of her psychotherapy. Several themes were vying for therapeutic attention:

- Louise had inadvertently allowed me to see her vulnerability; her superficial sophistication was on pause. I wanted to connect with her vulnerable self before she could put on a social facade. It was essential that I stay attuned to her affect and not get sidetracked into talking about her day-to-day activities. Perhaps Louise was ready to show me her secret self.
- Louise had exposed a bit of her self-criticism. I was certain that there was much more. I knew that it would be therapeutically necessary to uncover all of the self-imposed ridicule, much like a medical doctor opening and draining an abscess. We would then investigate the psychological functions of the self-criticism as a way to lessen their internal influence.
- Louise's transferential comments revealed a significant story about being devalued for being vulnerable. I already had some information about her mother's criticisms and harsh demands.
- Louise's shame was suddenly apparent; she no longer had an entitled and arrogant persona. It was time to attend to the sadness, fear, and compliance that were at the core of her shame.

Over the next several months we talked about shame, usually for several minutes in most sessions. I intentionally steered our dialogue away from spending more than a few minutes talking about her current life. At first she seemed confused when we talked about her intense fear of ridicule and her desperate attempt to conform to "the image of a daughter that my mother wanted." In a later session she exclaimed, "Shame … that's the same as I'm unworthy. Hell, UNWORTHY is what I have felt all my life." I made a quick retort, "It must be hell to live with a constant sense of not being worthy of a mother's love." She had tears in her eyes as she clutched the blanket.

In that session, and in following ones, I encouraged her to close her eyes in order to sense what was happening inside. She would alternately close her eyes for a few minutes and then open them briefly as if to see if I was still present. I responded with, "I am still here. Just take your time being inside." As we were ending a session she described her ten minutes of withdrawal as, "I go into the fog where everything is meaningless." When she returned to her "fog" in another session she added, "If I'm in a fog my mother can't nag me. All is quiet. I am hidden." I was reminded of Marye O'Reilly-Knapp's description of the schizoid conditions,

> In the withdrawn and hidden place there is only existence, with no true sense of self and no sense of self with another. The person remains uninvolved, unintegrated, and lives in quiet desperation. (2001, p. 48)

Homeostatic functions of self-criticisms

As Louise's psychotherapy progressed into the third and fourth year, our therapeutic work had two primary focal points: one, a lessening of her internal criticism; and two, therapeutic support to withdraw into her internal world. However, for her withdrawal to be therapeutic I would have to be fully present, watch over her like a parent may watch over a sleeping sick child, and be a witness of her feelings and memories—memories that had no defining pictures or descriptive words. To lessen Louise's internal criticism, we would first have to find a way for her to externalize what was secretly internal and to then discover and appreciate the homeostatic functions of the internal criticism. It seemed important to me that I focus our psychotherapy on diminishing Louise's internal criticism prior to supporting a therapeutic withdrawal.

She began one of our sessions with a realization, "I often reprimand myself … and then I spend time in self-pity." I encouraged her to say the internal criticisms aloud. It seemed important that she now externalize what she had been keeping internal. I had an idea that if Louise could diminish the self-criticism, much of her "depression" might also diminish. At first Louise had a difficult time articulating her various self-chastisements but with my patience and encouragement she was eventually able to say aloud, "I'm worthless," "I'm a fool for wanting," "I'm unlovable," and, "I won't make it." In several sessions I encouraged Louise to reiterate these criticisms aloud. Analyzing the various homeostatic functions of her criticisms was an important step in diminishing their intrapsychic effects.

I focused our therapeutic work on helping Louise understand the original purpose of her self-condemnation and the psychological functions it may still have in her life today. As we explored some of the events of her childhood, she remembered criticizing herself prior to going to high school and that, "I had perfected my self-criticism by the time I was sixteen. By then I did not need anything from anyone. I was better off alone, in my own quiet world." When we talked about her family interactions when she was a school-age child Louise added, "If I can criticize myself before my mother does, I escape her awful words … also my criticism makes me productive."

Together we identified four homeostatic functions of her continuous self-criticisms (Erskine & Moursund, 2022). First, her criticisms provided an archaic sense of *identity* that defined her place in relationship to other people; they provided an archaic organizing schema about herself, others, and the quality of her life. Second, the criticisms provided *consistency*. With self-criticism she maintained the same familiar sense of worthlessness that she had lived with throughout her childhood. Like most of us, familiarity was preferable to the unknown. Third, the self-criticisms provided a strategic *distraction* from the painful awareness of her mother's constant criticism. She heard the criticisms in her own voice, not in her mother's voice. Fourth, the self-criticisms functioned to provide *predictability* about what might occur; by criticizing herself first she could brace herself for any external criticism.

Together we devised a plan to help Louise stop the internal ridicule: each time she engaged in a self-condemnation, Louise would think about the functions of the criticism. I suggested that Louise ask herself if she still needed that old identity or still required a distraction from knowing what had occurred between herself and her mother. Louise realized that she no longer wanted either the consistency or predictability that the self-condemnations provided. Together we worked out a plan; each time Louise made a self-criticism she asked herself, "What is the function of this criticism?" This questioning of herself, particularly when she was at home, helped Louise become aware that the self-criticizing had an original purpose but that the original purpose was no longer a benefit to her. Through our constant attending to her self-condemnations and their various homeostatic functions, Louise's self-criticism largely diminished.

As the self-criticism diminished Louise became increasingly aware of her mother's influence. She was now able to have some vivid memories of her mother's caustic comments when she was in elementary school: "By the time I was an adolescent I could drown out her voice. She was constantly trying to make me the perfect daughter she wanted. Most of the time she did lovely things for me, but then it would all be spoiled by some criticism." Louise realized, "I learned to criticize myself to blot out her criticisms; and, it worked."

In the ensuing sessions I focused our psychotherapy on the quality of the relationship between Louise and her mother at various childhood ages. She cried with painful memories: of her mother's controlling demands about school work when she was eight and nine years old; of "my mother's great disappointment when I was six and I forgot my lines in a school performance"; of "my mother's control in how I dressed"; and, an implicit memory of "being forced to eat food that I didn't like." Throughout these sessions we were identifying and decommissioning the introjected attitudes of her mother. As a result, she increasingly allowed me to see her vulnerability.

Therapeutically supported withdrawal

During the third and fourth years, as we focused on externalizing the internal criticisms and deciphering the homeostatic functions of such criticisms, I watched for the moments in which Louise would lapse into her semi-concealed withdrawal. In some sessions she would avert her eyes, clutch the blanket to her chest, and have long pauses in her dialogue with me. When I picked up on those moments of Louise's partial retreat, I would encourage her to close her eyes and to remain quiet. In our discussion during the last ten minutes of our session she described her inner space as, "I just go into a thick, silent fog. I don't think about anything."

When we first began the supported withdrawal Louise would open her eyes every half-minute or so, as if she was checking to see if I was still present. I thought of Harry Guntrip's (1968) description of his client's half-in/half-out compromise: a seeking of relationship (as in her checking to see if I was present); and, a seeking of security (as in her repeated relational withdrawal). I would respond with "I am staying here with you. Just take your time to go to your quiet place," or "It's important to be silent," or "I am watching over you."

When I did speak, my voice was slow and reassuring. Louise, like other clients moving into relational withdrawal, required a particular sensitivity to her unique rhythm, fear of relationship, and possible loneliness. I provided time for her to make internal contact without having to talk. An important aspect of our psychotherapy was my continual self-reminder, "Don't try to make something happen, remain fully present and observant." I wanted to create the place and time for Louise to feel the security of her "fog," any possible loneliness that I suspected was at the core of her vulnerability, and perhaps a sense of security-in-relationship with me.

As our sessions continued over the next few weeks, she was able to stay in her "quiet" place for as long as fifteen or twenty minutes. As I watched her silently curled up under the blanket, I would relax into deep yoga-style breathing that helped me stay centered and sensitive to her little gestures and sounds. Louise's withdrawal engendered an unusual patience in me. Although I was periodically distracted by the over-detailed stories that Louise told me in the first couple of years, I was acutely present during this phase of the psychotherapy.

I kept my awareness on the *pregnant silence*—a silence that was gestating with emotions and implicit memories. It was essential that I be fully present in order to catch each nuance of her silent communication. I wanted to create a healing environment where she could make full internal contact without any requirement for interpersonal contact. Arnold Beisser's (1970) "paradoxical theory of change" served as a constant reminder that I needed to be calm and patient, to find her rhythm, to not attempt to effect any change within Louise, to just accept Louise as she was.

During this time, our psychotherapy sessions moved into a routine. The first ten or fifteen minutes were often spent either on some current event or in review of the previous session. Following this initial discussion, she would withdraw into silence for five to twenty minutes. I reserved the last ten to twenty minutes to have a therapeutic dialogue about what she experienced during her silence. The relational qualities of our interpersonal conversations before and after the supported withdrawal were an indispensable ingredient in Louise's psychotherapy.

In the first several weeks of our therapeutically supported withdrawal Louise would lapse into a quiet and restorative internal place. In most of our sessions in which I supported her withdrawal, Louise experienced a sense of calmness in her "fog," her muscles relaxed. Then, as the weeks went on, Louise gradually had emotional and body memories of intense fear—a fear that engulfed her whole body. I would reassure her that I was with her and watching over her. At one point she talked about descending into a dark, damp, and moldy smelling place. She cried for me to hold her hand. I moved near her and grasped her left hand between my two hands. She shook and wept with terror. After ten minutes she opened her eyes and was able to talk. As we reviewed what Louise had experienced, she realized that she was reliving being in the basement of the house where she lived as a child. As we talked in later sessions, she was aware of at least two occasions, perhaps more, when her mother had forced her into the basement as a punishment. She was terrorized by the darkness. She wept with a profound aloneness that she must have felt as a seven-year-old child.

We spent most of the following session talking about Louise's fear of being in the dark. She revealed that she always slept with the television on. In her words, "The TV is always on, silent, but always on ... I need the company." I thought about how the TV provided not only light but it also provided pseudo-companionship—a companionship that did not invade or criticize. Rather than make an interpretation as I might with other clients, I kept this idea to myself and used it to help me understand the increased dependency that Louise was displaying in our relationship (Price, 2016).

Another significant point in our work occurred when Louise called me on a Sunday morning to tell me about a nightmare. I urged her to come to the office immediately. When she arrived an hour later, she was shaking with fear and asked me to sit next to her and hold her hand. She told me about a dream, "I have no clear images, just these horrible body sensations. In my dream all is black. I am completely alone. I know it will get worse. I'm paralyzed. No one comes." As she squeezed my hand her whole body trembled. She cried like a desperate baby. After ten minutes of agony, she opened her eyes and looked at me. At that moment she reached out and grasped my arm to her cheek and chest. She then wept differently, as though her crying was releasing the tensions in her body.

When she had finished crying, I made what I hoped would be a useful interpretation. "You remind me of a baby who needs her mother to pick her up and comfort her." As I was saying these words her face, shoulders, and chest muscles constricted. She pulled back and screamed, "I don't want her awful touch." Later we talked at length about her repulsion at the thought of being physically close to her mother. In our follow-up discussions we assumed that Louise's dream, age regression, and physical repulsion were a reliving of presymbolic, procedural memories—memories that had no pictures, only intense affect and physiological reactions. However, rather than Louise's age regression being a mere reliving that may have been retraumatizing, my presence and touch were therapeutic because they provided a new experience that allowed her nervous system to relax (Porges, 2009; Porges & Dana, 2018).

We had several conversations about Louise's inner turmoil over her need for security-in-relationship and her fear of invasion and control. In a later discussion, Louise related her fear to a sense of "utter aloneness that I have felt all my life." As we explored her "utter aloneness," she realized that, "This loneliness is the depression I often feel. Whenever my mother didn't like how I was, I felt utterly alone."

On several occasions she wept with the sadness of "never feeling loved for who I am." After crying with loneliness, she would open her eyes and engage in conversation with me about her inner experiences. Now when she would talk with me after a fifteen or twenty minute withdrawal, I had the perception that she was fully present, engaging with me in a more authentic and lively way. Louise was changing: She related it to both her intense internal focus, facilitated by the therapeutically supported withdrawal, and the significance of our end-of-session discussions about her internal, nonverbal experiences.

As the months went on, she was less inclined to withdraw. She had many more impressions of her early life and how she coped with the relational disruptions by both criticizing herself and withdrawing from people. She was increasingly able to tell me memories of her childhood. It was as though previously non-visualized and never-spoken memories became more explicit. As Louise told me these stories of her early childhood, she was increasingly open and vulnerable in my presence. I felt a sense of fulfillment in that we were accomplishing a healing psychotherapy. At the same time I questioned my countertransference: "Was my sense of fulfillment my own quest it be important, or was I being therapeutically responsive to what Louise needed in order to heal from her history of neglect and criticism?" Or, both? I was certainly involved and invested in Louise's healing from the wounds of neglect and criticism.

Shifts in perspective

In the spring of our fourth year of psychotherapy Louise often complained of fatigue, no appetite, and that she was losing weight. I was again perplexed. I worried over the question, "Is the psychotherapy too intense for Louise to integrate her intense affect and physical reactions?" Louise, for the first time, canceled a session. I was then shocked when she again left a second phone message to say that she was canceling another session. She did not return my phone calls. I was distraught. What was I missing? What had I done wrong? Finally, Louise called to confirm her next appointment and said that she had "medical reasons" for missing her two sessions.

When Louise returned after three weeks' absence, I noticed immediately that her face was thinner and that there was a yellowish tint to her complexion. She said that she had been in Minnesota at the Mayo Clinic for a thorough medical evaluation. My worries that our psychotherapy was too intense and perhaps reinforcing the old patterns of self-stabilization were immediately replaced by concern for her health. Louise slowly told me that she had stage four pancreatic cancer and that it had already metastasized to her liver. She tightly gripped my arm as we wept together.

In our next session Louise surprised me when she said that she wanted to "continue my psychotherapy until I can't come any longer." She said that she had already quit her job and that she would work only until the end of the week. She had started to investigate home nursing care for when the time came. As she was leaving, she asked if she could come "much more often," and then she added, "I need you to be with me."

Louise continued to come for two, and sometimes three, sessions a week.

During these last three months she withdrew into her "fog" only a few times. There were no further age regressions to traumatic memories. We spent most of our time focusing on her saying good-bye to her sister and mother. In a couple of intense sessions, she talked to an image of her sister in an empty chair where she expressed her anger and sorrow. In doing so she revealed several "private resentments" that had prevented her from being close to her sister.

Then I asked her to express her appreciations to the image of her sister in the empty chair. At first she struggled; her resentments seemed to dominate. Eventually she was able to say to the image of her sister, "I'm grateful that you kept mother off my back." She went on to speak about several examples of how her sister "took the brunt of mother's demands."

Louise cried as she acknowledged her longing for a caring relationship with her sister. Following this work, she arranged a four-day weekend retreat with her sister. She was pleased with "our real conversation. We talked openly to each other for the first time since we were children. I now know that it was my resentment that prevented us from being close." In the following sessions she commented on talking to her sister "almost every day."

When talking about her sister, Louise made several comments that led me to think that she was living with a lot of resentment toward her mother. I suggested that she put her mother's image in the empty chair and to "tell your mother everything that you have always wanted to say." Louise said that my suggestion to talk to the image of her mother was "too difficult. I just hide inside at the thought of telling her anything about me." With this comment I assumed that she was telling me that I needed to do something differently. So, I relied on one of my guiding principles: *When in doubt about what to do, be relational.* I changed my approach and asked Louise to look me in the eyes and to tell me what she did not like about her mother's behavior.

Louise tensed up, "My mother has been dead for several years … but it's like she is still hovering over me, ready to boss me around." I asked about their mother–daughter interactions at various ages of her childhood: adolescence, school years, preschool years, and toddler years. Louise told me story after story of being "smothered … over-loved … without any freedom to be me." She was vehement in expressing her anger and resentment and very reluctant to speak of appreciations she felt for her mother. Eventually she told me that she appreciated her mother's work ethic and how her mother "tried to have perfect children … She tried so hard, but it just wasn't right for me. I withdrew from her and it broke her heart. And then she tried harder and harder to mold me into the image she wanted me to be … and I hid more and more." She cried deeply as she said, "I missed out on having a mother with whom I could confide, to be close." Our sessions in these last months were primarily focused on working with Louise's grief about the absence of any emotionally close relationship with her mother; it was her way of saying, "good-bye to what I never had."

While in this last phase of our psychotherapy Louise and I spent time addressing her regrets, resentments, and remorseful feelings toward her sister and mother, I also reserved time in many sessions to speak directly to Louise about her impending death and what she understood about life. Louise had changed; she was no longer resistant to my phenomenological inquiry; in fact, she seemed to welcome some of my inquiry. Now our psychotherapy was shaped by existential perspectives: "What is the meaning of life?"; "What happens when we die?"; "What influence have we made in this world?" (Becker, 1973; Frankl, 1959; Yalom, 1980). I was touched by a sense of the sacred that infused our interpersonal dialogue.

As these three months went on, Louise was continuing to lose weight and strength. When her sister invited Louise to live in her home near Boston we had only three more sessions in which to talk about our relationship with each other. We cried together—a cry of separation and a cry of joy—joy in having the rich interpersonal connection that we had created together and our mutual sorrow—an intense sorrow that we would never be with each other again.

Postscript

Writing this story of Louise's psychotherapy was a challenge because I would have liked to write about how our psychotherapy unfolded in an orderly sequence but that is not how our psychotherapy proceeded. The crucial therapeutic junctures did not happen in a timely order, one after another. Our psychotherapeutic work would suddenly move to a new theme, then we would return to a previous issue, then we would proceed to another focus. Often I had to keep several pertinent themes in mind. Yet, eventually, the fragmented, hidden, and split-off aspects of Louise's sense of Self became integrated into a new cohesive sense of Self.

Was Louise "narcissistic"? No, not any more. Perhaps she never was. Perhaps the arrogance, entitlement, and self-aggrandizement that I observed in the first year of Louise's psychotherapy were just a cover for her "fear of being controlled." Did she exhibit a schizoid pattern? Yes, most of the time during our years together; she continually relied on self-criticism and relational withdrawal as her way to self-stabilize. But Louise worked hard in her psychotherapy: we spent many sessions addressing her internal criticism, and many more in a therapeutically supported withdrawal.

Louise changed—the change occurred at a time when one might expect her to be more withdrawn. Instead, Louise's dialogue with me became intimate; she talked about having intimate conversations with her sister. I wish Louise was still alive because I would like to interview her these many years later in order to know her subjective version of our intense therapeutic interactions. My story of Louise's psychotherapy is from the point of view of a participant–observer, but it does not tell the whole story. It is Louise's subjective version of our psychotherapeutic journey that intrigues me. I am sure that we both would learn a lot if she could share her phenomenological experience with us.

References

American Psychiatric Association (2013). *Diagnostic and Statistical Manual of Mental Disorders* (5th edn.). Washington, DC: American Psychiatric Publishing. doi.org/10.1176/appi.books.9780890425596.

Bach, S. (1985). *Narcissistic States and the Therapeutic Process.* New York: Basic Books.

Basch, M. (1988). *Understanding Psychotherapy: The Science Behind the Art.* New York: Basic Books.

Becker, E. (1973). *Denial of Death.* New York: Free Press.

Beisser, A. (1970). The paradoxical theory of change. In: J. Fagan & L. Shepherd (Eds.), *Gestalt Therapy Now: Theory, Techniques, Applications* (pp. 77–80). Palo Alto, CA: Science and Behavior Books.

Erskine, R. G. (1991). Transference and transactions: Critique from an intrapsychic and integrative perspective. *Transactional Analysis Journal, 21*(2). doi.org/10.1177/036215379102100202.

Erskine, R. G. (1994). Shame and self-righteousness: Transactional analysis perspectives and clinical interventions. *Transactional Analysis Journal, 24*(2): 86–102. doi.org/10.1177/036215379402400204.

Erskine, R. G. (1995). A Gestalt therapy approach to shame and self-righteousness: Theory and methods. *British Gestalt Journal, 4*(2): 107–117.

Erskine, R. G. (2015). *Relational Patterns; Therapeutic Presence.* London: Karnac.

Erskine, R. G. (2021a). *A Healing Relationship: Commentary on Therapeutic Dialogues.* Bicester, UK: Phoenix.

Erskine, R. G. (2021b). *Early Affect Confusion: Relational Psychotherapy for the Borderline Client.* London: nscience.

Erskine, R. G., & Moursund, J. P. (2022). *The Art and Science of Relationship: The Practice of Integrative Psychotherapy.* Bicester, UK: Phoenix.

Erskine, R. G., Moursund, J. P., & Trautmann, R. L. (1999). *Beyond Empathy: A Therapy of Contact-in-relationship.* London: Routledge, 2023.

Fairbairn, W. R. D. (1952). *Psychoanalytic Studies of the Personality.* London: Routledge.

Frankl, V. E. (1959). *Man's Search for Meaning: An Introduction to Logotherapy.* Boston, MA: Beacon.

Guntrip, H. (1968). *Schizoid Phenomena, Object Relations and the Self.* New York: International Universities Press.

Johnson, S. M. (1987). *Humanizing the Narcissistic Style.* New York: W. W. Norton.

Johnson, S. M. (1994). *Character Styles.* New York: W. W. Norton.

Kernberg, O. F. (1975). *Borderline Conditions and Pathological Narcissism.* New York: Jason Aronson.

Khan, M. M. R. (1974). *The Privacy of the Self.* New York: International Universities Press.

Kohut, H. (1971). *The Analysis of the Self.* New York: International Universities Press.

Kohut, H. (1977). *The Restoration of the Self: A Systematic Approach to the Psychoanalytic Treatment of Narcissistic Personality Disorder.* New York: International Universities Press.

Laing, R. D. (1960). *The Divided Self.* London: Tavistock.

Little, R. (2001). Schizoid processes: Working with the defenses of the withdrawn child ego state. *Transactional Analysis Journal, 31*(1): 33–43. doi.org/10.1177/036215370103100105.

Little, R. (2011). Impasse clarification within the transference–countertransference matrix. *Transactional Analysis Journal*, *41*(1): 23–38. doi.org/10.1177/036215371104100106.

Masterson, J. F. (1981). *The Narcissistic and Borderline Disorders: An Integrated Developmental Approach*. New York: Brunner/Mazel.

Melniker, R. C. (1988). *The Narcissistic-Schizoid Bond: A British Object Relations View*. New York: Institute for Contemporary Psychotherapy.

O'Reilly-Knapp, M. (2001). Between two worlds: The encapsulated self. *Transactional Analysis Journal*, *31*(1): 44–54. doi.org/10.1177/036215370103100106.

Porges, S. W. (2009). The polyvagal theory: New insights into adaptive reactions of the autonomic nervous system. *Cleveland Clinic Journal of Medicine*, *76*(2): 86–90.

Porges, S. W., & Dana, D. (2018). *Clinical Applications of the Polyvagal Theory: The Emergence of Polyvagal-Informed Therapies*. New York: W. W. Norton.

Price, L. (2016). *Better Late than Never: The Reparative Therapeutic Relationship in Regression to Dependency*. London: Karnac.

Stern, S. (1994). Needed relationships and repeated relationships: An integrated relational perspective. *Psychoanalytic Dialogues*, *4*: 317–345.

Stolorow, R. D., Brandchaft, B., & Atwood, G. E. (1987). *Psychoanalytic Treatment: An Intersubjective Approach*. Hillsdale, NJ: The Analytic Press.

Wolf, E. S. (1988). *Treating the Self: Elements of Clinical Self Psychology*. New York: Guilford.

Yalom, I. D. (1980). *Existential Psychotherapy*. New York: Basic Books.

Yontef, G. (2001). Psychotherapy of schizoid process. *Transactional Analysis Journal*, *31*(1): 7–23. doi.org/10.1177/036215370103100103.

Index

Abram, J., 72
adapted child, 17 *see also* splitting
Aiken, C, 10
Ainsworth, M. D. S., 35
anxiety, 6, 50, 51, 55, 67, 85, 140, 159, 183, 184, 190, 194, 195, 198, 199, 229
    attachment, 18, 35, 46, 153
    hope and, 22
    schizoid personalities, 54, 56–58
Anzieu, D., 147
Arieti, S., 75
attachment, 18, 23, 25, 34–35, 46–47, 49, 51, 53, 59, 80, 88, 180 *see also* isolated attachment
    earned secure, 62
    relational, 22, 24, 35, 57
attunement in psychotherapy, 31–42
Atwood, G. E., 6, 32, 68, 70, 156, 160, 162, 226
autistic encapsulation, 48 *see also* schizoid compromise
avoidant *see also* isolated attachment
    attachment, 105, 107
    attachment style in mothers, 105
    and dependent personality disorder, 177–185
Axline, V. M., 4

Bach, S., 226, 229
Balint, M., 33, 66
Baruch, D. W., 4
Basch, M., 226
Bass, C., 178

Baumgardner, P., 117, 161
Beautiful Mind, A, 49–50 *see also* schizoid compromise
Becker, E., 239
Beisser, A., 235
Bergman, A., 47
Berne, E., 5, 17, 95, 102, 112, 128, 167, 169, 170
Bettelheim, B., 4, 66, 72
Bettles, L., 189–208
Bhui, K., 46
Bion, W. R., 53
Blehar, M. C., 35
Blumer, D., 178
Blyton, E., 189, 199
Bollas, C., 6
Bowlby, J., 16, 66, 147, 180
Brandchaft, B., 6, 32, 226
Brenner, C., 106
Bruch, H., 66

character structure, 80
child ego state, 69
Clancier, A., 71
Clark, N. H., 4
Clarkin, J. F., 47
Conner, K., 46
contact
    with client, 32–33
    initiation, 92–93, 159–160

inner safety to relationship, 209–222
-in-relationship, 162
within ourselves, 79
resisting, 161–162
in silence and withdrawal, 74–75
withdrawing from social, 45
continuity, 34, 52, 60, 68, 71, 72
Cooper, M., 169
coping strategies, xix, 4, 80, 81, 82, 214, 226
countertransference, 11, 28, 32, 47, 61, 62, 80–81, 85, 87, 93, 119, 123, 134, 142, 225, 237 *see also* transference
enactment, 106–107
reactions, 55, 60
Cozolino, L., 105
criticism *see also* psychotherapy of schizoid process; self-created criticism; self-criticism; shame
distraction from, 119–121
internal, 19, 24
cumulative trauma, 5, 25, 124, 147 *see also* schizoid process

Daellenbach, C., 45
Dana, D., 236
depersonalization, 5, 60
and derealisation, 86
depressive disorder, 102–103, 155–156 *see also* isolated attachment
case study, 225, 239
developmental theory, 46–47 *see also* schizoid compromise
DeYoung, P. A., 170
DID *see* dissociative identity disorder
dissociation, 4, 13, 60 *see also* schizoid compromise; schizoid process; silence and withdrawal
defensive structures, 71
dissociative identity disorder (DID), 70–71 *see also* silence and withdrawal
dream(s), 160, 236
analysis of, 128–129, 144–145, 168
revealing, 113–115
work, 167–168
dwelling, 160–161

Eagle, M., 46
effective therapy, 70
ego state, 5 *see also* schizoid process
child, 69
libidinal, 16
relational units, 46

Elliott, R., 169
encapsulated self, 20–21, 67–68 *see also* silence and withdrawal; splitting
Engel, G., 178
Erikson, E. H., 66, 148
Erskine, R. G., 4, 6, 12, 18, 24, 25, 28, 35, 36, 39, 45, 52, 55, 56, 69, 72, 79, 80, 81, 82, 83, 86, 87, 88, 93, 94, 102, 105, 106, 107, 118, 119, 124, 140, 147, 148, 151, 153, 155, 156, 157, 158, 161, 162, 163, 165, 167, 168, 170, 171, 172, 178, 181, 190, 207, 221, 228, 229, 230, 234
Evans, K., 157
external world, 70

Fairbairn, W. R. D., 5, 12, 16, 33, 45, 46, 47, 48, 55, 74, 79, 86, 88, 179, 184, 229
false self, 17, 34–35, 36, 57 *see also* attunement in psychotherapy; social facade; splitting; true self
Fine, C. G., 71
Finlay, L., 153, 154, 155, 157, 158, 159, 160, 161, 162, 163, 164, 166, 168, 169, 170, 171, 173
first split, 17–18, 22–23 *see also* psychotherapy of schizoid process; splitting
fourth split, 20–21, 25–28 *see also* psychotherapy of schizoid process; splitting
Fraiberg, S., 15, 17, 142
Frankl, V. E., 239
Freud, S., 106
functions, 34, 36, 57, 88, 111, 161
criticisms of others, 119, 120, 165
homeostatic, xvii, xix, 22, 126, 233–234, 235
introjection, 18
psychological, xviii, 82, 125, 234
self-criticism, 19, 21, 131, 232, 233–234

Galgut, D., 10, 117
Geller, S. M., 158
Gestalt therapy, 169 *see also* psychotherapy of schizoid process
contact and interruptions to contact, 36
dialogic approach, 158, 163
empty chair method, 22
and intrapsychic conflict, 117, 160–161
Gomez, L., 47
Goodman, P., 36, 140
Goulding, R., 6
Greenberg, E., 89
Greenberg, J. R., 33, 34
Greenberg, L. S., 158

Greenson, R. R., 106
Grotstein, J. S., 48
Guntrip, H., 6, 13, 14, 15, 33, 35, 46, 47, 67, 68, 74, 83, 86, 88, 89, 117, 180, 182, 229, 235 *see also* schizoid compromise

Hall, R., 46
Hazell, J., 6, 33, 35, 62, 67, 83, 103
healing, 25, 27, 95, 160, 170, 173
    of cumulative neglect *see* cumulative trauma environment, 235
    relational, 163
    relationship, 5–6, 14, 28, 35, 36, 58, 81, 107, 189, 192, 221
Hefferline, R. F., 36, 140
Heilbronn, M., 178
Heinmann, P., 106
Hesse, E., 106
Hesse, H., 10, 117
Hirsch, I., 61
historical
    detachment, 69
    events, 70
    experience, 163
    inquiry, 23, 26, 33, 41, 115, 116, 127, 153, 179, 210
    relational needs, 81
homeostatic *see* functions
Hossain, A., 46
Howard, R., 49
Husserl, E., 152
Hycner, R., 158, 159

idealization, 142
impingements
    impact of, 71–72
    settled state, undisturbed by, 72
    Winnicott's theory of, 72
inner safety to contact-in-relationship, 209, 221–222
    case study, 209–222
    client's reflective comments, 220–221
    organization of research, 210
    psychotherapy session, 211–220
    relational psychotherapy of client's schizoid process, 209–222
    relational space, 210
inner world, 70 *see also* psychotherapy of schizoid process
    and fantasy, 199–200

integrative psychotherapy, 116, 147, 165 *see also* isolated attachment
    principles of, 94
intensive psychotherapy, 70
internal *see also* psychotherapy of schizoid process; schizoid compromise; silence and withdrawal; splitting
    conflict, 202
    criticism, 19, 24
    saboteur, 20, 60, 88 *see also* saboteur
    sense of being, 69
    stability development and relational security, 147–148
    strategist, 19
    withdrawal to safe internal space, 168–169
    world, 49
interpersonal contact with client, 32–33 *see also* attunement in psychotherapy
interposition, 23
introjection, 18, 140 *see also* isolated attachment; splitting
    of mother's personality, 139–148
    psychotherapy of, 139–148
invisible fortress, 72
isolated attachment, 25, 101, 228 *see also* attunement in psychotherapy
    accommodating survival reaction, 105
    avoidant attachment, 105, 107
    case study, 101–108, 111–121
    countertransference, 106–107, 134
    distraction from criticism, 119–121
    emotion-filled moment, 132
    flow of psychotherapy, 115
    Gestalt therapy concept, 117
    healing relationship, 107
    homeostatic functions in silent quest for woman, 126
    idealization, 142
    infant developing internal stability and relational security, 147–148
    integrative psychotherapy, 116
    internal conflict, 131
    introjection of mother's personality, 139–148
    isolation, loneliness, and need to be loved, 123–130
    life half in relationship and half out, 117
    mothers with avoidant attachment style, 105
    pattern, 35, 151, 228
    patterns, 107–108
    phenomenological inquiry, 105

physical sensations, 112
psychotherapy of introjections, 139–148
revealing dream, 113–115
script, 112
self-criticism, 108, 117, 119–121, 123, 131, 136
self-criticism and shame, 115–118
shame, 112
social facade, 112
suicidal thoughts, 103
therapeutic withdrawal and painful memories, 131–137
transference–countertransference matrix, 106–107
trust issues, 118–119
uncertainty, 118
unconscious relational patterns, 105–106, 107
unhappy work situation, 104–105

Jacobs, L., 163
Jacobs, T. J., 106
Johnson, S. M., 80, 182, 226, 229
Jovanoska, K., 91

Kalmanovitch, J., 71
Kapitan, L., 159
Kernberg, O. F., 46, 47, 50, 229
Khan, M. M. R., 5, 33, 229
Klein, J., 88
Klein, M., 45, 46, 50
Klein, R., 46, 47, 48, 49, 51, 52, 53, 58, 60, 61, 90
Kluft, R. P., 71
Kobak, R. R., 106
Kohon, G., 33
Kohut, H., 226, 229
Kullander, J., 95
Kunz, G., 156

Laing, R. D., 12, 183, 229
Lambert, M. J., 157
Lee, T., 46
Levine, P. A., 164
Little, M., 67, 72
Little, M. I., 6, 33, 35
Little, R., 45, 46, 80, 229, 230 *see also* schizoid compromise
Loewald, H. W., 106
Lourie, J., 5

Mahler, M. S., 47
Main, M., 105, 106

Malkov, M., 46
Manfield, P., 48, 55, 57, 62, 85
mapping, 71 *see also* silence and withdrawal
Masterson, J. F., 48, 179, 229
May, R., 66
McFerran, K. S., 161, 162
McGilloway, A., 46
McWilliams, N., 46, 50, 51, 53, 60, 61, 158
Mearns, D., 169
Melniker, R. C., 229
Merleau-Ponty, M., 157
mind structure, 47–49
Mitchell, S. A., 6, 33, 34, 74
Modic, K. U., 147
Moursund, J. P., 6, 39, 72, 79, 83, 86, 88, 93, 102, 140, 147, 158, 162, 165, 167, 170, 178, 230, 234
Moustakas, C., 4
multiple parts of self, 169–171

narcissistic/schizoid matrix, 229
narcissistic style, 226–228
Nasar, S., 49, 50
Nash, J. F., Jr., 49–50
Nathanson, D. J., 181
neglect, 4, 13, 23, 34, 38, 41, 67, 81, 84, 105, 107, 124, 126, 136, 140, 144, 145, 147, 168, 171, 172, 173, 237
Newhill, C., 46
Newman, A., 72
Norcross, J. C., 155, 157, 164
Novellino, M., 107

object relations, 46, 48–49, 50, 53, 62, 68, 87–88, 89, 178, 229 *see also* schizoid compromise
Orange, D. M., 68, 70
Orcutt, C., 90
O'Reilly-Knapp, M., 14, 20, 48, 58, 60, 65, 68, 75, 84, 91, 94, 108, 226, 228, 233

pain, 56, 57, 172, 177–178, 182, 184
Perls, F., 22, 36, 66, 117, 140, 161
personality disorder *see also* isolated attachment
avoidant and dependent, 177–185
avoidant attachment, 105, 107
phenomenological
attitude, 152, 153
description, 154
phenomenological inquiry, 26–27, 105, 230 *see also* psychotherapy of schizoid process
non-invasive, 154–155
shame, 181

physical sensations, 112
Piaget, J., 46, 66
Pine, F., 47
Porges, S. W., 236
pregnant pause, xxiii, 215
pregnant silence, 235
presence
    psychotherapist's, 4, 26, 27, 38, 42, 55, 65, 72, 73, 74, 75, 92, 93, 118, 142, 148, 156, 157, 158, 159, 169, 207, 211–212, 221, 226, 231, 236, 237
    self in other's, 71, 108, 129, 209
    social, 9
Price, L., 236
prosody, xviii, xxv
Proust, M., 131
psychogenic pain, 178
psychotherapy *see also* integrative psychotherapy
    attunement in, 31–42
    with children, 4
    essential, 35–36
    flow of, 115
    integrative, 116
    intensive, 70
    of introjections, 139–148
psychotherapy of schizoid process, 6 *see also* attunement in psychotherapy; splitting
    analyzing, 209, 221–222
    client's perspective on, 189–208
    considerations for, 21–28
    first split, 22–23
    fourth split, 25–28
    Gestalt therapy methods, 22, 23
    inner world and fantasy, 199–200
    intense therapy session, 191–208
    internal conflict, 202
    internal criticism, 24
    phenomenological inquiry, 26–27
    positive outcomes of, 189
    script beliefs, 190–191
    second split, 23–24
    self-created criticism of saboteur, 24
    survival struggle, 205
    therapeutic description, 26
    third split, 24–25

Racker, H., 107
regulation, 34, 82, 126, 133, 168
relational *see also* schizoid compromise
    conflicts and therapeutic relationship, 230
    needs *see* relational needs

psychotherapy of schizoid process, 209–222
    space, 210
    themes, 163
    transactional analysis, 59
    units, 46
    withdrawal, 14, 225, 239
relational needs, 15–16, 22, 79, 80–81, 95–96
    anti-wanting self, 88
    case study, 81–95
    character structure, 80
    depersonalisation and derealisation, 86
    "devotion" to emergent self, 96
    false self, 17, 34–35, 36, 57
    impact on others, 85–88
    integrative psychotherapy principles, 94
    internal saboteur, 88
    interrelating needs, 91–92
    need for mutuality, 93–94
    need for survival, 94–95
    need to initiate contact, 92–93
    psychotherapy of schizoid process, 209–222
    schizoid compromise, 86
    security, 83–85
    self-definition, 88–91
    social facade, 83–84
    therapy within schizoid process, 95
    three-part continuum, 80
    transference, 80–81
    true self, 34, 36, 81, 87, 96, 195
relational withdrawal, 14–15, 25, 27, 40, 41, 45, 52, 79, 111, 124, 132, 207, 226, 228, 229, 230, 232, 235, 239 *see also* psychotherapy of schizoid process
Romanyshyn, R. D., 172
Rubens, R. L., 12

saboteur, 19–20, 24, 60, 88
Sayre, G., 156
Sceery, A., 106
schema(s), xix, 46, 49, 106, 234
schizoid, 9, 45
    in character, 5
    conditions, 233
    dilemma, 14, 55–57, 229
    disorder, 10, 75, 80, 228
    experience, 50–51
    organizing system, 68
    pattern, 10, 11, 16, 80, 81, 228–229, 239
    person, 183
    personality disorder, 3

personality's connection to external world, 48
person's behavior, 45
position, 47
relational psychotherapy, 209–222
role of shame in development of, 177–185
spectrum, 10
state, 50
style, 11–12, 16, 80, 81, 228
syndrome, 9
withdrawal, 52
schizoid compromise, 15, 33, 45, 57–58, 61, 86, 180, 190
 aloof from the crowd, 60
 "in and out program", 57
 anxiety, 58
 autistic encapsulation, 48
 case study, 49–50
 countertransference reactions, 55, 60
 developmental theory, 46–47
 dissociation, 60
 ego state relational units, 46
 experience of, 50–51
 maintaining withdrawal, 53–54
 "master–slave" relationship, 48
 nonattachment and attachment, 47–49
 object relations, 46
 rejecting behaviors, 54
 schizoid dilemma, 55–57
 splitting of self, 45
 structure of the mind, 47–49
 therapist's defensive compromise, 61–62
 therapist's stance, 58–59
 therapy of the compromise, 58–59
 withdrawal, 45, 51–53
 withdrawal during lockdown, 54
schizoid process, 3–7, 9, 12–16, 31, 79 see also splitting
 cumulative trauma, 5, 25, 124, 147
 dissociation, 4, 13
 ego state, 5
 healing relationship, 5
 isolation in quiet, 14
 "libidinal ego", 16
 metaphor of "splitting", 16
 parental relationship, 6
 psychotherapy, 4, 6
 relational dynamics of early childhood, 5
 relational withdrawal, 14
 schizoid compromise, 15
 schizoid dilemma, 14
 schizoid in character, 5

"secure self", 16
social self, 15
split in child's ego, 5
splitting, 12, 13
symptoms, 16
therapy within, 95
"turning away" from parent, 15
vital and vulnerable self, 15, 16
"whole self", 16
schizoid spectrum, 10
Schneider, K. J., 158
Schwartz, R. C., 169
script, 112 see also psychotherapy of schizoid process
 beliefs, 190–191
second split, 18–19, 23–24 see also psychotherapy of schizoid process; splitting
Seinfeld, J., 45, 46, 48, 51, 54, 56
self, multiple parts of, 169–171
self-created criticism, 19–20 see also psychotherapy of schizoid process; splitting
 of saboteur, 24
self-criticism, 108, 117, 119–121, 123, 136 see also isolated attachment
 functions of, 131, 233–234
 and shame, 115–118, 231–233
self-definition, 88–91
self-in-relationship, 34
self-stabilize, 13, 15, 18, 34, 35, 37, 40, 41, 111, 124, 164, 165, 207, 212, 229, 230, 237, 239
sequestered self see encapsulated self
shame, 11–12, 16, 19, 88, 112, 118, 120, 121, 124, 125, 140, 166, 168, 170, 178, 180, 190, 193, 215, 220, 232, 233
 criticism and, 231–233
 defenses against, 181
 to organize internal processes, 4
 personal, 151
 self criticism and, 115–118, 231–233
Shaun, M., 46
silence and withdrawal, 65, 75–76
 "between space", 70
 case vignettes, 65–67, 68–70, 70–71, 72, 73–74
 contact in, 74–75
 continuity of existence, 72
 detached spectator, 68
 dissociative identity disorder, 70–71
 effective therapy, 70
 encapsulated self, 67–68
 external world, 70
 impact of impingements, 71–72

inner world, 69–70
invisible fortress, 72
losing connection, 73–74
mapping, 71
remnants of person's past, 68–70
settled state, 72
spontaneous movement, 71
therapeutic presence, 72
therapeutic relationship, 65
trauma in, 72–73
Winnicott's theory of impingements, 72
"Silent Snow, Secret Snow", 10
social facade, 11, 35, 83–84 *see also* false self
case study, 225, 239
social self, 15, 17 *see also* schizoid process; splitting
splitting, 12, 17, 229 *see also* psychotherapy of schizoid process; schizoid process
adapted child, 17
as attempt to self-stabilize, 13
encapsulated self, 20–21
false self, 17
first split, 17–18, 22–23
fourth split, 20–21, 25–28
internal strategist, 19
introjections, 18
metaphor of, 16
organization towards invulnerability, 17
second split, 18–19
of self, 45
self-created criticism, 19
self-created saboteur/internal saboteur, 19–20
social self, 17
third split, 19–20
vital and vulnerable self, 17
stabilization, 82, 133, 151, 168, 218 *see also* self-stabilize
Steppenwolf, 10, 117
Stern, D. N., 4
Stern, S., 230
Stewart, A. L., 84, 92
Stiles, W. B., 169
Stolorow, R. D., 6, 32, 68, 70, 156, 160, 162, 226
Strange Room, 10
suicidal thoughts, 103
survival *see also* isolated attachment; psychotherapy of schizoid process
need for, 94–95
reaction, 105
struggle, 205
Sutherland, D., 33
Suttie, I. D., 33

therapeutically supported withdrawal, 235–237
therapeutic description, 26–27, 40, 41, 154, 207, 210, 212, 230
therapeutic presence, 72
therapy of compromise, 58–59
third split, 19–20, 24–25 *see also* psychotherapy of schizoid process; splitting
Thoreau, H. D., 101
three-part continuum, 80
titration, 164–165
tolerable nondefensive experiences, 46
transference, 39, 52, 80–81, 94, 160, 162, 192, 230 *see also* countertransference
–countertransference, 56, 59, 61, 106–107, 163
responses, 162–164
trauma, cumulative, 5, 25, 124, 147 *see also* schizoid process
Trautmann, R. L., 4, 6, 39, 72, 79, 80, 88, 102, 147, 158, 162, 165, 167, 178, 230
true self, 34, 36, 81, 87, 96, 195 *see also* attunement in psychotherapy; false self
trust issues, 118–119
Tustin, F., 75
Tyrer, S., 178

unconscious relational patterns, 105–106, 107 *see also* isolated attachment
unhappy work situation, 104–105

vital self, 36–39
vital and vulnerable self, 15, 16–20, 22–24, 35, 36, 42, 56–57, 81, 87–88, 90, 93–95, 156–157, 220, 221, 229
vulnerability, 9, 12, 13, 15, 16, 22, 34, 37, 38, 52, 58, 71, 82, 83, 84, 86, 91, 106, 108, 112, 116–118, 128, 129, 165, 168, 191, 227–228, 231, 232, 234, 235, 237

Wall, S., 35
Wallin, D. J., 60, 105
Wampold, B. E., 155, 164
Ware, P., 58
Warner, M., 169
Waters, E., 35
Watkins, H. H., 169
Watkins, J. G., 169
Wertz, F., 160
Winnicott, D. W., 6, 14, 17, 33, 34, 35, 58, 67, 71, 72, 81, 87, 88, 96, 111

withdrawal, 51 *see also* schizoid compromise; silence and withdrawal
    into different state of consciousness, 51
    enforced, 54
    home base, 51–53
    maintaining, 53–54
    as nonattachment, 48–49
    and painful memories, 131–137
    to safe internal space, 168–169
    schizoid, 52
    from social contact, 45
    therapeutically supported, 235–237
Wolf, E. S., 226
working creatively, 166 *see also* withdrawal
    being challenging, 166–167
    dream work, 167–168
    duplex transaction, 167
    withdrawal to safe internal space, 168–169

Yalom, I. D., 156, 166, 239
Yeoman, F. E., 47
Yontef, G., 90, 95, 117, 179, 229, 232

Zaletel, M., 93
Žvelc, G., 46, 91, 147
Žvelc, M., 91